INS Dictionary of Neuropsychology

INS

DICTIONARY

OF

NEUROPSYCHOLOGY

Edited by
DAVID W. LORING, PH.D.

Section Editors

Behavioral Neurology • Kimford J. Meador, M.D.

Developmental Neuropsychology • Ida Sue Baron, Ph.D

Etymology • Steven J. Loring, Ph.D

General Content • Kerry deS. Hamsher, Ph.D

Neurobehavioral Syndromes • Nils R. Varney, Ph.D

Neuroanatomy and Neuropsychiatry • Gregory P. Lee, Ph.D

General Content • Jordi Peña-Casanova, M.D.

Neuropsychological Assessment • Esther Strauss, Ph.D

Rehabilitation • Tessa Hart, Ph.D

New York   Oxford
OXFORD UNIVERSITY PRESS
1999

Oxford University Press

Oxford   New York
Athens   Auckland   Bangkok   Bogotá   Buenos Aires   Calcutta
Cape Town   Chennai   Dar es Salaam   Delhi   Florence   Hong Kong   Istanbul
Karachi   Kuala Lumpur   Madrid   Melbourne   Mexico City   Mumbai
Nairobi   Paris   São Paulo   Singapore   Taipei   Tokyo   Toronto   Warsaw

and associated companies in
Berlin   Ibadan

Copyright 1999 by International Neuropsychological Society

Published by Oxford University Press, Inc.,
198 Madison Avenue, New York, New York, 10016
http://www.oup-usa.org

Library of Congress Cataloging-in-Publication Data
INS dictionary of neuropsychology /
edited by David W. Loring ; section editors, Kimford J. Meador . . . [et al.].
p.   cm.
ISBN 0-19-506977-3 (cloth).—ISBN 0-19-506978-1 (paper)
1. Neuropsychology—Dictionaries.
I. Loring, David W.
II. Meador, Kimford J.
[DNLM: 1. Neuropsychology dictionaries.
WL 13 I59 1999]   QP360.I55   1999
612'.03—dc21   DNLM/DLC   for Library of Congress   98-23696

2 4 6 8 9 7 5 3 1

Printed in the United States of America
on acid-free paper

Foreword

Language and language usage evolve over time as new words are developed and old words are used in different ways. Terms may take on additional significance, their meaning may become narrower, or they may even fall into obscurity. The connotation of a word may vary across disciplines. Because the International Neuropsychological Society is an interdisciplinary organization involving professionals from a variety of educational and practice traditions, we thought that a dictionary might be a vehicle for standardizing terminology in our field. A common language could help to advance the science and practice of neuropsychology. Additionally, professionals and students entering the field would have a single source for the definition of terms they encounter in their readings. For these reasons, the dictionary-makers included entries not only from adult and developmental neuropsychology but also selected terms from clinical psychology, cognitive psychology, neurology, neurosurgery, neuroanatomy, neuroimaging, psychiatry, rehabilitation, psychophysics, genetics, and statistics as well as medical abbreviations that neuropsychologists sometimes come across. They hope that readers will provide comments to the editor pointing out acceptable alternative meanings or suggesting modifications of definitions for words already in the dictionary as well as recommending terms to be added to the next edition. In this way, the dictionary will continue to meet the needs of all our members and be the resource envisioned by its authors.

H. Julia Hannay, Ph.D.
President
International Neuropsychological Society
August, 1998

Preface

Neuropsychology is a diverse discipline with varied practice and application; this dictionary is intended to reflect that diversity. To some, it will contain too many tests, too much basic neurology, or too much history. One advantage of a dictionary, however, is that it is by definition athematic. Unlike textbooks that tend to be read in sections or chapters, dictionary entries that are not of interest can be easily ignored. We hope, however, that this dictionary will be a valuable resource to students, practitioners, and researchers in neuropsychology and related disciplines. It is intended to provide concise information about neurobehavioral abnormalities, diseases affecting the nervous system and clinical syndromes, neuropsychological and medical tests and procedures, basic neuroscience, and other matters relevant to neuropsychologists and professionals in allied fields.

The variety of approaches to neuropsychology as well as its different goals stemming from practice in different settings is reflected in this dictionary. Where geographic differences in meaning are present, they are noted in the definition, although a certain amount of North American bias is probably inevitable.

Plans for an INS dictionary project began to develop in 1987 during the INS presidency of Muriel D. Lezak, and the project has taken a somewhat circuitous route to completion. It has nevertheless benefited from that journey because, over the years, a wide cross-section of the INS membership has contributed to the project. The initial list of potential entries was compiled with the assistance of INS members under the direction of Kerry deS. Hamsher. During the final phases of the project, additional input was solicited from Section Editors with expertise in particular areas as well as volunteers from the INS membership. Both the Section Editors and INS contributors provided lists of potential entries and initial definitions, to which I made additions and deletions as I deemed appropriate.

The initial definitions were edited to be relatively homogeneous in content and style and to reflect the relative importance of each entry within neuropsychology. When faced with an entry for which additional clarification seemed necessary, I would contact at least one person with specialized expertise for assistance. At times, the feedback was obtained by posting questions to NPSYCH, an Internet discussion list for neuropsychology. Drafts of the dictionary were returned to contributors for rereview without specific instructions; consequently, the degree of participation was generally set by the contributor's interest. Persons who repeatedly reviewed the entire manuscript are identified as editorial consultants to reflect their significant contributions over an extended period. Most contributors, however, reviewed selected portions of the manuscript on multiple occasions.

My sources for entries included graduate school notes, reading lists for neuropsychology training programs, indexes from texts, and index entries from neuropsychology journals, including *Neuropsychology Abstracts*. I also kept an ear and eye open during meetings and conversations for words that simply seemed to be appropriate for a dictionary of neuropsychology. A rule of thumb was that the final set of entries should consist of material that a postdoctoral fellow in neuropsychology might be expected to have encountered during a 2-year training program. Decisions about the number of entries from related disciplines such as neuroscience, behavioral neurology, cognitive science, and clinical psychology were among the most difficult to make. Although the final list would be somewhat different under the direction of another editor, there should be few omissions that readers would consider "surprising" given the diversity of input from the Editorial Board and other INS members.

Many abbreviations and acronyms that appear in general medical charts and the clinical literature are included. Students in fields other than medicine are at a considerable disadvantage in learning these because they do not have clinical rotations in which terms are learned by repeatedly going on rounds. Words thought to be central to a definition and for which an independent dictionary entry exists are italicized.

This dictionary is not intended to be an encyclopedia sourcebook. Most definitions are 75 words or less. Neuropsychological assessment methods to detect malingering or symptom exaggeration are not discussed in detail. This kind of information is available elsewhere, and we do not want this volume to be regarded as a primary source that might subvert the validity of clinical neuropsychological testing.

Where there is controversy, as with some clinical syndromes which a consistent structural correlate has not been identified, space limitations usually have not allowed us to incorporate all viewpoints into the definition. Inclusion of a syndrome should not necessarily be taken as evidence that there is a consensus about its existence, only that it has attained some degree of visibility within professional or academic circles.

As Samuel Johnson observed, "Dictionaries are like watches; the worst is better than none, and the best cannot be expected to be quite true." We have tried to be as objective as possible in deciding on entries and writing the definitions. The etymologies and brief biographies, however, posed special difficulties. Since we are not experts in classical Greek or Roman languages, nor in the history of psychology and medicine, we have relied on a variety of sources for this material. Unfortunately, there were occasional discrepancies about word origins or specific dates in different source materials. The wording of these entries was based on consultation with the editorial board, but at times the choices had to be arbitrary. Although there was always a credible source, the dictionary should not be considered authoritative in these areas. Unless a person's name is associated with a clinical syndrome, biographic information is generally limited to individuals who are no longer alive.

I dedicate my portion of this work to the memory of two individuals who had very different, but nevertheless significant, effects on this project. Daniel E. Sheer, the founding director of the University of Houston Clinical Neuropsychology program, recognized the importance of formal multidisciplinary curriculum in neuropsychology that emphasized collaboration with colleagues in related fields. I have tried to be true to his multidisciplinary conceptualization of neuropsychology. Charles C. Matthews, of the University of Wisconsin, was the senior contributor to this dictionary and provided the wisdom and perspective that could only come from a rich, productive, and distinguished career in neuropsychology.

As is the case in all major projects, this one could not have occurred without the help of many individuals. I thank my MCG colleagues whose numerous hallway consultations significantly improved the quality of many dictionary entries. Thomas R. Swift, MCG Department of Neurology Chair, continues to provide the multidisciplinary environment that allows scholarly activity despite increasing pressures for clinical productivity. I also thank the members of the INS Publication Committee who provided thoughtful recommendations. Finally, I thank Jeffrey W. House, at Oxford University Press, not only for his helpful comments and advice, but also for his patience and tolerance.

Augusta, Georgia   D.W.L.
July 13, 1998

Contributors

PELAGIE M. BEESON, PH.D.
University of Arizona

THOMAS BENKE, M.D. †
Neurologische Klinic, Innsbruck

BROOKE CANNON, PH.D. †
Marywood College

NORMA COOKE, PH.D. †
Baylor College of Medicine

DAVID J. FRANCIS, PH.D.
University of Houston

LESLIE J. GONZALEZ-ROTHI, PH.D.
University of Florida

ROBERT L. HEILBRONNER, PH.D.
Rehabilitation Institute of Chicago

NANCY HELM-ESTABROOKS, SC.D.
Boston University

ELIZABETH WHITE HENRIKSON, PH.D. †
University of Massachusetts Medical Center

BRUCE P. HERMANN, PH.D.
University of Wisconsin

MALCOLM KAHN, PH.D.
University of Miami

ANDREW KERTESZ, M.D., F.R.C.P.(C)
University of Western Ontario

ANTHONY C. KNEEBONE
Flinders Medical Center

SHERRILL R. LORING, M.D.
Medical College of Georgia

LYNN M. MAHER, PH.D.
Georgia State University

CHARLES C. MATHEWS, PH.D. †
University of Wisconsin

GREGORY L. MAYER, PH.D.
Neurology Learning Behavior Center

FENWICK T. NICHOLS, III, M.D. †
Medical College of Georgia

CYNTHIA OCHIPA, PH.D.
James A. Haley Veteran's Hospital

ANDREW C. PAPANICOLAOU, PH.D.
University of Texas Medical School

ALAN J. PARKIN, PH.D.
University of Sussex

ANASTASIA RAYMER, PH.D.
Old Dominion University

FRIEDEL M. REISCHIES, M.D.
Freie Universität Berlin

JOSEPH H. RICKER, PH.D.
Wayne State University

DON ROBIN, PH.D.
University of Iowa

PAULA K. SHEAR, PH.D.
University of Cincinnati

LARRY S. SOLANCH, PH.D. [†]
Queens College

TOM SUTTON
Canberra Specialist Centre

MAX R. TRENERRY, PH.D.
Mayo Clinic Foundation

MICHAEL WESTERVELD, PH.D.
Yale University

DAVID J. WILLIAMSON, PH.D.
Columbus, Georgia

BARBARA A. WILSON, PH.D. [†]
MRC Applied Psychology Unit

GREIG DE ZUBICARAY
University of Queensland

[†] Also served as an Editorial Consultant

INS Dictionary of Neuropsychology

A

AAC. *See* Augmentative or alternative communication.

Aachen Aphasia Test. A linguistically oriented, standardized aphasia battery in German. Spontaneous speech is rated on six dimensions: communicative behavior, articulation and prosody, automatized language, semantic structure, phonologic structure, and syntactic structure. Performance on five subtests is also rated: token test, repetition, written language, confrontation naming, and comprehension. With the exception of the token test, which has a dichotomous scoring, responses on the subtests are rated on a four-point scale. The Aachen Aphasia Test is the most widely employed aphasia test for aphasia classification, patient description, and for treatment evaluation effects in German-speaking countries. (Huber, W., Poeck, K., and Willmes, K. 1983. *Der Aachener Aphasie Test*. Göttingen: Hogrefe.)

ABA design (reversal design). An experimental design to assess intervention effects in individual subjects. In the first A phase, baseline target behaviors are measured. An intervention is applied during the B condition while the same behaviors are assessed. The second A phase (i.e., reversal) measures the effect of withdrawing the intervention and is used to demonstrate that intervention does not simply reflect practice by allowing performance to return to or approach baseline levels. An ABAB design is a variant that studies the treatment effect on two occasions, and it has the clinical advantage of facilitating treatment beyond the experimental requirements of the study.

Abasia. The inability to walk. *See* astasia-abasia. [Gr. *a*, not; *basis*, a step.]

ABCs. Airway, breathing, and circulation (pulse).

Abiotrophy. A programmed loss of neurons in neurodegenerative diseases that reflects a genetic abnormality. Neural loss may begin at any age from infancy to old age. [Gr. *a-*, without; *bios*, life; *trophe*, nourishment.]

Ablation. Surgical removal or destruction of tissue. Ablation is performed in humans to eliminate abnormal function. Anterior temporal lobectomy, which is used to treat poorly controlled epilepsy, is an example of a surgical ablative procedure. Pallidotomy in Parkinson's disease, designed to interrupt excitatory motor pathways, is an example of ablation by electrical lesioning. [L. *ablatus*, past part. of *auferre*, to carry away.]

Abscess, brain. An encapsulated collection of pus in the brain associated with localized infection. Brain abscesses typically present with deficits similar to other space-occupying lesions. They are often difficult to treat with antibiotics because the encapsulation wall acts as a barrier, and surgical drainage is often necessary.

Absence seizure. *See* Seizure.

Abstract attitude. The capacity for abstraction characteristic of normal brain function. Loss of abstract attitude was used to describe the inability to see beyond the most simple or pedestrian concepts. Kurt Goldstein, an American neurologist born in Germany (1878–1965), considered loss of abstract attitude to be the cardinal feature of frontal lobe

1

damage and psychosis. The term is not in active use now, but it is still frequently encountered in older publications.

Abulia. Lack of initiative or drive, accompanied by a lack of spontaneity in speech, thought, and action. This condition appears in psychosis and in neurologic disease. In the latter, it is associated with bilateral lesions in the medial frontal lobe or orbital frontal lobe from tumor, severe traumatic brain injury, or degenerative processes such as Pick's disease. Social abulia is inactivity because of an inability to select a course of action, although a wish to participate may be present. Also spelled aboulia. [Gr. *a-*, without; *boulesis*, will.]

ACA. *See* Anterior cerebral artery.

Acalculia. Acquired disturbance of computational ability commonly associated with both alexia and agraphia for numbers. Both oral and written calculation are commonly impaired. Acalculia subtypes include primary acalculia (anarithmetria) and spatial acalculia. Milder forms of acalculia may affect division and multiplication more than addition and subtraction. The lesion classically associated with primary acalculia involves the left angular gyrus (Brodmann's areas 39 and 40), although computational impairment may be associated with aphasia resulting from any perisylvian lesion. [Gr. *a-*, without; L. *calculare*, to reckon, from *calculus*, a pebble.]

- **Anarithmetria.** *See* Primary acalculia.
- **Primary acalculia.** Acquired calculation impairment that cannot be explained by alexia or agraphia for numbers, or by spatial disorganization for numbers. Also known as anarithmetria.
- **Spatial acalculia.** Impaired ability to perform written calculations because of failure to process spatial aspects of written problems properly. In contrast to primary acalculia, spatial acalculia is more frequently associated with right hemisphere lesions (e.g., manipulating numerals across columns).

Acceleration–deceleration injury. Impairment associated primarily with *diffuse axonal injury* caused by rotational forces associated with rapid deceleration (e.g., high-speed accidents).

Acetylcholine (ACh). A major neurotransmitter of the central and peripheral nervous systems. Acetylcholine is an excitatory neurotransmitter that plays an important role in memory formation. Decreased ACh function has been demonstrated in Alzheimer's disease. It also plays a prominent role in involuntary movement disorders, which are often managed by pharmacologically decreasing caudate ACh. Because decreased ACh is associated with anterograde memory impairment, however, anticholinergic therapy may produce cognitive side effects. Acetylcholine is the principal neurotransmitter at the neuromuscular junction, and myasthenia gravis is characterized by a defect in ACh transmission.

Acetylsalicylic acid (ASA). Aspirin. Acetylsalicyclic acid is a nonsteroidal anti-inflammatory, analgesic, and antipyretic drug that is also used in the treatment of cardiovascular disease and ischemic (i.e., nonhemorrhagic) stroke because it decreases blood viscosity.

Achievement tests. Measures designed to assess school-based learning and competence for specific skills such as reading, spelling, or arithmetic. Achievement test performance is often contrasted with performance on intelligence tests, which is considered primarily a measure of learning potential.

Achilles tendon reflex. A *deep tendon reflex* in which a twitch-like contraction of the calf muscles and plantar flexion at the ankle is elicited by sharply tapping the Achilles tendon above the heel. This reflex may be abolished by either lesions of the first sacral root (S_1) or peripheral neuropathy. Also called ankle jerk.

Achromatopsia. Loss of color vision following temporal-occipital lobe damage. Color loss is usually restricted to one hemifield or one quadrant, although full-field achromatopsia may occur. In left occipital-temporal lobe lesions, patients may display alexia and hemi-anopsia in addition to achromatopsia. Clinically, patients may complain of washed-out colors or reduced brightness or vibrancy of colors. In severe cases, color perception may be completely lacking and patients may complain of seeing everything in gray. Achromatopsia differs from color agnosia, in which verbal color association is impaired because color discrimination is also affected. [Gr. *a-*, without; *chroma*, color; *opsis*, sight, vision.]

ACoA. *See* Anterior communicating artery.

Acoustic neuroma. A benign, slow-growing tumor arising from Schwann cells that surround the vestibular portion of the eighth (acoustic) cranial nerve. The tumor may displace and compress the pons and lateral medulla and obstruct cerebrospinal fluid (CSF) circulation. Symptoms include disturbance of hearing, headache, tinnitus, disturbance of balance, and unsteadiness of gait. [Gr. *akoustikos*, denoting sound; *neuron*, nerve; *-oma*, morbid growth, tumor.]

Acquired immune deficiency syndrome (AIDS). The late clinical expression of infection with human immunodeficiency virus (HIV), recognized as a distinct disease in 1981. AIDS is associated with reduction in CD4+ T lymphocytes. It is operationally defined as fewer than 200 CD4+ T lymphocytes per microliter, or a CD4+ T-lymphocyte percentage of < 14% of the total lymphocyte count with an accompanying AIDS-related condition. AIDS may affect the nervous system at any level, resulting in AIDs dementia, cerebral lymphoma, intracranial infectious processes such as cytomegalovirus (CMV), encephalitis, toxoplasmosis, meningitis, vacuolar myelopathy, neuromuscular transmission defects, peripheral neuropathy, or myopathy. *See* Dementia (AIDS dementia).

ACTH. *See* Adrenocorticotropin hormone.

Action tremor. A rhythmic intention or postural tremor that is often worse at the end of motor activity. It occurs with fine movements such as writing or lifting a cup for drinking. Patients with Parkinson's often have a combined resting tremor and a faster action tremor, particularly in the later stages of the disease.

Activities of daily living (ADLs). Skills necessary for independent or semi-independent living. Instrumental activities of daily living include the abilities to use the telephone, shop, prepare food, perform housekeeping tasks such as laundry and handling finances, and take medications responsibly. Physical self-maintenance activities of daily living (or "personal ADLs") include toileting, feeding, dressing, grooming, physical ambulation, and bathing. The first ADL scale with widespread acceptance was published in 1963. (Katz, S., Ford, A.B., Moskowitz, R.W., Jackson, B.A., and Jaffe, M.W. 1963. Studies of illness in the aged. The index of ADL: A standardized measure of biological and psychosocial function. *JAMA*, 185:914–919.)

AD. *See* Alzheimer's disease.

ADD. *See* Attention-deficit/hyperactivity disorder.

Adenoma. A benign epithelial tumor in which tumor cells arise from glandular structures, the most common of which in the CNS is the pituitary. [Gr. *aden*, signifying a gland or glands; *-oma*, morbid growth, tumor.]

ADHD. *See* Attention–deficit/hyperactivity disorder.

Adiadochokinesia. Deficit of rapidly alternating movements. This is commonly tested by having patients slap the palm and then the back of their hand repeatedly on their knee. Adiadochokinesia results from cerebellar lesions but may also be seen with cases involving frontal lobe or basal ganglia disease. Also called dysdiadochokinesia. [Gr. *a-*, without; *diadoche*, working in an orderly succession; *kinesis*, movement.]

Adipsia. The absence of thirst, characterized by an absence of drinking. The associated lesion is located in the lateral hypothalamus. [L. *a-*, without; *dipsia*, thirst.]

ADL. *See* Activities of daily living.

Adrenal glands. Triangular-shaped, ductless glands that sit above each kidney. They are subdivided into two broad regions: the adrenal cortex and the adrenal medulla.

- **Adrenal cortex**. The outer layer of the adrenal gland. It is stimulated from the pituitary gland by adrenocorticotropic hormone (ACTH) to produce steroid hormones. The adrenal cortex regulates metabolism, blood pressure, and sexual behavior.
- **Adrenal medulla**. The central portion of the adrenal gland. The adrenal medulla secretes epinephrine and norepinephrine.

Adrenergic system. The component of the autonomic nervous system that is composed of cells containing catecholamines (epinephrine, norepinephine, and dopamine).

Adrenocorticotropic hormone (ACTH). A hormone secreted by the pituitary that is the major regulator of adrenal activity. Levels of ACTH follow a circadian rhythm, with elevated levels in the early morning and depressed levels in the late afternoon and early evening. ACTH is increased in Addison's disease, congenital adrenal hyperplasia, ACTH-secreting tumors, stress, surgery, electroconvulsive therapy (ECT), and hypoglycemia, and it is decreased in panhypopituitarism and adrenal cancer. Also called corticotropin.

Adrenoleukodystrophy. A genetic disease of childhood transmitted as a sex-linked recessive trait marked by diffuse abnormality of the cerebral white matter and adrenal atrophy. It is characterized by cognitive impairment that progresses to dementia and by aphasia, apraxia, dysarthria, and impaired vision. [*adrenal* + Gr. *leuko*, white; *dys-*, hard, ill, bad; *trophe*, nourishment.]

Advance medical directive. A legal document that details one's wishes concerning life-sustaining treatments ("living will"), or assigns someone to make such decisions if one becomes incapacitated and is unable to provide such guidance (e.g., durable medical power of attorney). *See* Code.

Advanced Progressive Matrices. *See* Raven's Progressive Matrices.

Adverse event. In investigational drug trials, any untoward, noxious, or unintended event experienced by a subject, regardless of whether the occurrence is thought to be related to the investigational drug.

Aesthesiometer. A measure of tactile sensitivity that employs a compass-like device with nylon filaments of increasing thickness to assess the threshold or minimum spatial separation for two-point perception. [Gr. *aisthesis*, feeling; *metron*, measure.]

Affect. Observed behaviors that reflect underlying emotional tone or feeling state. This contrasts with mood, which is a more sustained and pervasive subjective emotional experience. Affect is revealed by facial expressions, tone of voice, speech content, and motor behaviors. Disturbed affect may be described as blunted, flat, inappropriate, labile, restricted, or constricted. [L. *affectus*, state of mind, from *afficio*, to have influence on.]

Affective disorder. *See* Mood disorders.

Afferent. Neural conduction toward the central nervous system. [L. *afferens*, past part. of *afferre*, to bear.]

Afterdischarge. Abnormal pattern of cell discharges that may appear at and above a specific electrical threshold during electrical cortical stimulation mapping.

Agenesis of the corpus callosum. A congenital condition in which the corpus callosum fails to develop. Patients typically present with mental retardation and epilepsy. However, agenesis of the corpus callosum has also been observed in healthy individuals. The agenesis may not be complete, and partial agenesis tends to involve the posterior corpus callosum. Also called callosal agenesis.

Ageusia. Loss of taste sense. Ageusia is common in Bell's palsy over the anterior two-thirds of one side of the tongue, and it may be associated with head injury if the first (olfactory) cranial nerve is severed. [Gr. *a-*, without; *gueusis*, taste.]

Agitation. A state characterized by extreme restlessness and heightened arousal. It may involve wringing of the hands, pacing, and poor emotional control, including increased irritability and crying or laughing without apparent cause. Agitation may be associated with psychiatric disease, such as schizophrenia, or neurologic conditions. In neurologic patients, agitation is common following acute lesions and with diffuse processes that are at least moderately severe (e.g., *closed head injury, Alzheimer's disease*). [L. *agitatio*, past part. of *agitare*, to put in motion.]

Agnosia. Impaired recognition of previously meaningful stimuli that cannot be attributed to primary sensory defects, attentional disturbance, or a naming disorder. Agnosia was described by Teuber (American psychologist born in Germany, 1916–1977) as a "normal percept stripped of its meaning." It can theoretically be present in each sensory modality, although clinically the most common agnosias are visual and auditory.

In his early descriptions of agnosia, Lissauer (1890) hypothesized that visual recognition could be disrupted either during visual perception (apperceptive agnosia) or during the process of associating the precept with meaning (associative agnosia). Although studies have demonstrated that Lissauer's description is not fully consistent with agnosia (e.g., associative agnosia may have some perceptual difficulty), it continues to accurately characterize stages at which the deficits are most pronounced. [Gr. *a-*, without; *gnosis*, knowledge.] (Lissauer, H. 1890. Ein Fall von Seelenblindheit nebst einem Beitrage zur Theori derselben. *Archiv für Psychiatrie und Nervenkrankheiten* 21:222–270.)

- **Apperceptive agnosia**. A form of visual agnosia in which the deficit is presumed to lie in the production of a stable percept arising from impaired visual perception. Patients have relatively intact acuity and other elementary visual functions but have impaired shape and object recognition. Recognition improves if the stimulus is in motion. Associated lesions are typically diffuse. [L. *ad*, to; *percipere*, to perceive; *gnosis*, knowledge.]

- **Associative agnosia**. Visual agnosia arising from disruption at the postperceptual stage of visual processing in which meaning is attributed. Perception is intact as demonstrated by the ability to draw the object, but it cannot be associated with semantic information for identification. Object recognition is demonstrated through other sensory modalities. Prosopagnosia is a specialized forms of associative agnosia.

- **Astereognosis**. Impaired ability to discriminate objects based on the physical characteristics of size, weight, shape, density, or textural cues. Astereognosis is classically associated with postcentral lesions. The term has been operationally defined in many ways, the most common being the loss of tactile object recognition in the absence of *hypesthesia*. Some have defined astereognosis as any disturbance in object recognition, perception, or discrimination. Astereognosis is usually unilateral, and in this respect it differs from tactile agnosia, which is an higher order impairment of tactile recognition that is present bilaterally. No study has demonstrated the existence of tactile agnosia in the absence of *hypesthesia*. [Gr. *a-*, without; *stereos*, solid; *gnosis*, knowledge.]

- **Auditory agnosia**. Impaired ability to recognize sounds despite normal auditory function. Two types of auditory agnosia have been described: auditory sound agnosia and pure word deafness.

- **Auditory sound agnosia**. The inability to recognize meaningful nonspeech auditory stimuli such as environmental sounds (e.g., train whistle). It occurs less frequently than pure word deafness. Subtypes consisting of either perceptual-discriminative impairments associated with right hemisphere lesions or semantic-associative impairment associated with posterior left hemisphere damage and aphasia have been described.

- **Autotopagnosia**. Disturbed body schema involving an inability to identify the parts of one's body, either to verbal command or by imitation. Gross autotopagnosia is rare and is not observed in isolation. Limited autotopagnosia includes impaired left-right discrimination and finger agnosia. [Gr. *autos*, self; *topos*, a place; *gnosis*, knowledge.]

- **Color agnosia**. The inability to recognize colors despite intact color discrimination ability. The impairment is distinct from color anomia, which is an inability to provide color names with normal color perception, and from achromatopsia, which is an impairment in color perception. Associated lesions are typically in the left or bilateral occipital-temporal areas. The term "color agnosia" has been applied to different phenomena in the literature, however, and it should be employed cautiously given the lack of a standard definition and usage.
- **Finger agnosia**. Bilateral loss of the ability to name or identify the fingers. The concept of finger agnosia is linked to that of the Gerstmann syndrome in which specific disorders of body schema are postulated to occur following left inferior parietal lobe/angular gyrus lesions. Failure on tests of finger recognition and finger localization may depend on the specific demands of the tasks employed (e.g., aphasic misnaming, sensory deficit, spatial disorientation, attentional disturbance). Finger agnosia may be considered a minor form of autotopagnosia.
- **Prosopagnosia**. The inability to recognize familiar faces that is unrelated to a primary visual disturbance. Familiar persons are recognized from their speech, articles of clothing, or gait. The recognition difficulty also often includes familiar buildings, landscapes, and automobiles, and patients may not recognize their own face. Color agnosia or achromatopsia is frequently associated with prosopagnosia. A left upper quadrantanopsia is commonly present. Lesions are typically bilateral infarctions in the territory of the posterior cerebral artery involving the inferior occipital-temporal junction or inferior parietal-occipital regions. Reports of prosopagnosia associated with unilateral lesions have been published, however, the lesions usually being in the right hemisphere. [Gr. *prosopon*, face; Greek *a-*, without; *gnosis*, knowledge.]
- **Pure word deafness**. Loss of aural language comprehension with preserved sound recognition that occurs in the absence of other language impairments. Comprehension of nonverbal sounds is relatively intact. The ability to copy written prose is normal although writing to dictation is severely impaired. The syndrome is thought to result from disconnection of Wernicke's area from auditory input. Lesions typically involve cortical/subcortical areas of the superior temporal gyri. Pure word deafness is often seen in the context of a resolving Wernicke's aphasia.
- **Simultanagnosia**. Impaired recognition of the meaning of a whole picture or object, with preserved ability to describe its parts. The failure to integrate the meaning of elements of a picture was interpreted by Gestalt psychologists as a failure of "simultaneous synthesis," although a defect in ocular scanning has been suggested as a more parsimonious explanation for this phenomenon. [L. *simul*, at the same time; Gr. *a-*, without; *gnosis*, knowledge.]
- **Static object agnosia**. Visual object agnosia, the effect of which is reduced when object is moved.
- **Tactile agnosia**. The inability to recognize objects by touch in the absence of *hypesthesia*. Patients can describe object qualities such as shape or texture but cannot recognize them by touch (*see* Astereognosis above). Tactile agnosia is a unilateral disorder affecting only a single hand. Associated lesions are generally in the inferior parietal lobe (Brodmann's area 39 and 40) and may include the posterior insula.
- **Visual agnosia**. Impaired ability to recognize visual information. *See* Apperceptive agnosia and Associative agnosia (above).

Agrammatism. A disturbance of the production or comprehension of grammatical structures such as function words (e.g., articles, prepositions, auxiliary verbs) and word endings (e.g., -ed, -ing). Although language does not adhere to conventional rules of grammar, meaning is generally preserved because of the presence of substantive words with high information content. Agrammatism is also called telegraphic speech (or telegrammatism) because of the absence of syntactical modifiers and the relative preservation of nouns, verbs, or substantive words, a pattern that was characteristic of telegrams in which charges were based upon the number of words transmitted. Agrammatism depends on characteristics of the specific language examined. [Gr. *a-*, without; gramma, letter, from *graphein*, to write.]

Agraphia. An acquired difficulty in writing or spelling. Agraphia is commonly associated with aphasia and alexia, although it may occur without other linguistic impairments. When seen in isolation, agraphia typically results from superior parietal lobe or the second frontal gyrus of the language-dominant hemisphere. Specific agraphia subtypes (e.g., apraxic, constructional, surface, and deep) have been distinguished depending on the motor mechanisms (writing disorder) and various linguistic features (spelling disorders) involved. [Gr. *a-*, without; *graphein*, to write.]

Agraphia spelling disorders.

- **Deep agraphia**. A syndrome that is similar to phonological agraphia in that there is an impairment of the nonlexical spelling route so that nonwords and unfamiliar words are misspelled. There is also damage to the lexical spelling route, resulting in semantic errors in writing. Spelling is strongly influenced by word class (content words are easier to spell than function words), frequency (high-frequency words are easier to spell than low-frequency words), and imagery/concreteness (high-imagery words are easier to spell than low-imagery words).

- **Jargon agraphia**. Agraphia characterized by senseless combinations of letters or words.

- **Lexical agraphia**. A selective impairment of the lexical (or whole-word) spelling route that results in an overreliance on spelling by sound-to-letter correspondences. This disorder is characterized by impaired ability to spell orthographically irregular or ambiguous words, with preserved ability to spell orthographically regular words and nonwords. Spelling errors typically include phonologically plausible attempts (e.g. "manshun" for "mansion"). Also called surface agraphia.

- **Phonological agraphia**. A syndrome that reflects an impairment of the nonlexical spelling route, that is, an impairment of spelling via sound-to-letter correspondences. The syndrome is characterized by markedly impaired spelling of nonwords and unfamiliar words but relatively spared spelling of real words. In many cases, some impairment of the lexical spelling route is evident so that effects of word class, frequency, and imagery are noted (as described in deep agraphia); however, semantic errors are not associated with phonological agraphia.

- **Semantic agraphia**. Loss of the ability to incorporate meaning into spelling and writing. Semantically incorrect but correctly spelled dictated homophones (e.g., "doe" for "dough") may be written. Irregular words and nonwords are written correctly, however, demonstrating intact lexical and phoneme-to-grapheme conversion.

- **Surface agraphia**. A spelling disorder in which sublexical spelling-to-sound correspondences are used to assemble the spelling of the word. Words may be phonetically plausible but misspelled. The reverse phenomenon is phonological agraphia.

- **Verbal agraphia**. The inability to combine single letters into words despite the ability to write individual letters.

Agraphia writing disorders

- **Afferent agraphia**. A writing impairment associated with impaired sensory feedback involving stroke or grapheme duplication or omission.

- **Allographic agraphia**. A writing impairment associated with poor written production characterized by frequent omission errors with well-formed letter production. Although well formed, the letter production may reflect the wrong letter. Copying and oral spelling are spared.

- **Apraxic agraphia**. A writing impairment characterized by poor letter formation. While copying is slavishly produced, oral spelling may be spared. It results from impaired ability to program the necessary motor movements for writing.
- **Peripheral agraphia**. A writing impairment characterized by distortion of written production reflecting motor/sensory system deficits.
- **Spatial agraphia**. A writing impairment due to spatial deficits that affect nonlinguistic aspects of writing. The term has been applied to a wide variety of phenomena such as writing on a slant, uneven spacing of letters or words and blank spaces, ignoring the left side of a blank page when writing, writing over other words, and duplicating strokes.

Agyria. *See* Lissencephaly.

AIDS. *See* Acquired immune deficiency syndrome.

AIDS dementia. *See* Dementia.

Akathisia. Inner restlessness and continual leg movement associated with *parkinsonism*. Patients feel compelled to walk or to pace to obtain relief. Akathisia may occasionally occur following medication reduction in the treatment of parkinsonism. It is also associated with neuroleptic therapy and may decrease over time after the dosage is reduced. [Gr. *a-*, without; *kathasma*, to sit, from *kata*, down; *hedra* from *hezesthai*, to sit.]

Akinesia. Decreased movement that occurs in the absence of paralysis. Unlike apraxia, akinesia is not associated with difficulty performing appropriate motor sequences but rather is a deficit in the initiation of movement (i.e., a disorder of motor intention). Parkinsonian akinesia is associated with decreased arm swing while walking and with a "masked face" (amimia or reptilian stare). More complete akinesia is seen with bilateral supplementary motor area and anterior cingulate gyrus lesions. [Gr. *a-*, without; *kinesis*, movement.]

Akinetic mutism. A state associated with decreased limb movements and absent speech, with preserved eye movements. Akinetic mutism is associated with large medial frontal lobe or basal forebrain tumors, or ruptured aneurysms of the anterior cerebral artery. It may also occur after thalamic injury. In contrast to locked-in syndrome, in which communication can be established with eye movements, cognition is not easily demonstrated in akinetic mutism because patients will not respond to requests.

Alcohol withdrawal syndrome. A syndrome of agitation, disorientation, and hallucinations that may be seen in alcoholics following alcohol withdrawal. This syndrome may progress to autonomic hyperactivity, delirium tremens, seizures, and death.

Alcoholic cerebellar degeneration. Cerebellar impairment from chronic alcoholism producing a wide-based stance and gait, varying degrees of truncal instability, and ataxia of the legs. Nystagmus and dysarthria are uncommon. In most cases, alcoholic cerebellar degeneration develops subacutely over several weeks or months and then remains unchanged. Alcoholic cerebellar degeneration is approximately twice as common as Wernicke-Korsakoff syndrome.

Alcoholic dementia. *See* Dementia.

Alcoholic Korsakoff syndrome. *See* Korsakoff's psychosis syndrome/disease.

Alexia/dyslexia, acquired. Loss or impairment of the ability to read caused by cerebral injury or illness (for developmental reading disorders *see* Dyslexia). Acquired dyslexias are typically observed as manifestations of aphasia, occurring with other language deficits such as agraphia and impaired comprehension and expression. Cases of relatively pure alexia occur and have contributed to theories of language processing and the cerebral localization of language. Acquired dyslexias are categorized according to clinical presentation, psycholinguistic features, neuroanatomical substrate, or historical convention.[Gr. *a-*, without; *lexis*, word.]

- **Alexia with agraphia**. Loss of the ability to read and write that is frequently associated with left parietal lobe (angular gyrus) lesions. Informally referred to by some as "acquired illiteracy." It was first described in 1891 (Dejerine, J.J. 1891. Sur un cas de cécité verbale avec agraphie, suivi d'autopsie. *Comptes Rendus Hebdomadaire des Séances et Mémoires de la Société de Biologie* 43:197–201).
- **Alexia without agraphia**. An acquired inability to read without a corresponding deficit in writing. Patients are unable to read their own written words. It is generally associated with large ischemic lesions in the posterior cerebral artery territory of the language dominant hemisphere that affects both the left visual cortex and the posterior corpus callosum. Visual information cannot be received by the damaged left occipital cortex. Because of the corpus callosum lesion, visual input to the right posterior cortex cannot be transmitted to the left perisylvian language areas (e.g., angular gyrus) involved in decoding written language. Although written language cannot be decoded, it can be generated because language and motor areas are unaffected. This syndrome was originally described in 1892. Also called pure alexia, Dejerine's syndrome. (Dejerine, J.J. 1892. Contribution à l'étude anatomoclinique et cliniques des différentes variétés de cécité verbale. *Comptes Rendus Hebdomadaire des Séances et Mémoires de la Société de Biologie* 44:61–90.)
- **Aphasic alexia**. A reading disorder associated with aphasia in which reading comprehension and oral reading are both impaired.
- **Attentional dyslexia**. A reading disorder characterized by gross disturbance in reading multiple words or text. Single-word reading is relatively preserved. Associated with disturbances of visual attention.
- **Central dyslexias**. Acquired reading disorders that affect processes by which word forms activate meaning or speech production mechanisms ("higher" language processes). These include deep, phonologic, and surface dyslexias, and alexia with agraphia. *Contrast with* Peripheral dyslexia (below).
- **Deep dyslexia**. A reading disorder affecting both the lexical (whole-word) and nonlexical (reading by letter-to-sound correspondences) reading routes. Deep dyslexia is characterized by semantic paralexias (e.g., reading "liberty" for "freedom"), and effects of word class (content words read better than function words), frequency (high-frequency words read better than low-frequency words), and imagery (high-imagery words read better than low-imagery words). Nonword reading is severely impaired.
- **Literal alexia**. A reading disorder characterized by an inability to recognize written letters.
- **Neglect dyslexia**. A reading disorder characterized by failure to identify the initial or left-most portion of a string of letters or words in text. Omissions and substitutions that preserve the overall length of the target are common errors. Errors can also be influenced by the lexical information contained in the stimulus, suggesting a root attentional disturbance at a relatively high level of representation. Although seen most commonly in patients with left-sided neglect, a few cases with right-sided neglect have also been described.
- **Peripheral dyslexia**. A reading disorder caused by visual processing deficits in which visual inputs cannot be associated with the stored representations of written words. They include attentional and neglect dyslexias, and alexia without agraphia. Term suggested by Shallice and Warrington (1980). *Contrast with* Central dyslexias (above).

(Shallice, T. and Warrington, E.K. 1980). Single and multiple component central dyslexic syndromes. In: M. Coltheart, K. Patterson, and J.C. Marshall (eds.), *Deep Dyslexia*. London: Routledge.)

- **Phonological alexia**. A reading disorder resulting from a selective impairment in the decoding of print to sound. Because words cannot be sounded out, they must be read as whole units. Thus, unfamiliar or nonsense words cannot be read, but recognition and pronunciation of familiar words is intact or only mildly impaired. Reading errors tend to involve visually similar words (e.g., "father" for "further"). This may be an isolated language impairment or it may be associated with fluent aphasia. Anatomic correlations have been inconsistent, although most cases include damage to superior temporal cortex and angular gyrus of the left hemisphere. *Contrast with* Surface dyslexia (below).
- **Pure alexia**. *See* Alexia without agraphia (above).
- **Semantic alexia**. Term describing surface alexia when it develops in dementia. Semantic alexia is used because stored representations of unusually pronounced words that reflect semantic knowledge are presumed lost.
- **Surface alexia**. A reading disorder in which words are read and understood only inasmuch as they can be "sounded out." Thus, in a pattern directly opposite that of phonological dyslexia, nonsense words are read accurately, as are words with phonetically regular spelling. Irregularly spelled words, however, are misread as regularly spelled ones (regularization errors; e.g., "busy" read as "buzzy"). A variety of cerebral lesions has been implicated; most cases have included injury to the left temporal-parietal cortex.

Alexithymia. Difficulty in recognizing and describing one's emotions. [Gr. *a-*, without; *lexis*, word; *thymia*, feelings, passion.]

Alien hand syndrome. A condition in which one hand, typically the left, either acts under its own volitional control or is perceived by the patient to be "foreign," "alien," or "uncooperative." Alien hand syndrome may result from large medial frontal lobe lesions, commissurotomy, or corticobasal ganglionic degeneration. It may occur in commissurotomy patients, although corpus callosotomy alone without additional cerebral involvement is considered insufficient to cause this syndrome. In most cases, the condition's severity decreases over several months.

Allesthesia. Commonly used to describe a condition in which the sensation of touch contralateral to the lesion is referred to the analogous location on the (opposite) side ipsilateral to lesion. This phenomenon, however, is more accurately termed *allochiria*. A more literal interpretation of allesthesia based on the term's Greek origins is the sensation of touch being experienced at a point remote from the point touched. Allesthesia is typically associated with right hemisphere lesions as part of the *neglect syndrome*. [Gr. *allaché*, elsewhere; *aisthésis*, perception.]

Allochiria. Sensation of touch contralateral to the lesion that is referred to the analogous location on the (opposite) side ipsilateral to the lesion. [Gr. *àllos*, other; *cheir*, hand.]

Allokinesia. Limb movement that occurs contralateral to the side of intended movement. Allokinesia is typically associated with right hemisphere lesions and seen as part of the *neglect syndrome*. [Gr. *àllos*, other; *kinesis*, movement.]

Alpha. The first letter of the Greek alphabet, α. **1**. The probability of *type I error* in making a decision about the tenability of a null hypothesis (e.g., P < .05 when α = .05). **2**. The EEG frequency band of 8–13 Hz that occurs maximally over posterior brain regions. Also called the alpha rhythm. **3**. A measure of a test's reliability (coefficient alpha) that reflects the internal consistency of an item.

ALS. *See* Amyotrophic lateral sclerosis.

Alternate forms. *See* Parallel tests.

Alternating sequences test. *See* Luria figures; Fist-edge-palm test.

Alzheimer's disease (AD). (Alois Alzheimer, German neuropathologist, 1864–1915). A primary degenerative dementia with characteristic pathology of *neurofibrillary tangles* and *senile plaques*. Alzheimer's disease is estimated to affect 1.2%–5.0% of the population older than age 65 years and its prevalence rises steeply with each decade (e.g., 30% by age 80–90 years). The clinical diagnosis requires a progressive loss of cognitive ability that interferes with social functioning when other causes of dementia are ruled out. Pathological analysis is necessary for a definite diagnosis, and in the absence of pathological examination, the syndrome is often called either probable Alzheimer's disease or dementia of the Alzheimer type (DAT). Neuropsychological assessment may be important for establishing a putative diagnosis in the early disease stages when cognitive impairment is mild to document memory impairment and other areas of neuropsychological difficulty (e.g., naming, visual-spatial function) that may not be easily recognized with a bedside examination. Patients with no family history of AD have approximately a 15% lifetime risk of the disease.

Alzheimer's Disease Assessment Scale (ADAS). A combined mental status examination and dementia rating scale for Alzheimer's disease. The scale has two parts, one for cognitive and the other for noncognitive function. The cognitive functions sampled include memory, language, and praxis, and the noncognitive functions include mood and behavioral changes. The ADAS is a commonly employed instrument in pharmaceutical research. (Rosen, W.G., Mohs, R.C., and Davis, K.L. 1984. A new rating scale for Alzheimer's disease. *Am J Psychiatry* 141:1356–1364.)

AMA. Against medical advice. This notation is made in a patient's hospital discharge summary, for example, to document that the discharge was neither ordered nor approved by the attending physician.

Amaurosis fugax. Transient monocular blindness resulting from a transient ischemic attack (TIA) of the ophthalmic artery. It is described by patients as a blanket of gray coming down slowly over one eye. Amaurosis fugax episodes indicate underlying atherosclerotic disease with an increased risk for stroke and myocardial infarction. [Gr. *mauros*, black; *amaurosis*, making something black; L. *fugare*, to cause to flee, chase.]

Ambidextrous. Having the ability to use either left or right hand for performing manual tasks. [L. *ambo*, both; *dexter*, the right hand.]

Amer-Ind. American Indian Sign Language. Amer-Ind is often used as a compensatory communication technique in aphasic patients.

Amimia. The inability to express ideas through gestures. This term is occasionally used to described the loss of facial expressiveness associated with parkinsonism. [Gr. *a-*, without; *mimos*, a mimic.]

Ammon's horn. Portion of the hippocampus that is a common site for scar tissue formation (i.e., sclerosis or gliosis), which often gives rise to temporal lobe seizures. Ammon was an ancient Egyptian god depicted as a ram; this area is so named because of its resemblance to a ram's horn.

Amnestic (amnesic) syndrome. Severe impairment in the ability to acquire and retain new information with otherwise preserved cognitive function. Common lesion sites include the hippocampus, hippocampal projections to the fornix and septum, and medial thalamic nuclei. Conditions associated with amnesia include Korsakoff's syndrome, herpes simplex encephalitis, posterior cerebral artery stroke, anoxia, trauma, and transient global amnesia (TGA). Memories that were encoded well before onset of the amnestic syndrome are relatively well preserved. Functional amnesia, which is a psychiatric disorder, usually involves failure to remember autobiographical material such as one's name. The ability to learn new information, however, is generally unaffected. [Gr. *mnéme*, memory; closely related to Gr. *amnestia*, forgiving (forgetting) a wrong, amnesty.]

Amobarbital. An intermediate-acting barbiturate used either as a sedative or to control seizures. It is the most common agent used in the Wada Test to induce hemispheric anesthesia.

Amorphognosia. The inability to identify an object by *proprioception* due to poor perception of its physical attributes that cannot be explained on the basis of concurrent *hypesthesia*. [Gr. *a-*, without; *morph*, form; *gnosis*, knowledge.]

Amorphosynthesis. Impairment of sensory integration that involves not only *tactile agnosia*, but also visual-spatial difficulties, *neglect*, and *dressing apraxia*. This is an old heuristic concept that is not currently used. [Gr. *a-*, without; *morph*, form; *synthesis*, composition.]

Amusia. An acquired deficit of music processing. Following right hemisphere lesions, amusia may involve impairment of melody recognition or difficulty in identifying musical elements such as rhythm. In left hemisphere lesions, music reading and music performance may be poor without impairment of either music recognition or the ability to judge music quality. [Gr. *a-*, without; *mousos*, song, music.]

Amygdala. The almond-shaped nucleus in the mesial anterior temporal lobe that plays a role in memory and emotional control. [Gr. *amygdale*, almond.]

Amyotrophic lateral sclerosis (ALS). A progressive motor neuron disease that affects neurons in the cerebral cortex, brainstem, and spinal cord. Amytrophic lateral sclerosis is not generally seen before 45 years of age. The disease ends fatally from respiratory complication, usually within 2–4 years of onset. Also called Lou Gehrig's disease in North America, named after the famous baseball player who developed the disease when he was 37 years old. Also known as motor neuron disease. [Gr. *a-*, without; *myos, mys,* muscle; *trephein,* to nourish; L. *latus,* side; Gr. *skleros,* hard.]

ANA. Antinuclear antibody. A positive ANA suggests collagen vascular disease such as systemic lupus erythematosus.

Anagram letters. Individual movable letters that are used to test spelling or orthographic competence without writing. [Gr. *ana,* back; *gramma,* from *graphein,* to write.]

Analogy theory. Theory proposing that the pronunciation of new words and nonwords is based on analogies with known words. *See* Rule-based reading.

Anaplasia. Loss of cell differentiation that is characteristic of most malignant tumors. [Gr. *ana,* again; *plasis,* a molding.]

Anarithmetria. *See* Acalculia.

Anarthria. Speech impairment, often used to describe impaired speech from bulbar paralysis. This term was originally used by Pierre Marie (French neurologist, 1853–1940) and was synonymous with pure motor aphasia or aphemia. [Gr. *an-*, without; *arthrosis*, articulation.]

Anastomosis. The anatomical connection of one set of blood vessels to another. [Gr. *anastomosis*, from *anastomoo*, to furnish with a mouth.]

Anencephaly. A congenital malformation resulting from failure of neural tube formation that involves degeneration of forebrain germinal cells and often results in spontaneous abortion. The cerebral and cerebellar hemispheres are often completely absent and there may be only a rudimentary brainstem and basal ganglia. [Gr. *an-*, without; *enkephalos*, brain.]

Anesthesia. Impaired tactile stimulus detection that may result from damage to the anterior parietal lobe, spinal injury, or peripheral causes. Anesthesia induced by pharmacological depression of neural function is used to minimize or eliminate pain associated with medical or surgical procedures. [Gr. *an-*, without; *aisthesis*, feeling.]

An aneurysm. An arterial bulge resulting from a weakened vessel wall. Most aneurysms are located in the subarachnoid space and pose a risk of hemorrhage. A dissecting aneurysm consists of layers of the artery separating. [Gr. *aneurysma*, from *aneurynein*, to widen; *ana*, throughout; *eurunein*, to dilate, widen.]

- **Berry aneurysm**. A sac-like or berry-shaped aneurysm that grows outward from an arterial wall. Intracranial aneurysms are commonly seen at bifurcations of cerebral vessels (e.g., at the internal carotid artery/posterior communicating artery junction, the anterior cerebral artery/anterior communicating artery junction, or the middle cerebral artery bifurcation). Ruptured berry aneurysms are the most common cause of nontraumatic subarachnoid hemorrhage. Because of the risk for bleeding or rupture, berry aneurysms are usually treated surgically. Also called saccular aneurysm.
- **Fusiform aneurysm**. A long segment of arterial dilation. Fusiform aneurysms typically develop secondary to atherosclerosis and pose a very low risk of bleeding.
- **Giant aneurysm**. An aneurysm that has expanded to greater than 25 mm in diameter. Giant aneurysms often present with mass effect rather than rupture.
- **Mycotic aneurysm**. Dilatation of an artery secondary to any infectious process, usually due to the lodgment of an infected embolus or from local spread of an infection (e.g., depressed skull fracture with local infection). Although "mycotic" refers to a fungal infection, the term was originally applied to describe infectious aneurysms without reference to fungal agents and is retained for historic continuity.

Angiography. A radiological technique for imaging cerebral vessels that involves the introduction of a contrast medium. Angiography is an invasive procedure that carries a risk of stroke and reaction to the contrast medium. Also called arteriography. *See* Magnetic resonance angiography. [Gr. *angeion*, a case, vessel, capsule; *grammein*, to write, draw.]

Angioma. A congenital vascular malformation involving blood vessel proliferation that resembles a tumor. Most angiomas are asymptomatic, and when present, symptoms are usually due to arteriovenous ventricular malformations (AVMs) or cavernous angiomas. [Gr. *angeion*, a case, vessel, capsule; *-oma*, morbid growth, tumor.]

Angular gyrus. Convolution of the inferior parietal lobe, arching over the posterior end of the superior temporal sulcus and continuous with the middle temporal gyrus; Brodmann's area 39. Angular gyrus lesions in the dominant hemisphere may produce various combinations of *Gerstmann syndrome* signs, which include agraphia, acalculia, finger agnosia, and right–left disorientation. Alexia may result from angular gyrus lesions.

Anhedonia. The inability to experience pleasure from events that are typically considered enjoyable. Anhedonia is a cardinal feature of affective disorders. [Gr. *an-*, without; *hedone*, pleasure.]

Ankle jerk. *See* Achilles tendon reflex.

Anomia (dysnomia). The impaired ability to name objects or retrieve words. Anomia refers to a pathological word-finding difficulty rather than normal word-finding difficulties or vocabulary limitations. Anomia has been historically associated with lesions of the temporal-parietal junction. It is, however, present to varying degrees with all forms of aphasia, is common in dementia of moderate severity, and by itself generally has little localizing significance. Anomia is often assessed through visual object confrontation although the term "anomia" is also used to characterize word-finding difficulty in spontaneous speech. These two types of word-finding difficulty, however, are dissociable. Although the terms "anomia" and "dysnomia" are often used interchangeably, dysnomia implies a less marked naming impairment than anomia. [Gr. *an-*, without; *onoma*, name.]

Anosmia. Impairment in the ability to smell. Anosmia is associated with facial bone injuries, olfactory nerve degeneration, head trauma, or frontal lobe tumors. Patients with anosmia often state that their sense of taste is also diminished, although this is an artifact of the way we derive food characteristics from odor. In anosmic patients, the ability to detect and recognize sweet, sour, salt, and bitter is preserved. [Gr. *an-*, without; *osmé*, sense of smell.]

Anosodiaphoria. Lack of concern for serious neurological impairments, without denying their existence. *La belle indifference,* which also describes a similar absence of concern for sensory or motor deficits, is commonly used in the context of psychogenic impairment (e.g., conversion symptomatology). [Gr. *a-*, without; *nósos*, disease; *diaphorein*, to disperse, dissipate (by perspiration): *dia-*, in different directions; *phorein,* from *pherein*, to carry or bear; *adiaphoría*, lack of interest.]

Anosognosia. Originally used to describe unawareness of hemiplegia following nondominant (right) hemisphere injury as part of the acute neglect syndrome, anosognosia is now used more broadly for commonly occurring unawareness of cognitive, linguistic, sensory, and motor deficits after focal injures (e.g., Wernicke's aphasia) or conditions affecting the CNS more diffusely (e.g., traumatic brain injury and dementia). Anosognosia consisting of denial of blindness is a cardinal feature of Anton's syndrome. The term was introduced by Joseph François Felix Babinski (French neurologist, 1857–1932). [Gr., *a-*, without; *nosos,* disease; *gnosis*, knowledge.]

Anoxia. Complete or nearly complete lack of oxygen supply to tissue. The most common cause of cerebral anoxia is cardiac arrest. Its greatest effects is on the hippocampus (Sommer sector), resulting in anterograde memory impairment. It also may affect the primary visual and visual association cortices, resulting in central visual disturbances (e.g., cortical blindness, visual agnosia). "Hypoxia" refers to lack of oxygen that is not as complete. [Gr. *an-* without; + *oxygen.*]

Anterior cerebral artery (ACA). *See* Arteries, cerebral.

Anterior commissure. An interhemispheric fiber bundle near the most anterior portion of the third ventricle that connects olfactory structures and lateral parts of the temporal lobe to each other. Commissurotomy as a treatment for intractable epilepsy may, but does not always, include transection of the anterior commissure in addition to the corpus callosum.

Anterior communicating artery (ACoA). *See* Arteries, cerebral.

Anterior communicating artery syndrome. A syndrome of dense anterograde amnesia, disorientation, and confabulation combined with disturbances of attention and behavior including distractibility, perseveration, and *utilization behavior.* Motor, sensory and linguistic functions remain intact. It is associated with rupture of anterior communicating artery aneurysms.

Anterior fossa. The cranial vault on which the frontal lobes rest.

Anterograde amnesia. The inability to acquire and retain new information regardless of the type of material presented (i.e., verbal or nonverbal) or the sensory modality in which it is presented (i.e., auditory, visual). *See* Amnestic syndrome.

Antianxiety drugs. Medications designed to reduce anxiety. Also called anxiolytics or minor tranquilizers. Benzodiazepines are the most commonly prescribed class of antianxiety agents.

Anticoagulation therapy. Drug therapy that decreases blood viscosity/coagulation and is often initiated following ischemic (i.e., nonhemorrhagic) stroke or transient ischemic attacks. The aim is to prevent thrombogenesis and recurrent embolism, and treatment may be administered on an acute or chronic basis, although different agents are used for the two modes.

Anticonvulsant drugs. An older term for antiepileptic drugs. This term has lost favor because some seizure types (e.g., absence seizures, simple complex seizures) are unaccompanied by convulsions, although it is still in active use. *See* Antiepileptic drugs.

Antidepressant drugs. Medications used to treat depression. The two most common classes of antidepressants include selective serotonin reuptake inhibitors (SSRIs) and tricyclic antidepressants.

Antiepileptic drugs (AEDs). Medications used to control seizures. Antiepileptic drugs may have cognitive side effects, primarily on psychomotor speed and rate of information processing, and the risk of cognitive impairment is generally increased with polydrug therapy.

Antihistamines. A class of drugs that reduces histamine action. Antihistamines have anticholinergic effects, which may cause sedation, although the sedating effects of newer antihistamines are significantly smaller than those of older antihistamines. In patients with dementia, the anticholinergic effects may exacerbate recent memory difficulty or confusion.

Antipsychotic drugs. Medications used to manage psychotic disorders. There are several chemical classes of antipsychotic agents that vary widely in potency and side effects (phenothiazines, thioxanthines, dibenzapines, butyrophenones, and indolones). Also called neuroleptic drugs.

Anton's syndrome. (Gabriel Anton, Austrian neurologist, 1858–1933). Denial of blindness, usually seen with bilateral occipital lobe lesions causing *cortical blindness*. Confabulation may be present. Anton's syndrome is a specialized form of *anosognosia*.

Anxiolytic drugs. *See* Antianxiety drugs.

Apgar score. (Virginia Apgar, American pediatrician/anesthesiologist, 1909–1974). A measure of neonatal status usually assessed at 1, 5, and 10 minutes after birth. It is based on heart rate, respiratory effort, muscle tone, skin color, and response to stimulation. Lower scores reflect poorer status with poorer prognosis.

Aphagia. Decreased eating, typically associated with hypothalamic lesions. Aphagia may also refer to swallowing difficulty, which in turn leads to decreased eating. [Gr. *a-*, without; *phagein*, to eat.]

Aphasia. Acquired disorder of symbolic language processing. Aphasia is characterized by a combination of naming, fluency, comprehension, and repetition deficits that are accompanied by reading and writing impairments. Characteristics of the language impairment include *paraphasias, circumlocution, anomia* or *conduite d'approche*. Different aphasia subtypes are classified according to the relative impairments of different language domains, and different names for the same constellation of deficits are often used. In addition, aphasia is commonly characterized by the mechanism of injury or by its relationship to underlying brain process. Aphasia does not include disorders of articulation such as dysarthria. Because most aphasia patients have disturbed language function rather than a complete absence of language, these disorders are more accurately classified as dysphasia. By tradition, however, the term "aphasia" is used.

The classic aphasia subtypes usually result from acute injury, which is usually vascular in etiology. Although slowly growing tumors may cause language disturbance, they produce much less impairment than stroke, given the brain area and volume of tissue involved. Aphasia may also be observed in a variety of other conditions such as traumatic brain injury. The quality of language impairments characteristically changes over the months following acute injury or as a function of disease progression. [Gr. *a-*, without, none; *phanai*, to speak; *phasis*, utterance.]

Aphasia related to clinical or atypical patient characteristics

- **Crossed aphasia**. Aphasia resulting from right hemisphere injury in right-handed individuals. Right hemisphere (or bilateral) language representation is inferred, and may be associated with complexly reversed cerebral language lateralization in which the left hemisphere is dominant for visual-spatial function (*situs inversus*).

- **Ictal aphasia**. Transient language impairment associated with seizure discharges from cortical language areas. Ictal aphasia suggests a seizure focus in the left hemisphere.
- **Optic aphasia**. The inability to name items despite preserved visual acuity and the ability to demonstrate their functions. Tactile examination of the same items results in correct naming. This rare syndrome is associated with parietal-occipital or occipital lesions.
- **Post-traumatic aphasia**. Impaired language following brain injury.
- **Primary progressive aphasia (PPA)**. Focal progressive decline in which aphasia develops and worsens without impairment of other higher cognitive functions. A variety of lesions involving the inferior frontal gyrus and temporal lobe has been described.
- **Subcortical aphasia**. Aphasia resulting from a subcortical lesion, as in the thalamus, basal ganglia, or afferent tracts to the auditory speech areas. Left thalamic hemorrhage is the most common cause of subcortical aphasia, which is associated with fluctuating language performance in which naming is impaired, speech is fluent with many paraphasias, and repetition is normal. Left basal ganglia lesions, if they are large, may produce a language impairment that resembles global aphasia.

Aphasia syndromes

- **Amnesic aphasia**. Aphasia subtype used in several early classification systems that is characterized by difficulty remembering words and names; synonymous with nominal (anomic) aphasia. It is seen with small left temporal lobe lesions. "Amnesic" aphasia implies that word-finding difficulty results from words being "forgotten."
- **Anomic aphasia**. Aphasia subtype characterized by impaired naming ability with circumlocutions, few paraphasias, good comprehension, fluent speech, and normal repetition. Anomic aphasia is not synonymous with anomia, although anomia is a feature of anomic aphasia. Also called nominal aphasia or amnesic aphasia, but anomic aphasia may be observed following lesions throughout the left hemisphere.
- **Anterior aphasia**. Nonfluent aphasia; Broca's aphasia. The term is used to contrast with posterior aphasia. Its name is derived from characteristic lesions anterior to the central sulcus.
- **Broca's aphasia**. (Pierre Paul Broca, French surgeon and anthropologist, 1824–1884). Nonfluent aphasia characterized by effortful, often agrammatic speech production with poor repetition and relatively preserved comprehension of single words and short phrases (although comprehension of syntax may be impaired, e.g., Token Test). Naming is generally impaired although either prompting with a context or with phonemic cueing may facilitate performance. Language lacks grammatical complexity, and similarly, reading comprehension is poor for sentences that require processing of grammatical words. Right hemiplegia is a common neighborhood neurologic sign due to the characteristic lesion of the posterior, inferior frontal lobe. The lesion typically results from infarction of the upper (anterior) division of the middle cerebral artery involving the upper and lower frontal operculum, insula, and adjacent regions surrounding the Sylvian fissure. Global aphasia following stroke commonly resolves into Broca's aphasia. (Broca, P. 1861. Remarques sur le siège de la faculté du language articulé; suivies d'une observation d'aphémie (perte de la parole). *Bull. Soc. Anat.* (*Paris*) 6;330–357, 398–407. Translated as Remarks on the set of the faculty of articulate language, followed by an observation of aphemia. In: G. von Bonin (ed). 1960. *Some Papers on the Cerebral Cortex.* Springfield, IL: Charles C. Thomas, pp. 49–72.)

- **Conduction aphasia**. Fluent aphasia with severely impaired repetition but relatively preserved language comprehension. Speech output is characterized by prominent phonemic (literal) paraphasias and word-finding difficulty. Patients with conduction aphasia have difficulty reading aloud because they make paraphasic errors, but they may have relatively good comprehension. Ludwig Lichtheim (German physician, 1845–1925) predicted the existence of this syndrome prior to seeing any clinical cases (*see* Wernicke-Lichtheim model). He further postulated the lesion to involve the arcuate fasciculus beneath the supramarginal gyrus, which disconnects the comprehension area of the temporal lobe from the language output area of the frontal lobe. Thus, the conduction of language information between these areas is disrupted. Current imaging studies have demonstrated that conduction aphasia is associated with lesions of the posterior perisylvian language areas, not the arcuate fasiculus, and it has been hypothesized as representing a Wernicke's aphasia that has largely resolved.
- **Dynamic aphasia**. Aphasia subtype proposed by Aleksandr R. Luria (Soviet neuropsychologist, 1902–1977) characterized by non-fluent output with preserved repetition and comprehension. Dynamic refers to difficulty in speech initiation; it is the equivalent of transcortical motor aphasia.
- **Expressive aphasia**. Aphasia subtype in which nonfluent output is the prominent feature; it generally arises from anterior lesions. The term is not commonly used because some degree of expressive difficulty is characteristic of most aphasias. The term is used in contrast with receptive aphasia.
- **Fluent aphasia**. Aphasia characterized by relatively normal prosodic variation and articulation with frequent paraphasias. Fluent aphasia includes Wernicke's aphasia, conduction aphasia, anomic aphasia, and transcortical sensory aphasia. The term is used in contrast with nonfluent aphasia.
- **Global aphasia**. Aphasia subtype that involves nearly complete loss of all core linguistic functions including fluency, comprehension, repetition, reading, and writing. Large lesions involving both Broca's area and Wernicke's area, as well as other perisylvian language regions, are generally found.
- **Jargon aphasia**. Aphasia subtype characterized by fluent paraphasic speech that may be incomprehensible and filled with neologisms. Speech contains numerous semantic (verbal) and phonemic (literal) paraphasias with significant perseveration. Jargon aphasia represents an acute expression of Wernicke's aphasia.
- **Mixed aphasia**. Aphasia that does not fit into classic nosology, or aphasia with both expressive and receptive features. This term is used informally and has no localization or heuristic value.
- **Mixed transcortical aphasia**. Rare aphasia subtype in which repetition is relatively intact despite significant aphasia. Spontaneous speech is nonfluent, and patients are unable to name, read, and write. Repetition, however, is normal up to standard span length and it may be echolalic. Norman Geschwind (American neurologist, 1926–1984) used the term "isolation of the speech area" since the pathology spares perisylvian language areas but involves the surrounding vascular watershed zones. (Geschwind, N., Quadfasel, F.A., and Segarra, J. 1968. Isolation of the speech area. *Neuropsychologia* 30:327–340.)
- **Motor aphasia**. Nonfluent aphasia; Broca's aphasia. The term is no longer in wide use and was used in contrast with sensory aphasia.
- **Nominal aphasia**. Anomic aphasia.
- **Nonfluent aphasia**. Aphasia that is characterized by effortful speech production and lacks normal prosody. Nonfluent aphasia includes Broca's aphasia, global aphasia,

transcortical motor aphasia, and mixed transcortical aphasia. The term is used in contrast with fluent aphasia.

- **Posterior aphasia**. Fluent aphasia; Wernicke's aphasia. The term is used to contrast with anterior, or Broca's, aphasia. Its name is derived from characteristic lesions posterior to the central sulcus. This term is no longer in wide use.
- **Pure motor aphasia**. Nonfluent speech with largely preserved language functioning, demonstrated by the ability to write. It is synonymous with aphemia. Also called apraxia of speech.
- **Receptive aphasia**. Aphasia subtype in which relatively impaired comprehension is the prominent feature. It is associated with more posterior lesions. The term is not commonly used because some degree of comprehension difficulty is characteristic of most aphasia. Contrasts with expressive aphasia.
- **Semantic aphasia**. Aphasia subtype described by Henry Head (British neurologist, 1861–1940) and Aleksandr Luria (Soviet neuropsychologist, 1902–1977) in which there is an impaired capacity to draw inferences beyond the literal meaning of the word. This classification is not in current use.
- **Sensory aphasia**. Wernicke's aphasia. The term was introduced by Carl Wernicke (German neurologist, 1848–1905), who based this classification on Theodor H. Meynert's (Austrian neurologist, 1833–1892) principle that motor function originates anterior to the central fissure and that sensory function is localized posterior to the central sulcus. This term is no longer in wide use; it was used in contrast with motor aphasia.
- **Transcortical motor aphasia**. Nonfluent aphasia characterized by preserved repetition and relatively preserved language comprehension. This aphasia is similar to Broca's aphasia except for the preserved repetition. Lesions are typically vascular and involve the area superior or anterior to Broca's area or the supplementary motor area.
- **Transcortical sensory aphasia**. Fluent aphasia in which language comprehension is severely impaired but repetition is relatively preserved. Speech is fluent and circumlocutory, often with semantic jargon. This aphasia is similar to Wernicke's aphasia except that repetition is preserved. Lesions have been reported to involve the posterior half of the brain from the occipital pole forward on both the medial and lateral surfaces, often reaching along the medial occipital lobe in the area of distribution of the posterior cerebral artery. Neighborhood signs include hemianopsia, visual agnosia, and sensory loss. Transcortical sensory aphasia has also been described in the later stages of Alzheimer's disease.
- **Wernicke's aphasia**. (Carl Wernicke, German neurologist, 1848–1905). Fluent aphasia with frequent semantic (verbal) paraphasias. Language comprehension and repetition are severely impaired. Naming is impaired, and in contrast to Broca's aphasia, prompting provides little benefit. Immediately after injury, patients often display jargon aphasia and may appear agitated, although agitation resolves over several days. Lesions usually involve the posterior-superior portion of the dominant hemisphere temporal lobe. The lesions are generally vascular and may result from occlusion of the posterior temporal branch, the angular branch, or occasionally, the middle temporal branch of the middle cerebral artery. There is no motor involvement present. (Wernicke, C. 1874. *Der aphasische Symptomenkomplex: Eine psychologische Studie auf anatomischer Basis.* Breslau: Cohn and Weigert. In: *Wernicke's Works on Aphasia: A Sourcebook and Review* (G.H. Eggert, trans.). The Hague: Mouton, 1977).

Aphasic alexia. *See* Alexia.

Aphasia Quotient (AQ). Summary score of the language subtests of the Western Aphasia Battery reflecting overall language impairment relative to a healthy control population. *See* Western Aphasia Battery.

Aphasia Screening Test (AST). Any test that samples language rather than comprehensively assessing major language domains.

Aphemia. Pure motor aphasia. Aphemic patients are nonfluent, although language functioning is largely preserved as demonstrated by the ability to write. Aphemia was Broca's original choice for what subsequently became known as aphasia. Also called apraxia of speech. [Gr. *a-*, without; *pheme*, speech, voice.]

Aphonia. Loss of voice. Patients can mouth words and whisper. In contrast to mutism, aphonia is a loss of voice associated with a peripheral etiology. *See* Hypophonia. [Gr. *a-*, without; *phanai*, to speak.]

Apnea. Absence or interruption of breathing. *See* Sleep apnea. [Gr. *apnoia*, want of breath.]

Apolipoprotein E (ApoE). A lipid-protein complex responsible for lipid transport in the blood. It is codified by a gene on chromosome 19. The ε4 allele has been linked to an increased risk of late-onset Alzheimer's disease (AD), although AD develops in the absence of the ε4 allele and patients with the ε4 allele may fail to develop the disease.

Apoplexy. Antiquated term meaning hemorrhagic stroke. The term is now reserved for pituitary apoplexy, an acute hemorrhage or infarction of a pituitary adenoma. [Gr. *apo*, from; *plexis*, stroke, from *plesein*, to strike.]

Appallic syndrome. Vegetative state.

Apperceptive visual agnosia. *See* Agnosia.

Apractagnosia. Older term for disorders of spatial recognition, constructional apraxia, spatial alexia, spatial agraphia, spatial acalculia, disorders of subjective visual coordinates, and hemi-asomatognosia. [Gr. *a-*, without; *praktos*, from *prassein*, to do, practice; *gnosis*, knowledge.]

Apraxia. The inability to perform learned purposeful movements for reasons other than impaired motor strength, sensation, coordination, or comprehension. The term "apraxia" was introduced by Hugo Karl Liepmann (German psychiatrist, 1863–1925), who described apraxia as a disconnection between the idea of the movement and its motor execution. The major subtypes of apraxia are constructional apraxia, ideomotor apraxia, and ideational apraxia. Although doubly dissociable, apraxia and aphasia frequently coexist. [Gr. *a-*, without; *praxis*, action, or a doing.]

- **Apraxia of eyelids**. An inability to volitionally open or close the eyelids. It is often associated with top-of-the-basilar syndrome.
- **Apraxia of speech**. An impairment of motor programming for speech production that results in relatively inconsistent articulation errors and difficulty with articulatory placement. Patients sound like they are struggling to articulate words.
- **Buccofacial apraxia**. An inability to perform voluntary motor movements of the face, lips, and tongue on command. It is tested by having patients perform non-speech oral gestures in the absence of objects (e.g., blowing out a match). The lesion commonly includes the left central operculum and anterior insula; consequently, buccofacial apraxia frequently coexists with Broca's aphasia. Also called oral apraxia.
- **Callosal apraxia**. A form of *ideomotor apraxia* associated with difficulty in executing motor sequencing tasks of the left hand following lesions of the corpus callosum. Callosal apraxia is thought to result from disconnection of the visuokinetic motor engrams of the left hemisphere from the motor area of the right hemisphere. It is seen, usually on a transient basis, in individuals with a lesion affecting fibers passing through the anterior corpus callosum. Also called unilateral apraxia.
- **Conceptual apraxia**. An inability to perform limb movements on command resulting from impairment in linking the meaning or intent of an action to the movement plan. Movements are well performed but inaccurate in content.

- **Constructional apraxia**. An inability to copy or assemble items in two- or three-dimensional space. Constructional apraxia differs from other forms of apraxia in that it is not a motor deficit but rather reflects visual-constructional impairment. Consequently, it is frequently not discussed in the context of other apraxias, and the more theoretically neutral term "visuoconstructional impairment" is often used to describe the impairment. Constructional apraxia is a common effect of right-sided parietal lobe lesions, although it may result from left-sided lesions that are often not associated with receptive language impairment. It is also one of the earliest neuropsychological findings associated with dementia and is common with diffuse cerebral impairment.
- **Dressing apraxia**. An inability to dress oneself. Dressing apraxia may be present as part of the neglect syndrome.
- **Frontal apraxia**. An inability to perform routine actions because of temporal or sequential disorganization. Verbal mediation does not improve performance. The links between the goal of action and the specific acts that must be "assembled" to serve the goal become destabilized, and the action sequence becomes a series of isolated fragments.
- **Gait apraxia**. An inability to walk despite the capacity to execute normal walking movements when lying in bed. Affected patients sometimes appear glued to the floor. Gait apraxia may be caused by frontal lobe lesions, normal pressure hydrocephalus, and Parkinson Plus syndromes, and it is often called frontal gait.
- **Graphomotor apraxia**. An inability to draw and write despite normal capacity to hold and manipulate pen or pencil. Graphomotor apraxias may exist independently from central agraphia and may accompany anterior or posterior lesions of either cerebral hemisphere. More commonly called apraxic agraphia.
- **Ideational apraxia**. An inability to perform a series of gestures due to a loss of the plan of action (ideation) for movement. A frequently given example of the type of movement series impaired with ideational apraxia is that of filling and lighting a pipe. Ideational apraxia is often seen in patients with moderately severe dementia.
- **Ideomotor apraxia**. An inability to perform transitive or intransitive gestures on command. Performance may or may not improve with imitation or with the actual object. A common error is using a body part as an object (or tool) in which part of the hand forms part of the object (tool) being demonstrated. Movements commonly used to assess ideomotor apraxia include the pretended use of common objects (e.g., hammer, scissors, key) and symbolic gestures (e.g., saluting, making the thumb-out gesture of a hitchhiker). Ideomotor apraxia is generally associated with left hemisphere lesions (inferior parietal lobe or supplementary motor area) or a lesion of the corpus callosum. Ideational apraxia and ideomotor apraxia frequently coexist.
- **Limb-kinetic apraxia**. Clumsiness of the hand that exceeds weakness or tone impairment. Limb-kinetic apraxia is thought to be related to pyramidal motor system lesions and is not considered a disorder of learned skilled movements per se; no difficulty in the selection or sequencing of motor programs is present. Limb-kinetic apraxia is typically asymmetric, greater for distal than proximal movements, and seen with pantomime, imitation, or the use of real objects. Transitive gestures are more affected than intransitive gestures. Also called innervation apraxia or melokinetic apraxia.
- **Melokinetic apraxia**. *See* Limb-kinetic apraxia (above).
- **Ocular apraxia**. Apraxia associated with visual scanning and volitional eye movements. Vestibular-induced saccades and optico-kinetic nystagmus are less severely impaired. Ocular apraxia is generally associated with bilateral frontal-parietal lesions.

- **Optic apraxia/optic ataxia**. Apraxia of ocular searching movements affecting visually guided hand movement. Optic apraxia/ataxia usually results from bilateral posterior parietal lesions. The symptoms are the same for both optic apraxia and optic ataxia; the different terms vary in their emphasis on the underlying neurobehavioral deficit that accounts for the phenomenon. Also called visuomotor apraxia. *See* Balint's syndrome.

Apraxia of eyelids. *See* Apraxia.

Apraxia of speech (aphemia). *See* Apraxia.

Aprosexia. A disturbance of attention and concentration associated with psychomotor inefficiency. Common complaints include difficulty remembering conversations, instructions, appointments and things to do, material just read, and keeping the mind on a task. Associated features include complaints of insomnia and fatigue. [Gr. *a-*, without or lacking; *prosexia,* from *prosechein,* to turn something (as one's mind or attention).]

Aprosodia (dysprosodia). An impairment in the prosodic or melodic component of speech. Aprosodia may be seen with either left or right hemisphere lesions. Left hemisphere lesions produce impairment in appropriate syllable stress, and right hemisphere lesions affect the emotional content of speech, often producing emotional flattening or lability. Also called motor aprosodia. *See* prosody. [Gr. *a-*, without; *prosodia,* a song sung to music, from *pros,* to; *ode,* a song.]

Aqueduct of Sylvius. (Franciscus Sylvius, Dutch anatomist, 1614–1672). *See* cerebral aqueduct.

Arachnoid (arachnoid mater). The middle of three meninges located between the dura and pia. The arachnoid and pia together form the leptomeninges. [Gr. *arachne,* spider, cobweb; *eidos,* resemblance; *mater,* mother, used as a metaphor for protector.]

Arachnoid villi. Granulations that function as one-way valves allowing the passage of substances from the cerebrospinal fluid (CSF) to venous blood in the superior sagittal sinus.

Arcuate fasciculus. The major association fiber bundle originating in the temporal lobe and terminating in the prefrontal cortex. It also forms part of the superior longitudinal fasciculus or dorsal pathway, and it connects Wernicke's area through the angular gyrus to Broca's area. *See* aphasia syndromes (conduction aphasia). [L. *arcucus,* a bow; *fascis,* a bundle.]

Areflexia. *See* Hyporeflexia.

Argyll Robertson pupil. (Douglas Moray Cooper Lamb Argyll Robertson, Scottish ophthalmologist, 1837–1909). Pupillary abnormality associated with normal pupillary convergence with loss of consensual pupillary reflex (eyes can accommodate but not react). This phenomenon often accompanies tabes dorsalis and is diagnostic of tertiary neurosyphilis.

Arhinencephaly. The congenital absence of the olfactory bulb and tracts. Arhinencephaly is associated with fusion of the cerebral hemispheres. [Gr. *a-*, without; *rhino, rhis,* nose; *enkephalos,* brain.]

Arnold-Chiari malformation. (Julius Arnold, German pathologist, 1835–1915; Hans Chiari, German pathologist, 1851–1916). A congenital anomaly in which the cerebellum and medulla protrude down into the spinal canal through the foramen magnum. It may be associated with many other defects, including spina bifida/meningomyelocele.

Arousal. The state of general alertness. Arousal may be divided into tonic arousal, which characterizes the general arousal state and includes the sleep-wake cycle, and phasic arousal, which refers to the sudden increase in attentiveness necessary for rapid response.

Arteries, cerebral. Blood vessels supplying the brain. [L. *arteria,* from Gr. *artēria,* the windpipe, later an artery as distinct from a vein.]

- **Anterior cerebral artery (ACA)**. An artery originating at the bifurcation of the internal carotid artery that supplies blood to the dorsolateral and mesial frontal regions.

- **Anterior communicating artery (ACoA)**. A small artery connecting the two anterior cerebral arteries and forming the anterior portion of the circle of Willis.
- **Basilar artery**. An artery formed by the union of the left and right vertebral arteries. The basilar artery runs from the lower to upper pons, where it bifurcates into the two posterior cerebral arteries.
- **Carotid artery**. One of the major arteries supplying blood to the brain. The carotid artery bifurcates to form the internal carotid artery (ICA) and external carotid artery (ECA). [Gr. *karotis*, pl. *karotides*, the two great arteries of the neck, from *karoun*, to plunge into sleep or stupor; compression of either artery causes unconsciousness.]
- **Internal carotid artery**. An artery beginning at the bifurcation of the common carotid artery that terminates in the middle fossa where it bifurcates into the anterior and middle cerebral arteries.
- **Lenticulostriate arteries**. Small penetrating arteries supplying the lentiform nucleus and striatum. They are prone to occlusion from chronic hypertension, producing small lacunar infarction. [L. *lenticula*, a lentil; *striatus*, grooved, furrowed, from *striare*, to groove, channel.]
- **Middle cerebral artery (MCA)**. A major cerebral artery supplying the temporal lobe, thalamus, striatum, and insula. Most strokes involve some aspect of the MCA distribution.
- **Posterior cerebral artery (PCA)**. An artery formed by the bifurcation of the basilar artery that supplies the thalamus, hypothalamus, cerebral peduncles, choroid plexuses of the lateral and third ventricles, and the temporal and occipital lobes.
- **Posterior communicating artery (PCoA)**. Arteries of internal carotid origin that connect with the posterior cerebral arteries to form the circle of Willis.

Arteriography. *See* Angiography.

Arteriolosclerosis. *See* Arteriosclerosis.

Arteriosclerosis. Vessel abnormalities in which walls of the arteries become thickened and lose their ability to stretch. There are two main forms of arteriosclerosis that affect cerebral vessels: arteriolosclerosis and atherosclerosis. Arteriosclerosis is a major risk factor for stroke. Literally "hardening of the arteries." [Gr. *arteria*, artery, *sklerosis*, hardness.]

- **Arteriolosclerosis**. Arteriosclerosis of the smaller arteries (arterioles) that is associated with chronic hypertension.
- **Atherosclerosis**. A buildup of fatty deposits (plaques) on the innermost layer of arterial walls resulting in narrowing of the vessel lumen. Thrombi may form over these plaques (localized atherosclerotic deposits). Atherosclerotic thrombi are often associated with myocardial infarction. [Gr. *athere, athera*, gruel; *sklerosis*, hardness.]

Arteriovenous malformation (AVM). A congenital vascular abnormality consisting of a direct connection between arteries and veins that bypasses the normal capillaries. Arteriovenous malformations typically present as a subarachnoid hemorrhage or seizures. Because of the high risk of hemorrhage, AVMs are treated by surgical resection, which is often preceded by embolization of the AVM to decrease its size. They may be associated with a *steal phenomenon* in which blood flow is diverted away from the normal circulation into the AVM, leading to decreased perfusion of neural tissue.

Arthur Point Scale of Performance Battery. A battery to assess intelligence. The battery includes several tests that are either precursors to current tests or have remained in active neuropsychological use, including the Knox Cube Imitation Test, the Seguin Form Board (*see* Tactual Performance Test), Porteus Mazes, and Kohs Block Design Test. (Arthur, G. 1943. *A Point Scale of Performance Tests.* Chicago; Stoelting Co.)

Articulation. The process of moving oral structures to produce the sounds for speech.

Articulatory loop. A component of *working memory* involved in the storage and manipulation of speech-based information. Also called phonological loop.

ASA. *See* Acetylsalicylic acid; abbreviation for aspirin.

Aseptic meningitis. *See* Meningitis.

Asomatognosia. Denial of one's own body part; this denial is commonly seen as part of the *neglect syndrome* resulting from acute right-sided cerebral lesions. When patients are confronted with their own arm and asked, "whose arm is this?," they will frequently answer "yours" or "I don't know." There is no similar impairment when identifying the contralateral, nonparetic arm. [Gr. *a-*, without; *soma*, body; *gnosis*, knowledge.]

Asperger's syndrome. A mild variant of *autism* characterized by social isolation and eccentric behavior in childhood. Two-sided social interaction and nonverbal communication are impaired. Though grammatical, speech is peculiar because of abnormalities of inflection and a repetitive pattern. Clumsiness is prominent in both speech articulation and gross motor behavior. This syndrome was broadened in 1981 to include arithmetic deficit, impaired humor, and gestural comprehension deficit. Hans Asperger (Austrian psychiatrist) originally defined this syndrome in 1944 as "autistic psychopathy."

Aspiration pneumonia. Pneumonia caused by saliva, food, or drink entering the lungs. It commonly occurs with impaired swallowing or oral motor control and diminished gag and cough reflexes.

Association cortex. Cortical areas other than primary sensory or motor regions involved with complex functions.

Associative agnosia. *See* Agnosia.

Astasia-abasia. An inability to stand (astasia) and walk (abasia). When used together and hyphenated, astasia-abasia typically refers to a psychogenic disorder of motor coordination characterized by the inability to stand or walk despite normal ability to move legs when lying down or sitting. Patients often sway wildly, stagger, and nearly fall, yet recover their balance at the last moment. The term is used less frequently in the context of genuine neurologic impairment (e.g., hydrocephalic astasia-abasia). [Gr. *a-*, without; *stasos*, stand, from *histanai*, to stand, a-, without; *basīs*, step.]

Astereognosis. *See* Agnosia.

Astereopsis. The inability to perceive the depth of objects. [Gr. *a-*, without; *optikos*, denoting sight.]

Asterixis. A motor disturbance characterized by a rapid, sporadic limb contraction followed by a slower return to extension. Asterixis is seen in toxic-metabolic encephalopathy or confusional states, and it is common in patients with impending hepatic coma. It is typically tested by having patients extend their arms and hands to motion "stop." [Gr. *a-*, without; *sterixis*, fixed position.]

Astrocyte. A large glial cell.

Astrocytoma. A primary brain tumor arising from proliferation of brain astrocytes. Astrocytomas in children typically are not infiltrating, and they are relatively benign and located in the posterior fossa. In adults, astrocytomas generally arise in the cerebrum, evolve into malignant tumors, and infiltrate extensively. Astrocytomas are graded from I (low) to IV (high) according to their degree of malignancy (grade I: high differentiation; grade II: astroblastoma; grade III; astroblastoma; grade IV: glioblastoma). [Gr. *astron*, a star; *cyto-*, combining form meaning "of a cell"; *-oma*, morbid growth, tumor.]

Asymbolia. Older term for impaired processing or recognition of symbolic material (e.g., language, pictures). It was often used to describe central cognitive or semantic disturbances, such as the inability to understand the significance of various signs and symbols or of environmental stimuli. [Gr. *a-*, without; *symbolon*, a mark or sign.]

Ataxia. Abnormal movement including errors in rate, range, direction, timing, and force ("coordination") of motor activity. Components of ataxia include decomposition of movement into component parts, dysmetria, dysdiadochokinesia, and tremor. [Gr. *a-*, without; *taktos*, from *tassein*, to order, arrange.]

- **Limb ataxia**. Incoordination of limb muscles associated with lesions of the cerebellar hemispheres.
- **Optic ataxic**. *See* Apraxia (optic apraxia).
- **Truncal ataxia**. Incoordination of the truncal musculature characterized by lurching, unsteady, and wide-based gait associated with tumors of the midline cerebellum (vermis) or chronic alcoholism.

Atherosclerosis. *See* Arteriosclerosis.

Athetosis. An involuntary slow, regular writhing movement resulting from kernicterus, hypoxia, and prematurity; it may also be present in many diseases of the basal ganglia. Distal limbs are usually more affected, although athetosis may be present in any muscle group. Willed movement of one hand may result in synkinesia, the contraction of distant muscles. Athetosis is commonly associated with mental retardation, although relatively normal IQs may be seen if damage is restricted to the basal ganglia. [Gr. *a-*, without; *thetos*, from *tithenai*, to place.]

Atonic seizures. Generalized seizures that result in a sudden loss of motor tone. These spells typically occur without warning, and patients run the risk of head or other physical injury. Also called drop attacks.

Atrophy. Tissue wasting associated with a reduction in the size and number of cells. [Gr. *atrophia*, from *a-*, without; *trophe*, nourishment.]

Attention. Processes that enable an individual to engage in certain cognitive operations while ignoring others. Thus, attention involves a selective awareness or responsiveness. Attention also refers to the ability to focus and maintain interest for given task or activity.

Attention deficit disorder (ADD). *See* Attention-deficit/hyperactivity disorder.

Attention-deficit/hyperactivity disorder (ADHD). A common disorder with childhood onset, characterized by excessive restlessness, impulsivity, distractibility, and low frustration tolerance. The onset of symptoms occurs before age 7 years, and symptoms disrupt social, academic, or occupational function. This disorder is diagnosed in the absence of any pervasive developmental disorder that can account for a similar constellation of findings. Methylphenidate is a widely used treatment that decreases hyperactivity by enhancing the release of norepinephrine and dopamine. Attention deficit disorder (ADD) is a common synonym for attention-deficit/hyperactivity disorder (ADHD), which is the presently preferred term.

Audiogram. A plot that displays hearing threshold in decibels as a function of sound frequency as presented by air conduction or bone conduction. [L. *audire*, to hear; Gr. *gramma*, a drawing.]

Audiometry. Measurement of hearing acuity across a range of frequencies (typically 125–8000 Hz). [L. *audire*, to hear; Gr. *metros*, to measure.]

Auditory agnosia. *See* Agnosia.

Auditory consonant trigrams. A memory test that employs the *Brown-Peterson distractor technique*. A consonant trigram (e.g., *d-w-l*) is presented, and the subject is asked to recall the three-letter sequence following distractor delays of differing lengths. Typically, the patient is instructed to count backward by 3's, and distractor intervals of 9, 18, and 36 seconds are employed. This is a procedure, not a formal test, however, and the above parameters can be modified to suit individual patient needs or the requirements of a particular experiment. Auditory consonant trigram testing has been demonstrated to be sensitive to certain types of frontal lobe impairment

Auditory evoked potentials. *See* Evoked potentials.

Auditory Verbal Learning Test. *See* Rey Auditory Verbal Learning Test.

Augmentative or alternative communication (AAC). Methods to support communication needs of patients who are unable to speak. The may include apparatuses such as a spelling board, Touch-Talker, or computer-based synthesizers.

Aura. The initial symptom of a neurologic event that precedes or "warns" of its imminent full-blown presentation. Auras are often present with seizures and migraine headaches. With seizures, the aura may be a sensation of inappropriate familiarity (*déjà vu*), fear, sensation of strangeness (*jamais vu*), unusual sensation, or a rising feeling from the epigastrium and nausea. Unpleasant smells are a common aura associated with uncinate seizures. [L. *aura*, a breeze, from Gr. *aura*, air, breeze, from *aenai*, to breathe, blow.]

Austin Maze. A push-button test involving the serial learning of a complex pathway embedded in a 10 x 10 button matrix. The test was developed by Brenda Milner (1965) as an experimental task and was subsequently popularized by Kevin Walsh in Australia as a clinical instrument for the assessment of topographical memory and error utilization. The Austin Maze is sensitive to nondominant hemisphere dysfunction, particularly when it affects the hippocampus or its afferents. (Milner, B. 1965. Visually guided maze learning in man: Effects of bilateral hippocampal, bilateral frontal, and unilateral cerebral lesions. *Neuropsychologia*, 3:317–338.)

Autism. A pervasive developmental disorder that appears in childhood before age 3 years. Autism is characterized by poor social interaction, communication deficits (e.g., delayed spoken language, echolalia), and peculiar behavior (e.g., stereotypic or ritualistic mannerisms). [Gr. *autos*, self.]

Autobiographical memory. *See* Memory.

Autobiographical Memory Interview. A semi-structured interview of events designed to assess retrograde amnesia. A Personal Semantic schedule assesses recall of facts relating to childhood (e.g., names of schools or teachers), early adult life (e.g., name of first employer), and more recent facts (e.g., holidays, previous hospitalizations). An Autobiographical Incidents schedule assesses recall of specific events or incidents in the same three periods (e.g., description of an incident from primary school, from first job). (Kopelman, M.D, Wilson, B.A., and Baddeley, A.D. 1990. *The Autobiographical Memory Interview.* Bury St. Edmunds, England: Thames Valley Test Company.)

Automatism. Simple, repetitive motor acts that are not mediated by conscious intention. Common automatisms associated with complex partial seizures include lipsmacking and repetitive hand movements. J. Hughlings Jackson (British neurologist, 1835–1911) used this term to describe normal complex behavior that occurred outside of conscious awareness. [Gr. *autos*, self; *matenein*, to strive to do.]

Autonoetic consciousness. The capacity to mentally represent and become aware of subjective experiences in the past, present, and future. [Gr. *autos*, self; *noetikos*, from *nous*, mind.]

Autonomic nervous system (ANS). A part of the nervous system involved in the maintenance of internal body functions and behavior. It consists of two major divisions, the sympathetic and parasympathetic nervous systems. In general, the ANS regulates smooth muscles and viscera. Walter Bradford Cannon (1871–1945) identified the important role of the ANS in emotions, stress reactions, and rage expression. Ivan Petrovitch Pavlov (1949–1936) demonstrated its role in conditioning. The ANS is involved with modulation of the four f's (feeding, fighting, fleeing, and sex). [Gr. *autonomia*, independence, from *autos*, self; *nemein*, to hold sway.]

Autotopagnosia. *See* Agnosia.

Axial amnesia. *See* Dementia (axial dementia).

Axial commands. Commands involving midline structures of the body (e.g., "touch your nose"). Comprehension of spoken axial commands is often preserved in individuals with severe auditory comprehension difficulty associated with aphasia.

Axial dementia. *See* Dementia.

Axon. Relatively long, single process of the neuron that conducts the action potential from the soma and dendrites to the presynaptic terminal. [Gr. *axon*, axis, axle.]

Axonal (also, dendritic) sprouting. Phenomenon in which injured axons regenerate or "sprout" new terminal connections. It has been shown to occur in mammalian CNS, but the typical extent and actual value to the organism are unknown.

B

B$_1$. Thiamine, a B-complex vitamin. Thiamine deficiency is associated with Wernicke-Korsakoff syndrome (Wernicke encephalopathy) in chronic alcoholics.

B$_{12}$. Cyanocobalamin, a B-complex vitamin. B$_{12}$ deficiency may be associated with a confusional state that can resemble dementia, and it is considered a cause of "reversible" dementia.

Babcock Story Recall. A test of prose passage memory. Unlike most paragraph memory tests, the story is presented a second time following immediate recall. Consequently, the test contains a learning component in addition to a memory component. This approach to story presentation was adopted by the Wechsler Memory Scale-III for one of the two paragraphs comprising the Logical Memory subtest. The Babcock Story Recall test contains a 20-minute delayed recall. (Babcock, H., and Levy, L. 1940. *The Measurement of Efficiency of Mental Functioning (Revised Examination). Test and Manual of Directions.* Chicago: Stoelting Co.)

Babinski reflex (Babinski sign). (Joseph François Félix Babinski, French neurologist, 1857–1932). A reflex involving extension (dorsiflexion) of the big toe after stimulation of the sole of the foot. The reflex is associated with functional or structural impairment of the corticospinal tract (upper motor neurons). The reflex is polysynaptic and may include fanning of the smaller toes. Babinski reflexes can be elicited early in infancy but usually disappear by the end of the first year, after which time the reflex is generally considered clinically relevant.

Backward chaining. Training technique in which the last step of an activity is practiced to criterion. This is followed by criterion training of each preceding step until the entire activity has been learned.

Bacterial meningitis. *See* Meningitis.

BAER. *See* Brainstem auditory evoked response.

Balint's syndrome. A syndrome in which elements in the visual field cannot be perceived as whole, despite variable perception of its elements. This syndrome was described by Rudolph Balint (Hungarian neurologist and psychiatrist, 1874–1934) as psychic paresis of gaze, referring to an apraxia of ocular searching movements. Two other features of Balint's syndrome are optic ataxia (optic apraxia), an impairment in using vision to reach, touch, or grab objects, and a disturbance in spatial attention characterized as difficulty in seeing into the periphery of the visual field. Lesions are usually bilateral, high in the parietal lobe, and over the posterior-lateral occipital and inferior temporal regions, although they are occasionally unilateral.

Ballismus. Intermittent, violent flinging actions associated with contraction of proximal limb muscles that resembles *chorea*. Ballismus usually affects only one side of the body (hemiballismus), is greater in the arm than leg, and results from a vascular lesion of the contralateral subthalamic nucleus. It usually resolves over several days and is not associated with cognitive impairment unless other lesions are present. As with most movement disorders, ballismus is not present during sleep. [Gr. *ballismos,* jumping.]

Barbiturate. Class of drugs derived from barbituric acid or thiobarbituric acid. These drugs produce central nervous system depression, and are used primarily in the treatment of seizures. Barbiturates are often associated with psychomotor slowing.

Barognosis. Inability to estimate weight when objects are placed in the affected hand. [Gr. *báros,* weight; *gnosis,* knowledge.]

Barona equation. *See* Premorbid estimation.

Basal forebrain. Region at the base of the frontal lobes that provides the major cholinergic innervation to the neocortex and medial temporal lobes. This group includes the nucleus basalis of Meynert, the diagonal band of Broca, and the septal nuclei.

Basal ganglia. Major components of the extrapyramidal motor system, generally regarded as consisting of the striatum (caudate nucleus and putamen), globus pallidus, substantia nigra, and subthalamic nuclei. The basal ganglia are involved in modulation of motor tone and involuntary motor activity. Basal ganglia disturbance may produce involuntary movements, muscular rigidity, tremor, and akinesia, which are important components of Parkinson's disease, Huntington's disease, and Wilson's disease. Some studies have suggested a role for the basal ganglia in aspects of cognitive functioning (e.g., procedural learning) and in limbic function through the nucleus accumbens, which is related to the amygdala and hippocampus.

Basilar artery. *See* Arteries, cerebral.

Bayes' theorem. An important theorem in probability and statistics frequently employed in decision analysis to allow the posterior probability of an event to be calculated. The probability of disease given a test sign, for example, is based on the probability of the test sign given the disease and the prior probability of disease.

Bayley Scales of Infant Development (BSID). (Nancy Bayley, American psychologist, 1899–1993). A developmental test for children between 1 and 42 months in age consisting of a Mental Development Scale, Motor Development Scale, and an Infant Behavior Rating Scale. The Mental Development Scale assesses sensory-perceptual abilities, object constancy, memory, learning and problem solving ability, communication and verbal skills, and early abstract reasoning. The Motor Development Scale measures fine motor and gross motor skill, and control of the body. Both development scales yield standard scores. The Infant Behavior Rating Scales (IBR) is based upon examiner observations during the assessment and is completed after the testing. The IBR measures qualitative aspects of the child's performance including motor control, responsiveness to the examiner and environment, and temperament (e.g., ability to be calmed when upset). The IBR provides centile ranks and category descriptions. The 1993 revision of the Bayley Scales significantly expanded the behaviors assessed and extended the upper age limit from 30 to 42 months. (Bayley, N. 1993. *Bayley Scales of Infant Development,* 2nd ed. (Bayley-II). San Antonio: The Psychological Corporation.)

BBB. *See* Blood-brain barrier.

Beck Depression Inventory (BDI). A 21-item questionnaire of dysphoria and stress-related complaints. Each item is rated by the patient on a 0–3 scale. Although not diagnostic for depression, the Beck Depression Inventory is commonly used to assess changes in emotional states. (Beck, A.T. 1987; Beck, A.T. and Steer, R.A. 1993. *Beck Depression Inventory.* Manual. San Antonio: The Psychological Corporation.)

Beery Visuo-Motor Integration Test. *See* Developmental Test of Visual-Motor Integration.

Behavioral medicine. An interdisciplinary field concerned with the role of psychosocial factors in disease related to etiology, prevention, compliance with medical therapy, patient's acknowledgment of medical diagnoses, and the methods of decreasing the stress associated with certain medical therapies.

Behavioural Assessment of the Dysexecutive Syndrome (BADS). A battery to test *executive function* that assesses the ability to establish priorities and to plan over relatively long periods. BADS is a collection of six tests that are similar to real-life activities (e.g., Zoo Map Test in which a route must be mapped to visit specific zoo locations, starting at the entrance and finishing at a designated picnic area, using designated paths only once). A Dysexecutive Questionnaire (DEX) that is also part of the battery and assesses changes in emotion and personality, motivation, behavior, and cognition. (Wilson, B.A., Alderman, N., Burgess, P.W., Emslie, H., and Evans, J.J. 1996. *Behavioural Assessment of the Dysexecutive Syndrome.* Manual. Bury St. Edmunds, England: Thames Valley Test Company.)

Behavioural Inattention Test (BIT). A measure of visual neglect and inattention. In addition to standard tests of inattention (e.g., cancellation tasks), multiple practical tests are used to assess the impact of inattention on daily function. The latter includes Picture Scanning, Telephone Dialing, Menu Reading, Article Reading, Telling and Setting Time, Coin Sorting, Address and Sentence Copying, Map Navigation, and Card Sorting. Two parallel forms are available. (Wilson, B.A., Cockburn, J., and Halligan, P. 1988. *Behavioural Inattention Test.* Manual. Bury St. Edmunds, England: Thames Valley Test Company.)

Bell's palsy. (Charles Bell, British surgeon and anatomist, 1774–1842). Facial paralysis from inflammation of the seventh (facial) cranial nerve causing motor paralysis with no sensory component. Bell's palsy is variably associated with changes in taste and *hyperacusis.* Seventh nerve involvement from other causes such as tumor is not generally referred to as Bell's palsy, but rather is called simply a peripheral seventh nerve palsy. Bell's palsy is usually benign and resolves within six months.

Bell's phenomenon. An outward and upward rolling of the eyeball when attempting eye closure. It is pronounced in patients with Bell's palsy.

Bender Visual Motor Gestalt Test. (Lauretta Bender, American child psychiatrist, 1897–1987). A collection of nine designs originally used to study the development of graphomotor (constructional praxis) skills in children. Each design is presented sequentially to be copied. The test may be used to assess visual spatial perception, visual-constructional ability, general organization, and with some approaches, visual memory. Many different scoring systems exist. The Cantor Background Interference Procedure is a modification in which the designs are copied on a special sheet with intersecting sinusoidal lines. This test is often called the Bender-Gestalt (Bender, L. 1938. A visual motor Gestalt test and its clinical use. *Am. Orthopsychiatr. Assoc. Res. Monogr.* 3; Canter, A. 1966. A background interference procedure to increase sensitivity of the Bender-Gestalt test to organic brain disorder. *J. Consult. Psychol.,* 30:91–97.)

Benign. In medical terms, a condition that is nonprogressive, nonmalignant, or nonfatal (e.g., benign neoplasm). [L. *benignus,* kind.]

Benign senescent forgetfulness. Mild forgetfulness and inefficiencies of learning and memory associated with normal aging.

Benton Visual Retention Test (BVRT). A measure of visual perception, short-term visual memory and visual attention, and visuoconstructional ability. Stimuli containing either two or three geometric designs are presented for either a 5- or 10-second exposure, after which the subject draws the designs shown on the cards from memory. In addition, the examiner may choose a delayed memory administration in which the figures are shown for 10 seconds, with a 15-second delay imposed before drawing. Multiple forms exist, each containing ten stimulus sets. Reproductions are scored both for the number designs correctly reproduced and for the number of errors produced. (Benton, A.L. 1974. *Revised Visual Retention Test: Clinical and Experimental Applications,* 4th ed. Sivan, A.B. 1992. *Benton Visual Retention Test,* 5th ed. San Antonio: The Psychological Corporation.)

Benzodiazepines. A class of psychoactive compounds classified as minor tranquilizers. Benzodiazepines are used to treat muscle spasms and seizures, and to calm patients undergoing minor surgery. Side effects may include drowsiness, confusion, and impaired coordination. Their effects are additive in combination with other central nervous system depressants (e.g., alcohol and barbiturates).

Bereitschaftspotential (BP). An *event-related potential* reflecting cerebral processing prior to movement. The wave appears for several hundred milliseconds before volitional movement, with the earliest onset recorded from the frontal-central midline (e.g., cingulate gyrus, supplementary motor area). Also called readiness potential.

Best performance method. A technique of estimating premorbid level of functioning by identifying the highest test score (e.g., from the Wechsler Intelligence Scales) or the highest level of functioning on everyday tasks. This level becomes the standard against which all other aspects of current performance are compared. The best performance method does not account for normal variability among tests, however, and tends to overestimate premorbid IQ.

Beta. The second letter of the Greek alphabet, β. **1**. The probability of making a *type II error* in statistical hypothesis testing. **2**. In signal detection theory, the perceptual threshold above which a signal is reported. **3**. EEG with frequencies greater than 13 Hz. Beta activity is associated with wakefulness, and beta activity of 18–24 Hz can be induced by barbiturates or benzodiazepines.

Beta-blockers. A class of drugs that blocks epinephrine. Beta-blockers are commonly used to treat hypertension and heart disease, and may be used to treat benign essential tremor.

bid. Shorthand notation for "twice a day." [L. *bis in die*.]

Binswanger's disease. (Otto Binswanger, German physician, 1852–1929). Periventricular subcortical demyelination resulting from uncontrolled, chronic hypertension; it is commonly associated with dementia. Ill-defined areas of demyelination occur, primarily in the temporal and occipital lobes. Cortex, subarcuate fibers, and the corpus callosum are spared. Binswanger's disease is associated with leukoaraiosis on CT or MRI, although these findings are not specific for Binswanger's disease. Binswanger considered this disease to be separate from atherosclerosis or infarction, but this distinction is not always made.

Bipolar disorder. A mood disorder consisting of cyclic episodes of mania, often alternating with periods of depression. Frank psychosis may be present.

Bitemporal hemianopsia. Loss of the outer halves of both visual fields that results from optic chiasm damage to both crossing fibers from the nasal portion of the retina. Bitemporal hemianopsia is classically associated with pituitary tumors that compress the optic chiasm.

Blepharospasm. Spasmodic blinking and intermittent involuntary eye closure associated with other dystonic contractions of the head and neck. [Gr. *blepharon*, eyelid; *spasmos*, from *span*, to draw, pull, wrench.]

Blessed Dementia Rating Scale. A mental status examination that was first used to study the a relationship between cognitive function and the number of neuritic plaques. It does not contain any measurement of language or visual-spatial function. *See* Dementia rating scales and mental status examinations. (Blessed, G., Tomlinson, B.E., and Roth, M. 1968. The association between quantitative measures of dementia and of senile changes in the cerebral grey matter of elderly subjects. *Br. J. Psychiatry* 114:797–811.)

Blind design. An experimental design in which information regarding the administration of a treatment or placebo, or which of several treatments, is withheld to maximize objectivity during data collection. In a single-blind design, the subject does not know which experimental condition is being received. In a double-blind design, neither the subject nor the experimenter is aware of which experimental condition is being received.

Blindsight. Visual disorder from primary visual cortex damage in which residual vision exists in the visual field associated with the damaged cortical area. Weiskrantz (1986) described a patient who was able to point to stimulus locations, detect movement, and discriminate line orientations and X's and O's, but insisted that he was unable to see the stimuli. (Weiskrantz, L. 1986. *Blindsight: A Case Study and Implications*. Oxford: Oxford University Press.)

Blood-brain barrier (BBB). A semi-permeable barrier that excludes many chemicals in the blood from entering the cerebrospinal fluid (CSF) and brain. This barrier is not absolute. The probable functions of the BBB include exclusion of blood-borne toxic substances and protection from systemic neurotransmitters and hormones. The BBB may break down in any nervous system condition in which significant histopathology is seen.

Boder Test of Reading-Spelling Patterns. A test designed to screen and diagnose subtypes of developmental dyslexia. It consists of word-recognition oral reading and a spelling-to-dictation subtests to categorize dysphonetic and dyseidetic dyslexia subtypes. A reading quotient can be calculated. (Boder, E. Jarrico, S. 1982. *Boder Test of Reading-Spelling Patterns*. Orlando: Grune & Stratton.)

Boston Diagnostic Aphasia Examination (BDAE). A language battery designed to assess a broad range of language and related functions often associated with impaired left hemisphere function. Language is tested through different perceptual modalities (e.g., auditory, visual, gestural), processing functions (e.g., comprehension, analysis, problem-solving), and types of response (e.g., writing, articulation, manipulation). The battery consists of five sections: Conversational and Expository Speech, Auditory Comprehension, Oral Expression, Understanding Written Language, and Writing. Performance on the language subtests can be plotted to facilitate aphasia subtyping. Supplementary language (e.g., Boston Naming Test) and non-language tests (e.g., three-dimensional block construction) may be administered. (Goodglass, H. and Kaplan, E. 1983. *Boston Diagnostic Aphasia Examination*. Philadelphia: Lea & Febiger.)

Boston Naming Test (BNT). A visual confrontation naming task in which line-drawn pictures range in difficulty from bed to abacus. The original version of this test contained 85 items, but the test has been shortened to 60 items in its current clinical version. Two types of stimulus cues may be administered depending on the nature of the subject's response. Semantic cues are provide if there is no response within 20 seconds, if there is indication that the patient does not know what the picture is, or if there is an obvious misperception. If the subject knows what the object is but provides a wrong answer within the semantic category, the initial sound of the object is provided as a phonemic cue. Correct responses following a stimulus cue are given credit whereas correct responses following a phonemic cue are not included in the total score. The BNT is a supplementary language test of the *Boston Diagnostic Aphasia Examination*. (Kaplan, E.F., Goodglass, H., and Weintraub, S. 1978. *The Boston Naming Test*, experimental ed. Boston: Kaplan & Goodglass; 1983. 2nd ed. Philadelphia: Lea & Febiger.)

Boston process approach. Method of assessment that emphasizes the qualitative aspects of how patients attempt to solve problems. This approach has been formalized in a formal WAIS-R modification (WAIS-R as a neuropsychological instrument).

Botulinum neurotoxin (botox). A chemical that blocks neural transmission, its most potent effects being on nerves that innervate striate muscles. Botox injections are used to treat blepharospasm, torticollis, and torsion dystonia.

BP. *See* Bereitschaftspotential. Also, abbreviation for blood pressure.

Bradykinesia. Abnormal slowness of movement associated with movement initiation difficulty. Bradykinesia is a common feature of Parkinson's disease and includes slowness of speech, chewing, and swallowing. It can be temporarily overcome during periods of intense excitement (kinesia paradoxica). [Gr. *bradys*, slow, delayed, tardy; *kinesis*, movement.]

Bradyphrenia. Abnormal slowness of mentation. Bradyphrenia is often associated with diffuse cerebral impairment, but it may also accompany advanced age, Parkinson's disease, and frontal lobe injury. [Gr. *bradys*, slow, delayed, tardy; *phrenos*, mind, thought.]

Brain death. A condition of extensive and permanent cortical and subcortical brain damage in which all integrative physiological activities are severely impaired and bodily functions are maintained by artificial means. Formal criteria for brain death exist, although they vary among states and countries. In general, however, there must be no response to noxious stimuli, and pupils must be fixed, with an isoelectric EEG.

Brain reserve capacity. A theory of residual cognitive function following neurologic compromise which proposes that patients with greater brain reserve, as inferred by level of education or premorbid intellectual status, have a higher threshold for developing cognitive impairment following injury.

Brain stem auditory evoked response (BAER, BSER). *See* Evoked potentials. Also called farfield potentials.

Brief Test of Attention (BTA). An attentional test in which numbers and letters are presented auditorially together in a single trial (e.g., M-6-3-R). Two tasks are included—one to count the numbers while ignoring the letters, and one to count the letters while disregarding the numbers. The trials increase in length from 4 to 18 items. (Schretlen, D. 1997. *Brief Test of Attention*. Technical manual. Odessa, FL: Psychological Assessment Resources.)

Broca's aphasia. *See* Aphasia syndromes.

Broca's area. (Pierre Paul Broca, French surgeon and anthropologist, 1824–1880). The posterior third of the inferior (third) frontal convolution in the language dominant hemisphere. This is the region that Broca postulated to be responsible for language impairment in his two original cases, although extensive perisylvian involvement was demonstrated in these patients at autopsy. Infarction limited to Broca's area does not result in Broca's aphasia but produces mutism with right face and arm weakness that quickly resolves over several days. Broca's aphasia typically involves a much larger territory of the upper (anterior) division of the middle cerebral artery.

Brodmann's areas. (Korbinian Brodmann, German anatomist, 1868–1918). Numbering system applied to surface brain areas for identification of histologically distinct cortical regions. The numbers reflect the order in which Brodmann studied the areas, and there are omissions in the numbering (e.g., 13–16) as these areas refer to nonhuman primate regions. Area 51 is not shown on many maps; it reflects the cortex of the prepiriform region and the olfactory tubercle. Brodmann numbering is the most commonly used approach for identifying surface brain areas.

Broken record syndrome. Tendency to repeat comments, questions, and topics of conversation over and over; this tendency is associated with a dense amnestic state (e.g., transient global amnesia).

Brown-Peterson distractor task. Memory procedure designed to assess retention of small amounts of information across a short distractor period (e.g., counting backwards by 3's or 7's). This is often considered a short-term memory task because it employs maximum retention intervals of 45–60 seconds and does not test for retention of information over longer delays. The Brown-Peterson technique has been a popular approach to investigate the memory impairment associated with Korsakoff's syndrome. This is the basic format for auditory consonant trigram testing, which is sensitive to certain types of frontal lobe impairment (*see* Auditory consonant trigrams). (Brown, J. 1958. Some tests of the decay of immediate memory. *Q. J. Exp. Psychol.* 10:12–21; Peterson, L.R. and Peterson, M.J. 1959. Short-term retention of individual verbal items. *J. Exp. Psychol.* 58:193–198.)

Bruit. A high-pitched noise generated by blood flow through arterial stenosis or over arterial roughening that suggests the presence of atherosclerosis. [F. *bruit*, noise.]

BSER. Brainstem evoked response. *See* Evoked potentials.

Buccofacial apraxia. *See* Apraxia.

Bulbar palsy. Dysarthria, difficulty in swallowing (dysphagia), and unresponsiveness of the gag reflex from injury to the bulbar (medullary) cranial nerves that innervate muscles of the soft palate, pharynx, larynx, and tongue (cranial nerves IX–XII). This condition superficially resembles *pseudobulbar palsy*, although the gag and jaw jerk reflexes are absent in bulbar palsy. Common causes of bulbar palsy include amyotrophic lateral sclerosis, vertebral artery stenosis, Guillain-Barré syndrome, chronic meningitis, tumors at the base of the skull, and myasthenia gravis.

Bulging fontanelles. A tightening or bulging of the skin above the skull openings in infants due to increased intracranial pressure. These soft areas disappear when sutures fuse. [F. *fontanelle*, diminutive of *fountain*.]

BUN. Blood urea nitrogen. Increased levels are sometimes associated with dehydration, renal insufficiency, and acute confusional states.

Burr hole. A surgical technique for gaining access to a limited area of brain. Burr holes are generally approximately 2–3 cm and are often used when draining subdural hematomas. In addition, burr holes are used to begin a craniotomy when greater brain access is necessary.

Buschke Selective Reminding Test. *See* Selective Reminding Test.

C

c̄. With. [L. *cum*, with.]

CA. Chronological age; cancer; or cardiac arrest.

CABG. Coronary artery bypass graft.

Cachexia. A profound and marked state of emaciation due to poor general health and malnutrition. [Gr. *kachexia*, from *kakos*, bad; *hexis*, habit.]

Cafe-au-lait spot. *See* Neurofibromatosis.

Calcarine cortex. *See* Striate cortex. [L. *calcar* spur, cock's spur.]

California Sorting Test. A test of concept generation and concept identification. The first task is to sort six cards, each of which contains a single word (e.g., "butterfly"), into two groups of three cards each and then to state the rule upon which the sort is based. Eight different sorting rules can be used. In a second condition, the examiner sorts the cards and the subject states which sorting rule has been applied. (Delis, D.C., Squire, L.R., Bihrle, A., and Massman, P. 1992. Componential analysis of problem-solving ability: Performance of patients with frontal lobe damage and amnesic patients on a new sorting test. *Neuropsychologia* 30:683–697.)

California Verbal Learning Test (CVLT). A serial word list learning task consisting of 16 words from four semantic categories (i.e., spices and herbs, fruits, tools, and clothing) constructed to examine the effects of semantic clustering in patient learning and recall. It is patterned in format after the Rey Auditory Verbal Learning Test. The CVLT involves five learning trials using the "Monday list." A single trial with a second list of words is administered ("Tuesday list"), followed by recall of the original Monday list. Semantic cues are then provided. After a delay of approximately 20 minutes, free and cued recall and recognition is tested. Consecutive recall of words from the same semantic category (semantic clustering) reflects organization based upon semantic word features. (Delis, D.C., Kramer, J.H., Kaplan, E., and Ober, B.A. 1987. *California Verbal Learning Test: Adult Version*. Manual. San Antonio: The Psychological Corporation.)

Callosal agenesis. *See* Agenesis of the corpus callosum.

Callosal apraxia. *See* Apraxia.

Callosotomy. *See* Commissurotomy.

Calvaria/calvarium. The upper domelike portion of the skull. [L. *calvaria*, skull, from *calva*, a scalp without hair.]

Cancellation tests. A family of tests to measure either sustained attention and vigilance or hemispatial neglect. An array of letters, numbers, or symbols is presented and the task is to mark each occurrence of the target item. Task variations include different targets for each row of stimuli, or two different targets throughout the test. Patients with attentional difficulty tend to make omission errors throughout the test whereas patients with hemispatial neglect will make errors primarily on the side of the page contralateral to their lesion.

Cantor Background Interference Procedure. *See* Bender Visual Motor Gestalt Test.

Capgras syndrome. (Jean Marie Joseph Capgras, French psychiatrist, 1873–1950). Delusional misidentification syndrome in which a familiar person is perceived as an impostor or as a double. Although Capgras syndrome is a psychiatric disorder, a similar disturbance of neurologic origin is *reduplicative paramnesia*, which is associated with nondominant parietal lobe lesions.

Carbon monoxide (CO) poisoning. Cerebral hypoxia from carbon monoxide inhalation that results in inadequate oxygenation. The initial damage occurs in the globus pallidus followed by generalized cerebral injury.

Carcinoma (CA). A malignant neoplasm. Brain carcinomas may be either primary, arising from brain tissue, or metastatic, spreading to the brain from other areas. The most common primary sites of brain metastases are lung and breast. [Gr. *karkinoma*, from *karkinos*, cancer; *-oma*, morbid growth, tumor.]

Carotid artery. *See* Arteries, cerebral.

Carotid stenosis. A narrowing of the carotid artery due to atherosclerosis. The degree of carotid stenosis is measured noninvasively by carotid duplex sonography. Significant stenosis, and at times, complete occlusion, can be compensated for by the collateral circulation from the ipsilateral external carotid and ophthalmic arteries or by intracranial cross-flow from the contralateral internal carotid artery.

Carphologia. Lint picking, or aimless plucking at clothing as if picking off thread, frequently accompanied by chewing movements. Carphologia is sometime seen in patients with Alzheimer's disease. Also called carphology or floccillation. [Gr. *karphologia*, from *karphos*, dry stalk, stick; *legein*, to speak.]

CAT. Computerized axial tomography; *see* Computed tomography.

Cataplexy. Abrupt attacks of muscle weakness and hypotonia triggered by emotional stimuli such as laughter, anger, fear, or surprise. The episodes typically last for 30–60 seconds or less. Cataplexy is often associated with narcolepsy. [Gr. *kataplexis*, to strike down.]

Catastrophic reaction. Excessive sadness, anxiety, or agitation following cerebral injury. Catastrophic reaction was first associated with left hemisphere lesions and aphasia, although it may accompany any brain injury that prevents a mature/adaptable response to stress. The term "catastrophic reaction" was introduced by Kurt Goldstein (American neurologist born in Germany, 1878–1965).

Catecholamines. Chemicals that share a common chemical structure consisting of a benzene ring and two adjacent hydroxyl groups with an ethylamine side chain. The catecholamines include dopamine, norepinephrine, and epinephrine.

Categorical perception. The perception of distinct sounds resulting from a continuous change in physical characteristics of speech. "Ba" and "pa" differ in voice onset time, but there is a threshold of voice onset time change that alters the perception of the syllables from one sound to the other.

Category fluency. *See* Semantic category fluency.

Category Test. *See* Halstead Category Test.

Cauda equina. Collection of spinal nerve roots descending the spinal canal below L_1-L_2 from their point of spinal cord attachment to their emergence between the vertebrae. [L. *cauda*, tail; *equina*, horse.]

Caudate nucleus. Long, horseshoe-shaped mass of gray substance of the basal ganglia that, with the lentiform nuclei, forms the corpus striatum. The caudate is closely positioned next to the lateral ventricle. Impaired caudate function is often associated with parkinsonism, and severe atrophy is seen in the head of the caudate nucleus in Huntington's disease. [L. *cauda*, tail; *nucleus*, a little nut.]

CBC. Complete blood count. The CBC indicates the number of white cells, which will indicate infection, and hemoglobin levels, which will indicate anemia.

CC. Chief complaint.

CCU. Coronary care unit or critical care unit.

CDC. Center for Disease Control (U.S.).

Ceiling effect. The inability to measure high performance resulting from limited test sensitivity at the upper end of the distribution because scores are already at the highest possible levels. True group differences between high-functioning subjects may be masked on measures where there is a ceiling effect, and the particular measure may not be considered sufficiently sensitive to the construct of interest. *See* Floor effect.

Centile. Score indicating the percentage of scores at or below the comparison value. The term "percentile" is often used for this score. *See* quantile. [L. *centum*, hundred.]

Central agraphia. A spelling disorder in both written and oral spelling that is related to linguistic disturbance and not to motor or sensory systems supporting written spelling.

Central nervous system. Brain and spinal cord.

Central sulcus. *See* Rolandic fissure.

Centrencephalic epilepsy. *See* Epilepsy.

CERAD Neuropsychological Test Battery. A brief battery of neuropsychological tests designed to assess functions affected by Alzheimer's disease (e.g., memory, language, praxis, general cognitive function). It is sensitive to cognitive decline in the early disease stages. The battery consists of Semantic Category Fluency (animals), a 15-item version of the Boston Naming Test, the Folstein Mini-Mental Status Examination, a word-list memory task with learning, free recall, delayed recall, and delayed recognition components, and constructional praxis. *See* Consortium to Establish a Registry for Alzheimer's Disease (CERAD).

Cerebellar gait. Lurching, unsteady, and wide-based ataxic gait in which a patient appears inebriated. Cerebellar gait is associated with dysfunction of the entire cerebellum or with lesions limited to its median lobe (vermis).

Cerebellum. The portion of *metencephalon* that occupies the posterior fossa behind the brainstem. It consists of a median lobe (vermis) and two lateral hemispheres and is connected with the brainstem by three pairs of peduncles, or white matter tracts. The cerebellum is important in the coordination of movements, and it may modulate higher-order behavior such as procedural learning and classical conditioning. [L. *cerebellum*, diminutive of *cerebrum*, the brain.]

Cerebral aqueduct. A canal approximately three-fourths of an inch long that drains cerebrospinal fluid (CSF) from the third ventricle to the fourth ventricle through the midbrain. This is a common site of obstruction causing childhood hydrocephalus. Also called Aqueduct of Sylvius.

Cerebral dominance. Superiority of one cerebral hemisphere for processing specific tasks. Cerebral dominance is frequently used synonymously with cerebral language dominance, although the term is applicable to other domains, such as visual-spatial dominance, praxis, or handedness. Cerebral language dominance is assessed in vivo with Wada testing and can also be demonstrated with functional magnetic resonance imaging. *See* lateral dominance.

Cerebral palsy (CP). Motor system impairment from cerebral injuries sustained in utero, perinatally, or during infancy or early childhood. Depending on the variety of CP, patients may have mental retardation, seizures, or other neurologic complications. Subtypes of CP include spastic (or pyramidal CP, the most common form), extrapyramidal CP, hypotonic or atonic CP, and mixed CP. The term *palsy* is a contraction of paralysis.

Cerebral thrombosis. Occlusion of a cerebral blood vessel by a clot, or thrombus.

Cerebral ventricles. Brain cavities that produce and contain cerebrospinal fluid (CSF). There are two *c*-shaped lateral ventricles, a midline third ventricle, and a midline fourth ventricle. [L. *venter*, stomach.]

Cerebrospinal fluid (CSF). Fluid produced in the choroid plexus that serves as a protective hydraulic system to cushion the brain and spinal cord from jarring injury. Cerebrospinal fluid is often examined as part of a neurological work-up since many CSF alterations may reflect nervous system impairment. Analysis of CSF is helpful in the diagnosis of bacterial meningitis, myelitis, multiple sclerosis, and subarachnoid hemorrhage. In addition, many germ-cell tumors secrete characteristic hormones, such as chorionic gonadotropin and alpha-fetal protein, into the CSF. Samples of CSF are obtained by lumbar puncture (LP). [L. *cerebrum*, brain; *spina*, spine.]

Cerebrovascular accident (CVA). Stroke.

Ceruloplasmin. Copper-containing protein that is the primary vehicle for copper transport and maintenance of the optimal levels of copper in the tissues. Low ceruloplasmin is associated with the excessive copper accumulation of Wilson's disease (hepatolenticular degeneration). [L. *ciruleus*, dark blue; Gr. *plasma*, from *plassein*, to form, mold.]

Charpentier's illusion. (Augustin Charpentier, French physician, 1852–1916). Illusion created by squeezing objects of different size, followed by holding two objects of the same size. The illusion is that the object in the hand that previously squeezed the larger object feels as if it were now squeezing the smaller object (and vice versa). Aleksandr Luria (Soviet neuropsychologist, 1902–1977) claimed that this illusion was lost following nondominant parietal lobe lesions, but most investigators have not found this relationship reliable. Charpentier described an additional illusion that occurs when a small, dimly illuminated object appears to move in a darkened room. This movement illusion has subsequently become known as the autokinetic effect.

Chelation. Treatment for heavy metal poisoning. Chelation is usually performed by introduction of an oral agent containing a substance for which the toxin has a chemical affinity. The purpose is to cause the toxin to bind with the chelating agent so that the toxin may be excreted. [Gr. *chele*, claw.]

CHI. *See* Closed head injury.

Chiasm. Decussation or crossing of two tracts; most often refers to the optic chiasm. Compare with decussation. [Gr. *chiasma*, two lines crossed, from *chiazein*, to mark with the Greek letter χ (chi).]

Child Behavior Checklist. A rating checklist that is completed by parents or teachers to provide a measure of personality function, social competencies, and behavior problems in children. Different forms of the test are available for use with children between 2–18 years of age. (Achenbach, T.M. 1991. *Manual for the Child Behavior Checklist/4–18 and 1991 Profile*. Burlington, VT: University of Vermont, Department of Psychiatry.)

Children's Category Test. A shortened version of the Halstead Category Test. Level 1 is intended for children 5–8 years of age and consists of 80 items. Level 2 is given to children aged 9–16 years and contains 83 items. *See* Halstead Category Test.

Children's Depression Inventory. A self-rated scale of depression designed for school-age children and adolescents. Each item consists of three choices, with higher scores indicating increasing severity. A 10–item short form is also available. (Kovacs, M. 1992. *Children's Depression Inventory*. North Tonawanda, NY: Multi-Health Systems.)

Children's Memory Scale. A battery of tests designed as a downward extension of the Wechsler Memory Scale. It consists of six core subtests to assess verbal and visual learning and memory, as well as attention. Two supplemental subtests may be given. The test is intended for children aged 5–16 years. (Cohen, M.J. 1997. *Children's Memory Scale*. San Antonio: The Psychological Corporation.)

Chimeric figures. Figures created with differing stimuli in each hemifield (e.g., a face with each half from a different person) or in each quadrant that are used in the study of hemispheric processing and specialization. The stimuli are often faces, but complex designs and patterns have also been used. [Gr. *chimaira*, a goat, a monstrous beast; *chimera*, mythical being.]

Chin reflex. *See* Jaw jerk.

Choice reaction time. *See* Reaction time.

Chorea. Involuntary, intermittent jerky movement of muscle groups that may involve the arms or legs, trunk, neck, or face that is associated with basal ganglia dysfunction. Choreic movements occur randomly and are often incorporated into more elaborate movements to make the choreoform activity less noticeable. As with most involuntary movement disorders, choreic movements subside during sleep. The most commonly encountered chorea is associated with Huntington's disease. [Gr. *choreos*, a dance.]

Choreoathetosis. Combined choreic and athetoid movements, usually consisting of an involuntary writhing (athetosis) of the face, tongue, hands, and feet, with occasional jerking movements (chorea) of the trunk, arms, and legs. Choreoathetosis is typically symmetric and has a variety of causes (e.g., neuroleptics, cerebral palsy, Huntington's disease).

Choroid plexus. Epithelial tissue in the ventricular system that secretes cerebrospinal fluid (CSF). The choroid plexus is a major component of the blood-brain barrier.

Chronic Fatigue Syndrome (CFS). A syndrome characterized by unexplained fatigue that does not result from exertion, is not alleviated by rest, and results in a reduction of activity. Difficulties with memory and concentration often arise, although for diagnostic purposes these must not precede the onset of fatigue. There is considerable overlap with the diagnostic criteria of fibromyalgia.

Chronic Obstructive Pulmonary Disease (COPD). Diseases with poor expiratory airflow. Chronic obstructive pulmonary disease may cause chronic hypoxia, resulting in cognitive decline.

Chronotaraxis. Inability to identify the date, time of day, or season of the year. [Gr. *chrono-*, time; *taraxis*, confusion.]

Chunking. The process of reorganizing materials in working memory to increase the number of items successfully recalled. As described by Miller (1956), most individuals have a span of immediate recall of approximately seven items. Combining items into chunks, however, permits an increase in the number of items recalled. For example, the eight-digit sequence 3-9-4-1-6-5-2-7 may exceed many peoples' span, but when recoded into 39-41-65-27, all eight single digits may be recalled. (Miller, G.A. 1956. The magical number seven: Plus or minus two. Some limits on our capacity for processing information. *Psychol. Rev.* 9:81–97.)

Cicatrix, brain. Scarring of the brain that results from injury. The scarring consists of both vascular and glial components. [L. *cicatrix*, a scar.]

Cingulate gyrus. Arch-shaped cortical gyrus lying above the corpus callosum. Lesions of the cingulate gyrus often produce akinesia. [L. *cingula*, girdle; L. *gyrus*, convolution.]

Cingulotomy. Surgical technique that sections the cingulum to treat chronic pain or to control obsessive compulsive disorders.

Cingulum. Bundle of association fibers in the white matter under the cingulate gyrus on the medial surface of the cerebral hemisphere. This fiber bundle contains afferent and efferent axons, and axons of passage from other cortical regions. [L. *cingula*, girdle.]

Circle of Willis. (Thomas Willis, British physician and anatomist, 1621–1675). A ring of arteries at the base of the brain surrounding the optic chiasm and pituitary stalk that allows for blood circulation from one internal carotid artery to the other, and from the vertebrobasilar to carotid circulation. The circle consists of the anterior communicating artery (ACoA), which connects the two anterior cerebral arteries (ACAs), and two posterior communicating arteries (PCoAs), which connect the internal carotid arteries (ICAs) with the posterior cerebral arteries (PCAs). Normal variants in this system are so common that only 50% of the population has a complete circle of Willis.

Circuit of Papez. *See* Papez, circuit of.

Circumlocution. Discourse that begins with a specific subject, wanders to various other topics, and returns to the original subject matter. It is not synonymous with tangentiality, which is characterized by wandering speech that never returns to the original subject matter. Circumlocution also refers to verbal behavior characterized by talking around word-finding difficulties as if to avoid using specific words. Word substitution is frequently attempted, but speech is often empty. Circumlocution is common with fluent aphasias.

Classical conditioning. The process in which a neutral stimulus becomes capable of eliciting a response by its frequent pairing with an unconditioned stimulus. Classical conditioning is considered a form of nondeclarative (or implicit) memory.

Clinical Evaluation of Language Fundamentals-Revised (CELF-R). A measure of expressive and receptive language for children aged 5 to 16 years. It consists of three receptive and three expressive language tests plus five supplementary tests. The receptive tests are Linguistic Concepts, Sentence Structure, and Oral Directions. The expressive tests are Word Structure, Formulated Sentences, and Recalling Sentence (sentence repetition). The supplementary tests include Listening to Paragraphs, Word Associations, Word Classes, Semantic Relationships, and Sentence Assembly. (Semel, E., Wiig, E.H. and Secord, W. 1987. *Clinical Evaluation of Language Fundamentals—Revised*. San Antonio: The Psychological Corporation.)

Clock drawing. *See* Draw-a-clock test.

Clonus. Rapid repetitive alternating muscle contraction and relaxation. Clonus may be observed in a variety of contexts such as seizures (e.g., generalized tonic-clonic seizures or myoclonic seizures), hyperactive tendon reflexes (e.g., ankle clonus), or myclonic jerks associated with involuntary movement disorders. [Gr. *klonos*, a tumult; hence, a confused movement.]

Closed class words. *See* Function words.

Closed head injury. Injury to the head in which the skull is not penetrated, although a linear skull fracture may be present. The term is used in contrast with open, or penetrating, head injury.

Closing-in. A phenomenon in which an individual seems pulled toward a stimulus. A design, for example, may be copied inappropriately close to or on top of the stimulus figure. This phenomenon is occasionally called crowding. *See* Stimulus-boundedness.

Closure picture. Incomplete silhouette picture on which the subject must impose perceptual completion for identification. Closure pictures are often considered to reflect right hemisphere processing. Also called Gestalt completion tests.

Cluster analysis. Multivariate technique of classifying variables into groups or clusters. A cluster consists of variables that correlate highly with one another and have relatively low correlations with variables in other clusters. Cluster analysis is used for subjects or variables, and there is considerable flexibility in how "similarity" between objects is defined and in the rules for grouping objects into clusters.

Clustering. In memory recall, the tendency to group similar items together during the process of recall. Clustering is often semantic, with words recalled together from similar semantic categories.

CMV. *See* Cytomegalovirus.

CNS. Central nervous system.

CNV. *See* Contingent negative variation.

Code. Life-threatening patient situation in which an emergency response is necessary. A patient's code status (i.e., whether to perform or withhold medical treatment such as intubation, cardioversion) is based upon the patient's overall medical condition in combination with the wishes of the patient through an advance medical directive (living will) or the patient's family. Patients who are "no code" will have no life-sustaining intervention. No-code status is sometimes referred to as DNR, or do not resuscitate.

Coefficient alpha. *See* Alpha.

Cognistat. An extended cognitive mental status examination that assesses function in five areas: Language, Memory, Calculations, and Reasoning. Four areas of language are tested: Spontaneous Speech, Comprehension, Repetition, Constructional Ability, and Naming. A *screen and metric* approach is employed. Also called the Neurobehavioral Cognitive Status Examination. The Northern California Neurobehavior Group. (1995. *Manual for Cognitstat: The Neurobehavioral Cognitive Status Examination.* Fairfax, CA: The Northern California Neurobehavior Group.)

Cognition. Mental processes associated with attention, perception, thinking, learning, and memory. [L. *cognitio,* knowledge, from *cognitus,* past part. of *cognoscere,* to know, from *co-,* together; *noscere,* to know.]

Cognitive Estimation Test. A test of the ability to make mental projections and evaluate conclusions without complex computation. An example from the test is "What is the average length of a man's spine?". A North American version of the test contains 10 questions. (Axelrod, B.N. and Millis, S.R. 1994. Preliminary standardization of the Cognitive Estimation Test. *Assessment* 1:269–274; Shallice, T. and Evans, M.E. 1978. The involvement of the frontal lobes in cognitive estimation. *Cortex* 14:292–303.)

Cognitive map. Mental representation of a known spatial location.

Cognitive rehabilitation (cognitive remediation, cognitive retraining). Any systematic program directed at modifying cognitive function or cognitively oriented activities following acquired brain injury. Two broad rehabilitation approaches exist. The restorative approach consists of reinforcing previously learned patterns of behavior. The compensatory approach establishes new patterns of cognitive activity or compensatory mechanisms for impaired systems. The term is also used to refer to more comprehensive, holistic programs that offer compensatory skills training along with psychotherapy, vocational counseling and training, and individual/family adjustment counseling.

Cogwheel rigidity. The muscle rigidity associated with parkinsonism. It is characterized by ratchet, or cogwheel, resistance to joint movement resulting from *lead pipe rigidity*/hypertonia combined with tremor.

Colloid cyst. A benign neoplasm that is composed of epithelial cells surrounded by a capsule and that is filled with a gelatinous substance. They commonly arise from the roof of the third ventricle. Although colloid cysts are a congenital abnormality, symptoms are usually not present until adulthood when the cyst blocks the cerebral aqueduct and produces an obstructive hydrocephalus. [Gr. *kolla,* glue; *kystis,* fluid-filled sac, bladder.]

Color agnosia. *See* Agnosia.

Color amnesia. Loss of knowledge about color in the context of normal color vision or color perception. Central to the disorder is "forgetting" how objects with intrinsic color should be colored (e.g., broccoli is green).

Color anomia. A loss of color naming ability. It often occurs in conjunction with alexia without agraphia. The color naming loss must be selective without similar impairment in object naming. Color anomia is thought to result from lesions of the lingual gyrus of the occipital lobe.

Colorado Malingering Tests. A series of computerized memory tests that employs both forced-choice methodology and implicit memory tasks. (Davis, H.P., King, J.H., Bajszar, G.M., Jr., and Squire, L.R. 1995. *Colorado Malingering Test Package.* Colorado Springs: Colorado Neuropsychology Tests Co.)

Colorado Neuropsychology Tests. A battery of computerized tests that includes Memory Cards (similar to the card game "Concentration"), Tower of Hanoi, Repeat Test (a serial reaction time test of implicit memory), Mirror Reading, Priming (word priming), Recall (with serial position effects, proactive interference, release from proactive interference), Recognition, Paired Associates, Temporal Order Test, and Visual and Digit Span Tests. Because the tests are computerized, the stimulus parameters can be modified to accommodate individual patient requirements. (Davis, H.P., Bajszar, G.M., Jr., and Squire, L.R. 1995. *Colorado Neuropsychology Tests*. Colorado Springs: Colorado Neuropsychology Tests Co.)

Coloured Progressive Matrices. *See* Raven's Progressive Matrices.

Columbia-Greystone Project. The principal study examining the effectiveness of frontal topectomy. The findings, published in 1949, indicated a beneficial effect of psychosurgery on social adjustment. Neuroleptics were introduced in the early 1950s, which led to a relatively rapid decline in the number of psychosurgery procedures preformed. (Columbia-Greystone Associates, F.A. Mettler, ed. 1949. *Selective Partial Ablation of the Frontal Cortex: A Correlative Study of its Effects on Human Psychotic Subjects*. New York: Paul B. Hoeber.)

Coma. State of unconsciousness and decreased responsiveness associated with neurologic injury, most often to the reticular activating system in the upper pons and midbrain. Definitions of coma are often imprecise. The Glasgow Coma Scale is commonly used to measure the degree of nonresponsiveness by assessing the ability to open the eyes, utter words, and obey commands. [Gr. *koma*, deep sleep.]

Coma stimulation. Systematic, repetitious sensory stimulation administered to comatose or vegetative patients to shorten coma or improve arousal level. It has not been subjected to controlled empirical trials.

Coma vigil. *See* Locked-in syndrome.

Combined system disease. Disorder associated with either pernicious anemia or with vitamin B_{12} deficiency without anemia. It is manifested by subacute development of myelopathy, dementia, posterior spinal column dysfunction, and peripheral neuropathy. Folic acid can reverse anemia while allowing neurologic complications to worsen.

Commissure. White matter fiber tract that connects the two cerebral hemispheres and transfers information from one hemisphere to another. The largest commissure is the corpus callosum, which connects large cortical regions of one side of the brain to homologous contralateral areas. The other major commissure is the anterior commissure, which connects olfactory structures and lateral parts of the temporal lobe to each other. [L. *commissura*, a joining together, from *comittere*, to put together.]

Commissurotomy. Surgical procedure to separate the hemispheres and thus decrease the severity of generalized tonic-clonic seizures. The corpus callosum, the primary interhemispheric fissure, is severed often with the anterior commissure. Commissurotomy allows each cerebral hemisphere to function relatively independently and has provided great insight into hemispheric specialization because each hemisphere can be tested in isolation. A complete corpus callosotomy is performed infrequently because of the risk of producing permanent disconnection symptoms. In most patients an anterior corpus callosotomy, which spares interhemispheric sensory communication, is performed. Also called split-brain procedure, or corpus callosotomy.

Communicating hydrocephalus. *See* Hydrocephalus.

Communicative Abilities in Daily Living. A test of communication abilities, including nonverbal communication, for aphasic adults. The range of communications includes gestures, writing, and drawing, and it is assessed using a variety of everyday contexts (e.g., making telephone calls, visiting a doctor's office). (Holland, A. 1980. *The Communicative Abilities in Daily Living*. Manual. Austin, TX: Pro-Ed.)

Community re-entry. Model of outpatient rehabilitation emphasizing the resumption of community roles (within work, school, family) rather than the restoration of specific skills.

Comorbidity. The coexistence of two or more diseases. [L. *morbidus*, sickly, diseased, from *morbus*, disease.]

Compensation neurosis. Exaggeration of symptoms in pursuit of financial gain.

Compensatory strategy. An alternate means of task performance that is used because the preferred approach has become more difficult or impossible because of impairment or disability. A patient unable to learn a work routine, for example, may use a palm-top computer to provide a reminder of tasks that need to be accomplished daily.

Competency. Capacity to make personal decisions and manage one's financial affairs. Legal competency is determined by the courts, usually with input from healthcare professionals in cases of neurologic impairment.

Complex Figure Test. A test of visual-spatial constructional skill and visual memory developed by Rey (1941) and standardized by Osterrieth (1944). The figure is first copied and this provides information about constructional ability. Memory is assessed by using immediate recall, delayed recall, or both. There are many different approaches to scoring, both quantitative and qualitative, and to testing administration. There is also considerable variability in the interpretation of the standard 18 scoring units so that scores should not be generalized across institutions uncritically. In addition, recognition memory can be assessed with some administration versions. An alternative complex figure was developed by Taylor (Taylor Complex Figure). Most studies have not found the memory components of Rey-Osterreith and Taylor Complex Figures to be equivalent, with performance generally higher on the Taylor Figure. Also called the Rey Figure or the Rey-O. *See* Denman Neuropsychology Memory Test. (Osterrieth, P.A. 1944. Le test de copie d'une figure complex: Contribution a l'etude de la perception et de la memoire. *Arch. Psychol.* 30:286–356; Rey, A. 1941. L'examen psychologique dans les cas d'encephalopathie traumatique. *Arch. Psychol.* 28:286–340; Taylor, L.B. 1969. Localization of cerebral lesions by psychological testing. *Clin. Neurosurg.* 16:269–287.)

Complex partial seizure (cps). *See* Seizure.

Computed tomography (CT). Imaging technique using ionizing radiation that permits noninvasive depiction of brain and other structures. Brain CT reveals ventricular enlargement, differentiates gray from white matter, reveals the basal ganglia, and can identify certain parenchymal changes. Computed tomography was originally called computed axial tomography (CAT) because images could be acquired only in the axial plane. The spatial resolution of CT is superior to that of conventional magnetic resonance imaging (MRI), but the contrast resolution of MRI is superior to that of CT. Computed tomography is superior to MRI in detecting blood and thus in identifying image acute hemorrhage. Computed tomography was introduced in 1972. [Gr. *tomos*, a cut section, from *temnein*, to cut.]

Conation. A constant willing or desire, volition, or striving. It includes instincts, drives, wishes, and cravings. [L. *conatio*, an attempt, from *conari*, to undertake, attempt.]

Concentration Endurance Test (d2 Test). A cancellation test that assesses vigilance, sustained attention, and visual scanning (hemispatial neglect). The target items are d's with two quotation marks, and are part of a series containing distractors of the letter p with 1–4 quotation marks and the letter d with 1, 3, or 4 quotation marks (See Cancellation tests). (Brickenkamp, R. 1981. *Test d2: Aufmerksamkeits-Belastungs-Test*. Handanweisung, 7th ed. [Test d2: Concentration-Endurance-Test. Manual, 7th ed.]. Gottingen, Toronto, Zurich: Verlag für Psychologie Dr. C.J. Hogrefe.)

Concussion. Mild traumatic brain injury characterized by at least a brief loss of consciousness or brief post-traumatic amnesia. [L. *concutere*, to shake violently.]

Conditional probability. The probability of an event or outcome, given that a different event has occurred. See Bayes' theorem.

Conduction aphasia. *See* Aphasia syndromes.

Conduite d'approche. Successive phonemic approximations toward a target word. It is seen in conduction aphasia. [F. "approach behavior".]

Confabulation. Narration of *paramnesias* as true events, usually seen in the context of an amnestic syndrome. Confabulation involves information that may be implausible (i.e., fantastic confabulation) and is a prominent feature of the acute Wernicke-Korsakoff syndrome and Anton's syndrome. [L. *confabulari*, to talk together or converse.]

Confidence interval. Interval around a statistic (e.g., observed test score, sample mean) that reflects its expected sample-to-sample variability. Confidence intervals are usually expressed in standard deviation units (±1 SD or 2 SD) or percentages (95% or 99%).

Confirmatory factor analysis. Multivariate technique for studying the dimensionality of a set of measures. In contrast to exploratory factor analysis, relations between variables and the underlying dimensions are posited in advance of the analysis. This allows an explicit hypothesis testing approach to studying the psychometric properties of measures and the consistency of these properties across time, populations, or other domains of interest.

Confrontation naming. Naming task in which the stimuli (objects or pictures) are presented visually. This contrasts with responsive naming, in which the object is described. Two examples are the Visual Naming Test from the Multilingual Aphasia Examination and the Boston Naming Test. Also called nominal speech.

Confusion. Disorientation to time and place.

Confusional state. Condition involving alterations in level of arousal, disturbances of attention, and impairment in the logical stream of thought. It typically has a short time course and is commonly associated with disturbance in the sleep-wake cycle, disorientation to time and place, rambling or incoherent speech, illusions, visual hallucinations, and either increased or decreased psychomotor behavior. Onset is generally rapid, with a fluctuating course in which the delirium is worse at night (sundowning). Common etiologies include metabolic disturbances, toxic exposure, medications, infection, trauma, increased intracerebral pressure, focal stroke, or seizures. On testing, patients often display neuropsychological impairments on measures of attention and concentration, memory, language comprehension (e.g., Token test), and visual spatial functions. Also called delirium.

Conners' Rating Scales. Rating scales of problem behavior (e.g., conduct problems, hyperactivity) designed for children 3–17 years or age. The rating scale has two parts, Conners' Parent Rating Scales (CPRS) and Conners' Teacher Rating Scales (CTRS), both of which have short and long forms. All four measures include a 10-item Hyperactivity Index, which is a general index of child psychopathology rather than a special scale for Attention-deficit/hyperactivity disorder. (Conners, C.K. 1989. *Conners' Rating Scales*, Manual. Tonawanda, NY: Multi-Health Systems.)

Consciousness. State of awareness of both self and environment. Consciousness implies being fully responsive to stimuli so that behavior and speech reflect awareness of self and of the environment. Normal consciousness fluctuates from alertness and concentration with a focused field of attention, to mild general inattentiveness and drowsiness. It has two main aspects: arousal and content. Duration of loss of consciousness following cerebral injury is often used as a measure of the injury's severity.

Consortium to Establish a Registry for Alzheimer's Disease (CERAD). A consortium established to develop, standardize, and test the reliability of brief clinical evaluation and neuropsychological assessment for patients with presumptive diagnoses of Alzheimer's disease. In addition, CERAD developed a protocol for postmortem examination of brain tissue to provide standardized neuropathologic criteria for the diagnosis of Alzheimer's disease. *See* CERAD Neuropsychological Test Battery.

Construct validity. Degree to which scores on a measure support inferences about a dimension of interest. Construct validity of tests can be established with factor analysis by demonstrating high correlations with tests measuring similar constructs and low correlations with tests measuring different constructs, by examining test performance in patient groups that have a high frequency of impairment for the construct being studied, or by studying the effects of intervention known to impact the specified construct.

Constructional apraxia. *See* Apraxia.

Content validity. Measure of the adequacy with which a specific domain of content is sampled.

Content words (open class words). Words that have semantic and referential meaning, consisting primarily of nouns, verbs, adjectives, and adverbs. Because new lexical words continue to be invented (e.g., "fax"), content words are sometimes referred to as open class words. Also called contentives.

Contextual encoding deficit. Theoretical account of amnesia in which the memory deficit lies in the encoding of contextual information.

Contingent negative variation (CNV). A slow, negative potential shift in the EEG that occurs in anticipation of a stimulus following a warning or alerting signal. The CNV occurs maximally over the frontal lobe. Also called an expectancy wave.

Continuous Performance Test (CPT). A vigilance task that requires the focusing of attention on one or more sources of information for relatively long periods during which subjects must detect and respond to target stimuli. Most CPT versions are patterned after the original two tasks developed by Rosvold et al. (1956). In the simpler condition, letters of the alphabet are individually presented, and the task is to respond each time that the letter *X* is seen. In the more demanding condition, the patient is to respond only to those *X* presentations that have been immediately preceded by the letter *A*. In other variations using similar designs, the modality, type of stimuli, and the way responses are analyzed have been altered (omissions, commissions, interstimulus interval, d' and β derived from signal detection theory). In more substantial variations, a subject responds to all letters except *X*, thereby increasing the demand for response inhibition. (Conners, C.K. and Multi-Health Systems Staff. 1995. *Conners' Continuous Performance Test.* North Tonawanda, NY: Multi-Health Systems; Rosvold, H.E., Mirsky, A.F., Sarason, I., Bransome, E.D., Jr., and Beck, L.H. 1956. A continuous performance test of brain damage. *J. Consult. Psychol.* 20: 343–350.)

Continuous Visual Memory Test. A test of recognition memory in which abstract designs are presented individually for 2 seconds. The procedure consists of 7 target figures that are repeated with 112 other stimuli. The task is to determine whether each stimulus is a new or repeated design. A 30–minute delay and recognition are assessed. (Trahan, D.E. and Larrabee, G.J. 1988. *Continuous Recognition Memory Test.* Odessa, FL: Psychological Assessment Resources.)

Contracture. A permanent tightening of muscle, tendons, ligaments, or skin that prevents normal movement and often results in permanent deformity of the associated body part. Contractures occur primarily in the skin, underlying tissues, muscle, tendons, and joint areas and develop from immobilization or inactivity. [L. *contractura*, from *con-traho*, to draw together.]

Contralateral. Relating to the opposite side. The term is often used to refer to the affected side opposite a cerebral lesion, although its use is not restricted to clinical description. [L. *contra*, opposite; *latus*, side.]

Contrast agents. Chemical agents administered during radiologic procedures to enhance structural imaging. Contrast agents for angiography and CT contain radioactive material whereas those for MRI are paramagnetic.

Contrecoup contusion. Cerebral contusion appearing opposite to the point of impact after a blow to the head; for example, a left parietal-occipital contusion following a focal blow to the right frontal region. [F. *contre*, against, opposite; *coup*, a stroke, blow.]

Controlled Oral Word Association (COWA). A test of verbal fluency in which words beginning with a specific target letter of the alphabet are generated. The COWA differs from the Thurstone Fluency Test, which involves writing words that begin with a target letter, in that the responses are given orally. The COWA is sometimes called the FAS test after the letters that were originally used. Age and education corrections are used in clinical applications, but not always in research designs. Also called letter fluency. (Benton, A.L. and Hamsher, KdeS. 1989. *Multilingual Aphasia Examination.* Iowa City: AJA Associates; Spreen, O. and Benton, A.L. 1977. *Neurosensory Center Comprehensive Examination for Aphasia.* Victoria, B.C.: University of Victoria, Psychology Laboratory.)

Contusion, brain. A bruise, typically of the brain surface, without cerebral hemorrhage. [L. *contusus,* past part. of *contundere,* to bruise, beat together.]

Conversion disorder. A disorder characterized by apparent neurologic symptoms involving voluntary motor or sensory function without neurological pathology. Although psychogenic in origin, conversion symptoms are not intentionally produced and are often detected because they are inconsistent with motor and sensory organization (*See* Astasia-abasia, Splitting the midline, Give way weakness, Face-hand test).

Convulsion. Generalized involuntary muscle contraction associated with generalized tonic-clonic seizures. *See* seizures. [L. *convulsio,* from *convello,* past part. of *vulsus,* to tear up.]

Cookie theft picture. A stimulus card from the Boston Diagnostic Aphasia Examination designed to elicit conversation and expository speech. The picture contains multiple activities that can be described, and the instruction given is to "tell me everything you see going on in this picture." Responses are rated on melodic line, phrase length, articulatory agility, grammatical form, paraphasias in speech, and word-finding ability. The stimulus card may also be used to elicit a sample of narrative writing ability with the direction to "write as much as you can about what you see going on in this picture."

COPD. *See* Chronic obstructive pulmonary disease.

Coprolalia. Vocal tic consisting of either a vulgarity or its initial phoneme. [Gr. *kopros,* filth, excrement; *lalein,* to speak.]

Copula. In the English language, forms of the verb "to be" that are used to link subject to predicate (e.g., "he is happy"). [L. *copula,* a bond, tie.]

Coronal. Dividing the body (or brain) into anterior and posterior portions. The coronal plane is a vertical plane at right angles to a sagittal plane. [L. *corona,* a crown.]

Corpus callosotomy. *See* Commissurotomy.

Corpus callosum. The major interhemispheric commissure connecting the two cerebral hemispheres. This structure is severed during some types of epilepsy surgery or for surgical access to the third ventricle. [L. *corpus,* body; *callosum,* large.]

Corpus striatum. Region of the basal ganglia consisting of a subcortical mass of gray and white matter anterior and lateral to the thalamus. The gray matter is arranged in two principal masses, the caudate and lentiform nuclei; the latter includes the putamen and globus pallidus. [L. *corpus,* body; *striatus,* furrowed or striped.]

Corsi Block Tapping Test. Spatial learning task, similar to spatial span, in which a series of same-length block spans is presented. The span length of the trials exceeds the patient's normal spatial span by one block. The same spatial sequence is repeated every third trial although no warning is given that there are repeated sequences. The task is to see how quickly the patient learns the repeated spatial sequence. This test was developed as a spatial analog of Hebb's Recurring Digit Test. (Corsi, P.M. 1972. Human Memory and the Medial Temporal Region of the Brain. Doctoral thesis, McGill University, Montreal, Quebec, Canada.)

Cortex, cerebral. Outer layer of the brain consisting of gray matter. Its surface area is greatly increased by being folded into convolutions called gyri, which are separated by furrows, or grooves, called sulci. The cortex has been mapped and divided into a number of distinctive areas that differ in total thickness, cell density, patterns of myelinated fibers, and cellular arrangement. The most famous cytoarchitectural map is that of Korbinian Brodmann (German anatomist, 1868–1918). [L. *cortex*, bark or outer covering.]

- **Archicortex**. The dentate gyrus and hippocampus. The archicortex is phylogenetically the oldest region of the cerebral cortex and consists of three cortical layers. [Gr. *archos*, chief, from *archein*, to be first, to rule (in biology, it usually means "primitive").]
- **Neocortex**. The major portion of the cerebral cortex, consisting of six layers. Also called isocortex, homogenetic cortex, and neopallium. Called neocortex because of its phylogenetically recent development. [Gr. *neos*, new; L. *cortex*, bark.]
- **Paleocortex**. The subiculum, piriform cortex, and the cingulate gyrus. It consists of three to five cortical layers. [Gr. *palaios*, ancient; L. *cortex*, bark.]

Cortical blindness. Loss of vision due to occipital lobe damage. Despite the name, cortical blindness may also result from purely subcortical lesions, which are usually bilateral optic radiation lesions. Direct and indirect pupillary reflexes are preserved. Optokinetic nystagmus cannot be elicited, visual evoked potentials cannot be demonstrated, and Anton's syndrome is common. The most frequent etiology is bilateral infarction of the posterior cerebral arteries.

Cortical dementia. *See* Dementia.

Cortical dysplasia. A neuromigrational disorder of cortical neurons that is associated with a high incidence of mental retardation and epilepsy.

Cortico-basal ganglionic degeneration (CBGD). A progressive disease of the basal ganglia characterized by apraxia, rigidity, dystonia, and postural abnormality. Patients with GBGD display moderate generalized cognitive deterioration and a *dysexecutive syndrome*. Apraxia is common. Explicit learning deficits may be compensated by using semantic cues for encoding and retrieval. CBDG is a parkinson-plus syndrome, and it is also called corticostriatonigral degeneration.

Corticobulbar. Motor tracts from primary motor cortex to cranial nerve nuclei in the brainstem.

Corticofugal. Proceeding, conducting, or moving away from the cortex.

Corticopetal. Proceeding, conducting, or moving toward the cortex.

Corticospinal. Motor tracts from primary motor cortex to spinal cord nuclei in the ventral horns.

Corticostriatonigral degeneration. *See* Cortico-basal ganglionic degeneration.

Corticotropin. *See* Adrenocorticotropic hormone.

Coup contusion. Brain contusion beneath the area of impact in head injury. Contrasts with contrecoup contusion. [F. *coup*, a blow; L. *contusus*, past part. of *contundere*, to bruise, beat together.]

COWA. *See* Controlled Oral Word Association Test.

CPR. Cardiopulmonary resuscitation.

CPT. *See* Continuous Performance Test; also Current Procedural Terminology.

Cranial nerves. Twelve paired nerves arising from the brainstem that innervate muscles of the head and receive sensory information, primarily from the head.

Craniopharyngioma. A tumor arising from cells derived from the pituitary stalk that often increases intracranial pressure. Also called suprasella cyst.

Craniosynostosis. A condition in which the cranial sutures fuse prematurely, resulting in deformity of skull growth. Untreated, it may result in developmental delay and learning disability, and it may affect psychosocial development.

Craniotomy. A surgical opening of the skull for access to the brain. The bone-flap is the portion of skull that is temporarily removed, and it is often left attached to overlying scalp and muscle tissue (osteoplastic flap) to maintain bone vascularization.

Creutzfeldt-Jakob disease (CJD). (Hans-Gerhard Creutzfeldt, German neuropathologist, 1885–1964; Alfons M. Jakob, German neuropathologist, 1884–1931). A rare, subacute cerebral degeneration characterized by a rapidly progressive dementia. This disease is associated with varying degrees of myoclonus, ataxia, derangement of posture and movement, disturbance of vision, and seizures. It generally affects individuals 65 years of age and older, and the course is usually fatal within 6 months. Creutzfeldt-Jakob disease is transmitted by prions, which contain no nucleic acids but are otherwise similar to viruses, and which are the infectious agents of scrapie and bovine spongiform encephalopathy (mad cow disease). In most CJD patients, there is a characteristic EEG abnormality that consists of periodic runs of sharp wave complexes, and biopsy reveals characteristic spongiform encephalopathy. Also called Jakob-Creutzfeldt disease.

Criterion-related validity. The ability of to predict specific variable behavior for measures external to the measuring instrument itself (e.g., the presence or absence of a specific disease).

Critical flicker fusion. Temporal frequency at which a rapidly flashing visual stimulus appears to be a steady light. This test was part of Halstead's original test battery but was deleted because of poor sensitivity to brain damage.

Crowding. **1.** A decline in visual-spatial abilities associated with a shift in language dominance to the right cerebral hemisphere following left hemisphere damage early in life. This shift occurs at the expense of visual-spatial abilities that are typically associated with right hemisphere function. The term was introduced by Hans-Lukas Teuber (American psychologist born in Germany, 1916–1977), who argued that the decline in cognitive abilities occurs when "one hemisphere tries to do more than it had originally been meant to do." **2.** The tendency to copy several stimuli into a space intended for a single item. It is often associated with unilateral visual neglect. Patients with diffuse generalized impairment may also display a type of crowding in which a shape is "copied" on top of the stimulus figure, or the original stimulus is incorporated into the copy (closing-in).

CRT. *See* Reaction time.

Crystallized intelligence. Intelligence that reflects information acquired through education, experience, and socialization. The division of intellectual skills (generalized intelligence, or g) into crystallized (Gc) and fluid (Gf) dimensions was made by Cattell (1963), who suggested that Gc reflects the appropriation of a culture's collective intelligence for individual use. Because Gc is heavily based upon experience, it is strongly age dependent and increases throughout the normal life span (e.g., vocabulary). The Stanford-Binet Intelligence Scale (4th ed.) applies the crystallized/fluid distinction in its approach to intelligence assessment. (Cattell, R.B. 1963. Theory of fluid and crystallized intelligence: A critical experiment. *J. Educat. Psychol.* 54:1–22.)

CSF. *See* Cerebrospinal fluid.

CT. *See* Computed tomography.

Cued recall. Memory recall in which information about items to be recalled is provided. Common cues include the semantic category or the initial phoneme of the word.

Current Procedural Terminology (CPT). A listing of descriptive terms associated with digit codes that is used or reporting medical services and procedures. It is published by the American Medical Association.

Cushing's disease. (Harvey W. Cushing, American neurosurgeon, 1869–1939). A disorder associated with increased adrenocortical secretion of cortisol, caused by ACTH-dependent adrenocortical hyperplasia or tumor. Psychiatric manifestations are common.

Cutaneous sense. The sense of pressure, pain, cold, warmth, and touch. Cutaneous receptors lie beneath the skin or in the mucous membranes. [L. *cutis*, skin.]

CVA. Cerebrovascular accident.

CXR. Chest x-ray.

Cyanosis. A dark slate blue color of the mucous membranes, lips, nail beds, and skin, due to deficient blood oxygenation. [Gr. *kyanosis*, dark blue color, from *kyanos*, dark blue.]

Cysticercosis. Larval or intermediate stage of infection with the pork tapeworm *Taenia solium*. Infection occurs from eating fresh vegetables and raw legumes contaminated by feces or from eating undercooked pork. In India, Central and South America, and in some southern border regions in the U.S., cysticercosis is a major cause of epilepsy (generalized tonic-clonic seizures). Increased intracranial pressure is also common. [Gr. *kystis*, bladder; *kerkos*, tail, used to describe form of tapeworm.]

Cytomegalovirus (CMV). A herpes virus that is a common cause of intrauterine infection. It is often associated with congenital malformations and growth retardation. Cytomegalovirus may occur as an independent viral syndrome, but is also frequently seen with Guillain-Barré syndrome or AIDS.

D

d' (d prime). A measure derived from *signal detection theory* that represents the discriminability of the signal (target stimulus) from background stimulation without regard to the threshold or response bias.

d2 test. *See* Concentration Endurance Test.

DA. Developmental age; dopamine.

DAT. *See* Dementia of the Alzheimer type (DAT).

dB. Decibel; one-tenth of a bel. Decibels express the relative loudness of sound on a logarithmic scale. Also abbreviated db.

Debridement. Removal of unhealthy damaged tissue and foreign matter, including bone fragments, from a wound. [F. *debrider*, to unbridle.]

Decerebrate rigidity. Bilateral, marked, rigid extension of the legs, with internal rotation of the arms and extension of the arms. This posture is produced by bilateral cerebral dysfunction that extends to the upper brainstem near the red nucleus.

Declarative memory. *See* Memory.

Decorticate rigidity. Bilateral, marked, rigid flexion of the arms to the chest and of the legs that is associated with bilateral dysfunction of the cerebral cortex. The lesions may involve gray and white matter, internal capsule, or thalamus bilaterally.

Decubitus ulcer. Skin breakdown, or bedsore, commonly occurring on sacrum, heels, and back of the head from constant pressure that restricts blood flow. Decubitus ulcers may develop from continuous exposure to chemical or mechanical irritation (e.g., urine, plaster casts). Bed-ridden patients are at risk for developing decubitus ulcers because of absence of movement. Also called pressure ulcer. [L. *decumbo*, to lie down; *ulcus*, a sore, ulcer.]

Decussation. Crossing of paired fiber tracts across midline. *Compare with* Chiasm. [L. *decussare*, to intersect; from *decussin*, ten, represented by the symbol X.]

Deep agraphia. *See* Agraphia spelling disorders.

Deep brain stimulation. An approach to the treatment of chronic pain and parkinsonism in which constant high-frequency stimulation (100–180 Hz) is applied to thalamic nuclei. A pulse stimulator, similar to a pacemaker, is implanted near the collarbone and used to deliver the electrical stimulation.

Deep dyslexia. *See* Alexia.

Deep structure. The underlying meaning of a spoken or written expression as opposed to its exact linguistic form. Deep structures contain no words; meaning is conveyed to others through words and their order, called *surface structure*. Term introduced by Chomsky. (Chomsky, N. 1965. *Aspects of the Theory of Syntax*. Cambridge, MA: MIT Press.)

Deep tendon reflexes (DTRs). Involuntary muscle contraction that is seen after a tendon is percussed. Hyperactive reflexes indicate *upper motor neuron* impairment; hypoactive reflexes indicate *lower motor neuron* disease.

Déjà vu. Sense of inappropriate familiarity characterized by the feeling that an experience has been lived through before. Déjà vu episodes may represent a seizure aura or manifestations of a psychiatric disorder such as schizotypal personality disorder. This is a normal, infrequent phenomenon, especially during childhood and adolescence. [F. *déjà*, already, *vu*, seen.]

Dejerine's syndrome. (Joseph Jules Dejerine, French neurologist, 1849–1917). *See* Alexia/ dyslexia, acquired (alexia without agraphia).

Delayed response tasks. Tasks developed to assess memory in primates in which the animal is required to remember the location of a reward until a response is permitted.

- **Delayed match-to-sample**. A memory task for primates in which the animal first observes in which of two food wells food is placed. A screen is introduced to prevent the food wells from being seen for a specified period. The screen is then removed and the two locations are displayed. The animal obtains a food reward if its choice of wells is correct.
- **Delayed response alteration**. The same conditions apply as the delayed match-to-sample task but the location of the food is changed to the opposite side; the animal must learn this alternating location to obtain the food reward. Performance on this task declines following dorsolateral frontal lesions.

Delirium. *See* confusional state. [L. *delirium*, madness, from *delirare*, to rave, be crazy.]

Delirium tremens (DTs). A condition associated with agitation, tremor, confusion, and vivid hallucinations that develop several days after sudden alcohol cessation in alcoholics. DTs may last up to 1 week, and patients are at risk for developing generalized status epilepticus.

Delta. The fourth letter of the Greek alphabet, δ or Δ. **1.** EEG frequencies less than 4 Hz. **2.** A capital delta (Δ) is used to represent the amount of change between repeated measurements.

Delusion. A false belief about external reality that is firmly maintained despite contrary evidence or proof. Common delusions include the following: persecutory delusions that others are cheating, conspiring against oneself, or threatening harm; grandiose delusions, an inflated sense of self-worth, power, or knowledge; delusions of being controlled by an external force; delusions of reference, beliefs that surrounding events have particular and unusual personal significance; thought broadcasting, which are delusions that one's thoughts are being broadcast aloud so that others can know them; and thought insertion, delusions that some thoughts are being implanted into one's mind from an external source. [L. *delusio*, delusion, from *delusus*, past part. of *deludere*, to cheat, delude.]

Dementia. Generalized loss of cognitive functions resulting from cerebral disease occurring in clear consciousness (i.e., in the absence of a confusional state). According to the DSM-IV, the decline must be of sufficient magnitude to impair social or occupational function. Memory impairment is required for diagnosis, with at least one additional area of impairment present such as aphasia, apraxia, agnosia, or impaired executive function. The DSM-IV definition of dementia does not suggest a progressive course or irreversibility, although these factors were part of previous definitions. The disease processes underlying dementia may have many causes, including static lesions, such as head injury, and rapidly or gradually progressive neurodegenerative disorders, including Alzheimer's disease, Pick's disease, Creutzfeldt-Jakob disease, Parkinson's disease, and Huntington's disease. The course of dementia is variable and depends on etiology. [L. *de-*, signifies separation, cessation; *mens (mentis)*, mind.]

- **AIDS dementia**. A dementia syndrome resulting from direct HIV involvement of the brain. The characteristic features of AIDS dementia include apathy, impaired concentration and memory, psychomotor slowing, and decreased cognitive performance on many "frontal lobe" tests. Because of this constellation of neuropsychological impairments, AIDS dementia is viewed by some as a subcortical dementia. Dementia usually occurs in the later stages of HIV infection but may be the initial manifestation. As it progresses, patients often develop myoclonus or parkinsonism. Formerly referred to as AIDS encephalopathy or AIDS encephalitis.

- **Alcoholic dementia.** A condition of cognitive decline associated with chronic ethanol abuse of approximately 15–20 years duration. Patients tend to display neuropsychological deficits associated with frontal lobe impairment, including decreased interest, poor personal hygiene, poor judgment, decreased cognitive efficiency, poor attention and recent memory, and flattened affect. This condition is associated with enlarged cerebral ventricles, frontal cortical atrophy, and thinning of the cerebral cortex. Previously called alcoholic pseudoparesis because of its clinical similarity to general paresis (neurosyphilis).
- **Axial dementia.** Dementia associated with loss of recent memory due to impairment of midline (axial) brain structures, which may include thalamus, hippocampus, fornix, mammillary bodies, and hypothalamus. The prototype disease associated with axial dementia is Korsakoff's syndrome. Also called axial amnesia.
- **Cortical dementia.** Dementia characterized by a loss of higher cortical function, such as aphasia, apraxia, or agnosia, and introduced to contrast with subcortical dementia, which is characterized by slowed mental processing. Alzheimer's disease is the prototype of cortical dementia. The distinction between cortical and subcortical dementia, however, is not universally accepted because the terms "cortical" and "subcortical" are imprecise and both cortical and subcortical histologic changes are associated with most causes of dementia.
- **Dementia of the Alzheimer type (DAT).** A description of dementia that behaviorally appears to be Alzheimer's disease given that there is absence of pathological verification. Senile dementia of the Alzheimer type (SDAT) may be used for patients who are at least 65 years of age.
- **Dementia paralytica.** *See* Neurosyphilis.
- **Dementia pugilistica.** Condition characterized by forgetfulness, slowness in thinking, dysarthric speech, and a wide-based, unsteady gait that occurs in boxers who have histories of many boxing matches over a long period. A flattened affect and parkinsonian extrapyramidal symptoms are common.
- **Dialysis dementia.** A condition that may develop following years of hemodialysis for chronic renal failure characterized by subtle personality change, speech impairment, and cognitive impairment. The condition initially appears at the end of a dialysis session and rapidly resolves over the next day. Over the course of 6 months, however, the changes progress to include general cognitive impairment, asterixis, mutism, myoclonus, and occasionally, seizures. The etiology may be related to aluminum or chronic renal insufficiency. The incidence has declined following removal of aluminum from the dialysate and purification of the water used in dialysis. [Gr. *dialyein*, to separate, from *dia*, through, apart, and *lyein*, to loose.]
- **Lewy-body dementia.** A Parkinson Plus syndrome that may appear clinically to be either Alzheimer's disease or Parkinson's disease. The cortical neurons contain Lewy bodies (intracytoplasmic inclusion bodies) but neurofibrillary changes or senile plaques are not present. The typical clinical picture is a combination of parkinsonian extrapyramidal disorder and dementia with delusions, visual hallucinations, and fluctuations.
- **Multi-infarct dementia.** Dementia that arises from repeated small cerebral infarctions. There are often associated physical impairments, including paresis, clumsiness,

rigidity, and reflex abnormalities. In contrast to Alzheimer's disease, there is usually an abrupt onset followed by a stepwise deterioration of cognitive function. Multi-infarct dementia is often operationalized using the Hachinski ischemia scale. A form of vascular dementia.

- **Presenile dementia**. Dementia that develops during the presenium, which is variably defined as before 60 or 65 years, as distinct from senile dementia, which develops after age 60–65 years. Both terms have decreased in usage following the demonstration of similar neuropathologic change in presenile and senile dementia of the Alzheimer type. Pick's disease, however, is still often called a presenile dementia since it characteristically begins between 55 and 60 years of age.
- **Semantic dementia**. Dementia characterized by a selective impairment in semantic memory, with the relative sparing of other nonsemantic language components and of perceptual and spatial skills. Semantic dementia is thought to result from focal cortical degeneration that predominantly affects the temporal lobes.
- **Senile dementia**. Dementia developing during the senium, commonly defined as age 60 or 65 years and older. This term has become less popular after the demonstration of similar neuropathologic changes associated with progressive dementia independent of age of dementia onset.
- **Senile dementia of the Alzheimer type (SDAT)**. A term for patients who behaviorally appear to have Alzheimer's disease but in whom pathological verification has not been established (i.e., at autopsy or from biopsy) and who develop dementia after 65 years of age. The term dementia of the Alzheimer type (DAT) is employed for patients appearing to have Alzheimer's disease without regard to age at disease onset.
- **Subcortical dementia**. A clinical syndrome characterized by slowing of cognition, memory disturbances, visual-spatial abnormalities, disturbances of mood/affect, and difficulties with complex intellectual tasks such as strategy generation and problem solving. Although subcortical dementia should not be taken to imply that there is no cortical component to the clinical presentation, it does suggest that "higher cortical function" is relatively spared. However, the distinction between cortical and subcortical dementia is not universally accepted. Examples of subcortical dementia include Huntington's disease, Parkinson's disease, progressive supranuclear palsy, and HIV dementia.
- **Vascular dementia**. Dementia resulting from cerebrovascular disease. Vascular dementia may result from a variety of causes including repeated cerebral infarction (i.e., multi-infarct dementia), a single vascular insult to a critical brain region, or chronic ischemia without discrete infarction.

Dementia rating scales. Tests that screen for dementia and assess its severity. This term is often a misnomer since most dementia rating scales are extended mental status examinations, and few behavioral characteristics of dementia are actually rated. In the context of standardized approaches to assessing the elderly, the terms "dementia rating scale" and "mental status examination" are often used interchangeably.

Demographic characteristics. Population attributes that provide sample characterization. Demographic information is important in neuropsychological assessment since many factors, such as age, education, and sex, are known to influence performance on a variety of cognitive tasks.

Demyelination. Destruction of the myelin sheath surrounding a nerve fiber that disrupts neural conduction. The most common demyelinating disease is multiple sclerosis, but various leukodystrophies, viruses, and toxins may produce demyelination. The most common peripheral demyelinating disease is Guillain-Barré syndrome.

Dendrite. The receptive process of the neuron on which axons or other dendrites terminate. Dendrites are extensions of the cell body that receive synaptic inputs. [Gr. *dendrites*, relating to a tree.]

Denervate. A block of a nerve from its normal connections.

Denervation supersensitivity. Phenomenon in which receptors in an area partially cut off from normal neural connection become hypersensitive to remaining inputs, resulting in partial sparing or restoration of function.

Denman Neuropsychology Memory Scale. A clinical memory test that contains eleven subtests to evaluate immediate and delayed verbal and nonverbal memory. It is similar in format to the Wechsler Memory Scale (WMS), but contains several tasks without a WMS analogue, including a memory for faces subtest, a musical tone differentiation task, and the Rey-Osterreith Complex Figure. The Denman Neuropsychology Memory Scale contains a comprehensive scoring system for the *Complex Figure Test*. (Denman, S.B. 1987. *Denman Neuropsychology Memory Scale*. Charleston, SC: Sidney B. Denman.)

Dependent variable. The outcome measure of interest in an experimental design.

Depression. A mood disturbance characterized by sadness, loss of pleasure or interest, and psychomotor retardation. It is often associated with difficulty in attention and concentration, and loss of energy and feelings of worthlessness are common. DSM-IV differentiates between dysthymic disorder, which consists of depressed mood for at least one-half of the days for at least 2 years duration, and major depressive disorder, which consists of nearly daily depressed mood and has occurred for at least 2 weeks' duration.

Depressed skull fracture. Cranial injury associated with protrusion of bony fragments into the dura and brain, causing laceration of the dura and underlying cortex.

Derivational error. A reading, writing, or speaking error at the single word level in which the correct morphemic root is retained but differs in part of speech (e.g., "confuse" for "confusion," "deflate" for "inflate").

Dermatome. The area of the skin supplied with afferent nerve fibers by a single posterior spinal root. Neighboring dermatomes may overlap slightly.

Design fluency. *See* Figural fluency.

Developmental dysphasia (aphasia). Failure to develop language skills normally in the absence of an identifiable neurologic etiology or other medical problems. Subtypes may be primarily expressive, primarily receptive, or mixed expressive/receptive. Development dysphasia is classified by DSM-IV as a communication disorder and uses the term "language disorder" rather than "aphasia."

Developmental Test of Visual-Motor Integration. A test of visual-constructional ability assessed by copying geometric designs. The test has a developmental gradient of difficulty, beginning with a vertical line for 2-year-olds and progressing to three-dimensional cube and star designs for 14- and 15-year-olds. (Beery, K.E. 1997. *The Visual-Motor Integration Test*, 4th ed. Administration, Scoring, and Teaching Manual. *Austin, TX: Pro-Ed.*)

Deviation quotient. Standard score that expresses performance relative to the mean of a reference group. In addition, deviation quotients are scores derived from combinations of other scores and transformed into a standard score similar to the intelligence quotient. This approach was advocated by Tellegen and Briggs (1967) so that Wechsler Intelligence Scale (WIS) subtests could be combined into "quotients" that are more homogeneous in content. (Tellegen, A. and Briggs, P.F. 1967. Old wine in new skins: Grouping Wechsler Subtests into new scales. *J. Consult. Psychol.* 31:499–506.)

DEX. Dysexecutive questionnaire. *See* Behavioral Assessment of the Dysexecutive Syndrome.

Dexamethasone suppression test. A procedure used in the diagnosis of Cushing's disease. Dexamethasone is administered in the late evening, and the normal response is suppression of cortisol secretion for 24 hours. Patients with Cushing's disease, however, fail to show the normal suppression. The test is also used in some research application studying depression.

Diagnosis-related group (DRG). An approach to the classification of hospitalized patients by diagnosis that correlates each group with the level of care needed and the average length of hospitalization. Diagnosis-related groups are widely used in the U.S. to establish reimbursement parameters.

Diagnostic and Statistical Manual of Mental Disorders (DSM). Diagnostic criteria that catalog and code more than 300 psychiatric, psychological, and neurologic disorders published by the American Psychiatric Association. Each DSM-IV disorder contains specific diagnostic criteria, the essential features and clinical information associated with the disorder, and differential diagnostic considerations. Information concerning diagnostic and associated features, culture, age, and gender characteristics, prevalence, incidence, course and complications of the disorder, familial pattern, and differential diagnosis are included. Many diagnoses require symptom severity ratings (mild, moderate, or severe) and information about the current state of the problem (e.g., partial or full remission). DSM-III was the first edition to incorporate the multiaxial system to ensure appropriate description of biopsychosocial factors related to patient classification, treatment, and outcome. Axes I and II comprise traditional psychiatric and psychological disorders, Axis III represents physical disorders, and Axes IV and V refer to the severity of psychosocial and environmental stress and the global assessment of function respectively. DSM-IV was published in 1994.

Dialysis dementia. *See* Dementia.

Diaschisis. A temporary loss of function produced by acute focal brain damage in an adjacent region or in a region connected through fiber tracts. Constantin Von Monakow (Russian/Swiss neurologist, 1853–1930) postulated that functional continuity between various centers is disrupted beyond the direct effects of the permanent lesion and that the resolution of diaschisis partially accounts for functional recovery after focal injury. The term "diaschisis" is also used to describe cerebellar hypometabolism contralateral to a large hemispheral infarct (crossed cerebellar diaschisis). [Gr. *diá*, through; *schizein*, to tear.] (von Monakow, C. 1911. Lokalisation der Hirnfunktionen. *J. Psychol. Neurol.* 17:185–200. Translated as Localization of brain functions. In: Von Bonin, G. 1990. *Some Papers on the Cerebral Cortex.* Springfield, IL: Charles C. Thomas, pp. 231–250.)

Dichotic listening. A technique involving binaural presentation of independent information in each ear that was developed by Donald E. Broadbent (British psychologist, 1926–1993). The subject may be instructed to monitor information from one ear while competing information is presented concurrently to the other ear. Dichotic listening is used to study divided attention and vigilance, and auditory processes. Verbal stimuli presented to the right ear typically are identified more accurately and faster than those presented to the left ear; this is referred to as the right ear advantage, which presumably reflects left hemisphere dominance for language. [Gr. *dichotiké*, of both ears; *dicha*, in two, from *dis*, twice, from *dyo*, two.]

Diencephalon. Inferior portion of the *forebrain*, composed of the thalamus, hypothalamus, subthalamus, and lenticular nucleus. *See* Basal ganglia. [Gr. *dia* through, across; *enkephalos*, brain; between brain.]

Differential reinforcement of appropriate behavior. Behavioral modification technique by which social attention and praise are provided for prosocial behaviors while uncooperative, disruptive, or antisocial behaviors are ignored (extinguished).

Diffuse axonal injury (DAI). Widespread, patchy macroscopic and microscopic injury to brain tissue associated with the rotational forces of traumatic brain injury sustained at high speed (*see* Acceleration-deceleration injury). A DAI is produced mechanically by shear strains between brain tissue of differing densities and neurochemically by released cyto-toxic factors (e.g., free radical). It also occurs hours after injury from secondary cell degeneration.

Digit span. Span task assessing the ability to repeat a series of numbers of increasing lengths. The ability both to repeat numbers immediately following their presentation and to re-peat them in reversed serial order are typically tested. Digit span, particularly backward digit span, is regarded by many as the prototypic test of mental tracking or working mem-ory. Digit span tasks are part of a variety of procedures including many mental status ex-aminations, Wechsler Intelligence Scales (WIS), and the Wechsler Memory Scale.

Diplegia. Bilateral paralysis of corresponding extremities (e.g., both arms, both legs).

Diplopia. Double vision.

Disability. According to the World Health Organization, the restriction or inability to per-form a skill or activity that results from pathology or impairment. This may turn into a handicap.

Disability Rating Scale (DRS). Ordinal outcome scale designed to reflect the range of out-comes in traumatic brain injury; produces quantitative index of disability in self-care and of social and occupational function across 10 levels of severity. (Rappaport, M., Hall, K.M., Hopkins, K., Belleza, T., and Cope, D.N. 1982. Disability rating scale for severe head trauma: Coma to community. *Arch. Physical Med. Rehab.* 63:118–23.)

Disconnection syndrome. Any disorder in which cortical areas that normally work in con-junction become isolated, usually because of white matter lesions. In some cases, this is an accurate description, as in alexia without agraphia in which there is a lesion of the dominant hemisphere visual cortex combined with disruption of the callosal pathways from the nondominant hemisphere. In other cases, although not anatomically accurate, it is maintained for historical continuity (e.g., conduction aphasia).

The concept of disconnection was used in the late nineteenth century to account for a variety of aphasia subtypes, and the *Wernicke-Lichtheim model* (1885) describing the neural basis of language is still useful in conceptualizing aphasia subtypes. After the holistic ap-proach to understanding brain function became dominant in the early twentieth cen-tury, the concept of disconnection remained dormant until it was formally reintroduced in 1965 by Norman Geschwind (American neurologist, 1926–1984). Geschwind argued that many neurobehavioral syndromes, including aphasias, agnosia, apraxias, syndromes of the corpus callosum, memory impairment, and behavioral disturbances seen with lim-bic lesions, were not simply the result of lesions of specific brain areas but were due to the interruption of information transfer from one brain region to another. (Geschwind, N. 1965. Disconnexion syndromes in animals and man. *Brain* 88:585–644.)

Discriminant analysis. Multivariate statistical technique used to describe differences be-tween two or more groups on a set of measures (descriptive discriminant analysis) or to classify subjects into groups on the basis of a set of measures (predictive discrimi-nant analysis).

Disorientation. Confusion or loss of information about one's location in time, space (place), social surroundings (person), and recent events leading to all three (circumstances). The historical and neurologically valid use of the phrase "disoriented to person" refers to loss of the ability to appreciate the significance of the persons in one's immediate surround-ings (e.g., that the presence of medical personnel implies one is in a hospital and may be ill or injured). This same phrase is sometimes mistakenly used to mean orientation to one's own personal identity (e.g., name). Most often, impaired orientation to self-iden-tity in a conscious and conversant person is due to a psychological disturbance. Also, "dis-orientation to person" is sometimes applied to awake but nonresponsive patients who fail to respond when their name is called (e.g., fail to show directed eye movement and head turning toward the speaker). This latter phenomenon may be seen in psychosis, cerebral disease, and various sensory or motor deficits. [L. *orire, orientem,* to rise; literally not knowing in what direction the sun rises, or in which direction is east (the orient).]

Displacement. Memory process by which information is lost from one's attention span or short-term memory because of the arrival of new information. Displacement is the rationale for providing distracting information in certain memory procedures such as the Brown-Peterson distractor task.

Dissociation. Loss of mental integration in which mental processes become separated from normal consciousness and function on their own. For example, a driver may be listening to the radio, pass the intended destination, and then recall the radio broadcast but not the driving experience. In some psychologic and neurologic conditions, the term may be used to describe incongruity between emotional responses and cognitive content or between verbal expression and actions.

Distinctive feature. Binary system for characterizing all the elements of language sounds into distinguishable patterns; aspect of speech articulation that allows phonemes to be discriminated. The place feature, for example, provides discrimination based on the position of the lips and tongue (*b* vs. *d*). The voice feature differs depends on whether the sound is aspirated (*b* vs. *p*). See Categorical perception.

Distractor task. A task administered as part of some memory tasks (e.g., Brown-Petersen) to prevent rehearsal. A commonly employed distractor technique is to count backward by 3's or by 7's before memory is tested.

Divided attention. The ability to attend to more than one stimulus at a time, or to multiple elements or operations within a task.

DNR. Do not resuscitate. *See* code.

Doll's eye reflex/maneuver. Reflexive eye movement in the direction opposite to that in which the head is moved (e.g., eyes looking up while the head is lowered). Absence of this response indicates a brainstem lesion.

Dominance. *See* Cerebral dominance.

Doors and People. A face valid measure of visual and verbal memory containing four subtests. The Doors Subtest measures visual recognition using photographs of various doors. The Shapes Test assesses visual recall; simple line drawings of crosses are studied for 5 seconds and then drawn from memory. The Names Test is a measure of verbal recognition in which names are presented, and then name recognition is assessed. The People Test is a measure of verbal recall in which photographs of individuals containing a name and occupation are presented to the patient and then their recall of the occupation is tested. (Baddeley, A., Emslie, H., and Nimmo-Smith, I. 1994. *Doors and People.* Manual. Bury St. Edmunds, England: Thames Valley Test Co.)

Dopamine (DA). A neurotransmitter associated with involuntary movement disorders and several neuropsychiatric syndromes. Decreased DA in the nigrostriatal pathway causes *rigidity, tremor,* and *akinesia.* Excess DA levels, which may be associated with levodopa therapy during later stages of Parkinson's disease, produce *dyskinesia.* Dopamine has been implicated in the pathogenesis of schizophrenia, attention deficit disorder, and Gilles de la Tourette's syndrome. The clinical potency of antipsychotic (DA antagonist) drugs is closely correlated with their ability to block DA (D2) receptors in the striatum. DA is a precursor of norepinephrine and epinephrine.

Doppler. (Christian J. Doppler, Austrian/American mathematician and physicist, 1803–1853). A technique of measuring speed of sound through different media that is based upon the transmission and reflection of high-frequency or ultrasonic waves and is used in *ultrasound.*

Dorsiflexion. Backward bending and turning upward of the hand/fingers or foot/toes.

Double dissociation. A technique described by Hans-Lukas Teuber (American psychologist born in Germany, 1916–1977) in which two functions are found to be selectively and independently affected. Such demonstrations are important in the development of modular theories of cognitive function. (Teuber, H-L. 1955. Physiological psychology. *Ann. Rev. Psychol.* 6:267–296.)

Double simultaneous stimulation. A procedure in which bilateral receptive fields (e.g., left and right visual fields; left hand and right face) are stimulated simultaneously to assess sensory suppression or extinction. *See* Neglect syndrome; Extinction; Imperception.

Down syndrome. (John Langdon H. Down, British physician, 1828–1896). A genetic syndrome resulting from a defect in which there are three chromosomes rather than the normal pair of chromosome 21 (trisomy 21). A higher risk is associated with increasing maternal age at time of conception. Down syndrome is associated with moderate mental retardation and characteristic physical features of a face with epicanthal folds, open mouth, short stature, and abnormal palmar crease and fingerprints. Behavioral and pathological changes associated with Alzheimer's disease (neurofibrillary tangles and senile plaques) develop in patients with Down syndrome at a relatively early age (30's to 40's). The syndrome was previously referred to as mongolism, but in 1965, representatives of the Mongolian People's Republic asked the World Health Organization to abandon the term.

Draw-a-clock test. A test of visual-constructional skill that is often used as a screening measure for dementia or hemispatial inattention. Patients are instructed first to draw a clock face with standard numbering and then to draw the clock hands set at a particular time. Many different times may be requested, but those that require both left and right visual fields or have the potential for semantic ambiguity are often used ("20 to 4," "10 after 11").

Dressing apraxia. *See* Apraxia.

DRG. *See* Diagnosis-related group.

Drop attacks. *See* Atonic seizures.

Drug holiday. Withdrawal of a drug, usually for a period of 3–14 days, to reverse or minimize side effects. Drug holidays have been used in Parkinson's disease, but they are rarely prescribed because of risks to the patient.

Drug potentiation. The synergistic action of two or more drugs that is greater than their additive effects.

DSA. Digital subtraction angiography.

DSM-IV™. Diagnostic and Statistical Manual of Mental Disorders *(4th ed.)*. See *Diagnostic and Statistical Manual of Mental Disorders*.

DTRs. *See* Deep tendon reflexes.

DTs. *See* Delirium tremens.

Dual code theory. Memory theory that concrete words can be represented by an *imaginal code* and a *verbal code*, whereas abstract words give rise only to a verbal code.

Dual task performance. Experimental technique in which two tasks are simultaneously performed. Subjects may perform a finger tapping task, for example, while concurrently performing a cognitive test (e.g., digit span). Two tasks sharing common resources will interfere with each other and will be performed less quickly and with more errors than two tasks that have nonoverlapping demands.

Duchenne muscular dystrophy. (Guillaume Benjamin Amand Duchenne, French neurologist, 1806–1875). A sex-linked genetic disorder that begins with weakness of the thighs and shoulders and progresses steadily. By the end of childhood, patients are wheelchair bound and have respiratory insufficiency. Duchenne muscular dystrophy is one of the few myopathies that is associated with mild mental retardation. [Gr. *dys-*, hard, ill, bad; *trophe*, nourishment.]

Dura (dura mater). The outermost and strongest layer of the meninges that forms a protective sheath around the brain and spinal cord. [L. *durus*, hard; *mater*, mother; used as a metaphor for protector.]

Dysarthria. A type of speech disorder resulting from disturbances of muscular control of the speech mechanisms, including paralysis, weakness, or incoordination of the respiratory muscles, larynx, tongue, lips, jaw, and other articulators. The origin of dysarthria may be peripheral (e.g., facial paralysis, loss of teeth) or central (e.g., basal ganglia disease, cerebellar disease). Dysarthric speech is characterized by slurring, breathiness, wetness, or straining. Articulation errors in dysarthria are produced consistently in voluntary and involuntary speech activities, and this distinguishes them from inconsistent articulation errors associated with apraxia of speech. A variety of dysarthria subtypes has been distinguished on the basis of their different presentation and different lesions. [Gr. *dys-*, hard, ill, bad; *arthron*, a joint.]

- **Ataxic dysarthria.** Impaired articulation and prosody characterized by slurred speech; the patient may appear inebriated. Ataxic dysarthria results from cerebellar lesions.
- **Flaccid dysarthria.** Hypotonia and weakness in the speech muscles; this disorder results from damage to the motor units of the cranial or spinal nerves.
- **Hyperkinetic dysarthria.** Abnormal rhythmic speech associated with involuntary movements (e.g., choreaform, athetoid, ballistic). Hyperkinetic dysarthria is usually associated with basal ganglia lesions but may result from lesions of the basal ganglia and subthalamic nucleus.
- **Hypokinetic dysarthria.** A disorder characterized by speech monotone and reduced range of speech that is associated with lesions of the basal ganglia.
- **Spastic dysarthria.** A disorder characterized by slow speech that further deteriorates with rapid fatigue. It is associated with bilateral *upper motor neuron* lesions.
- **Unilateral upper motor neuron dysarthria.** A mild motor speech disorder resulting from weakness of the tongue and lower facial muscles that is associated with acute upper motor neuron lesions. Speech symptoms frequently diminish or resolve completely.

Dysconjugate gaze. The inability of both eyes to move together in alignment. Dysconjugate gaze may result from congenital disorders, injury to the brainstem or the cranial nerves that control the extraocular muscles, or disease of the extraocular muscles (e.g., myasthenia gravis). The result is an uncoupling of the fixation point, causing diplopia.

Dyseidetic dyslexia. *See* Dyslexia.

Dysexecutive syndrome. *See* Frontal lobe syndrome (dorsolateral frontal syndrome).

Dysfluent speech. Disturbed speech rhythm. Most commonly associated with stuttering.

Dyskinesia. Impairment of voluntary movement involving an excess of movement. Dyskinetic movements may be choreic, ballistic, dystonic, or stereotypic, and they are typically very disabling. Dyskinesia is often seen in patients with Parkinson's disease whose response to levodopa levels fluctuates, and it may develop in psychiatric patients from neuroleptic therapy. [Gr. *dys-*, hard, ill, bad; *kinesis*, movement.]

Dyslexia. This term is used in North America to refer to a primary, congenital, or developmental disability in learning to read and spell that does not result from mental retardation, aphasia, cultural deprivation, lack of motivation to learn, or a psychologic disorder. The term "alexia" is generally reserved for acquired reading impairment. In Europe (UK), "dyslexia" refers to both developmental and acquired reading disability. Authors have proposed different subtypes of dyslexia, although overlap exists in the different models. *See* Alexia/dyslexia, acquired, for acquired reading disorders.

- **Dyseidetic dyslexia.** Developmental dyslexia subtype characterized by an inability to read words as a whole or as gestalts. Children read phonetically, sounding out even familiar words as if they had not been previously encountered. Spelling errors tend to be phonetic (e.g., "laf" for "laugh").

- **Dysphonetic dyslexia**. Developmental dyslexia subtype in which reading is heavily dependent on sight vocabulary; children respond to words as individual configurations. Word attack and phonetic decoding/coding skills are weak. Spelling errors are nonphonetic, and they may make semantic substitutions (e.g., "funny" for "laugh").
- **Mixed dysphonetic-dyseidetic dyslexia**. Developmental dyslexia subtype characterized by an inability to develop phonetic-word synthesis skills and an inability to perceive letters and words as visual gestalts. This subtype consists of the deficits associated with both dyseidetic and dysphonetic dyslexia subtypes.
- **L-type dyslexia**. Dyslexia subtype in which there is a premature reliance on a left hemisphere linguistic strategy through which semantic and syntactic strategies are generated. L-type dyslexics have fast and inaccurate reading and produce many substantive errors.
- **P-type dyslexia**. Dyslexia subtype in which there is too much reliance on a right hemisphere bias that emphasizes perceptual strategies. This approach is normal during the early stages of reading development, but P-type dyslexics do not develop semantic and syntactic strategies employed by more advanced readers. P-type dyslexics read slowly and in a fragmented fashion, although their reading tends to be accurate.

Dysmetria. Disordered measuring of distance in muscular acts (i.e., a disturbance in the control of the range of movement in muscular action). Dysmetria is often tested with the finger-to-nose test. It is one of the cardinal signs of cerebellar disease and cerebellar ataxia. [Gr. *dys-* hard, ill, bad; *métron*, measure.]

Dysnomia. *See* Anomia.

Dysphagia. An impaired ability to chew or swallow food or liquid. Dysphagia may be due to impairment of corticobulbar tracts or lesions of the fifth (trigeminal), seventh (facial), ninth (glossopharyngeal), tenth (vagus), or twelfth (hypoglossal) cranial nerves. Dysphagia is a prominent component of bulbar palsy. [Gr. *dys-*, hard, ill, bad; *phagein*, to eat.]

Dysphonetic dyslexia. *See* Dyslexia.

Dysphonia. An impairment of phonation, or sound generation, from the larynx. Dysphonias reflect abnormal vocal fold vibration and may result in breathiness, hoarseness, or harsh vocal quality. [Gr. dys-, hard, ill, bad; *phoné*, voice or animal sound.]

Dysphoria. Unpleasant *mood* or *affect* including anger, irritability, sadness, jealousy, anxiety, fear, restlessness, or malaise. Contrasts with euphoria. [Gr. *dys-*, hard, ill, bad; *pherein*, to bear.]

Dysplasia. Abnormal tissue development. [Gr. *dys-*, hard, ill, bad; *plasis*, a molding.]

Dysprosodia. *See* Aprosodia.

Dysthymic disorder. A chronically depressed *mood*. Dysthymic disorder is usually less acute and less disabling than major depression, but it often persists from an early age. [Gr. *dys-*, hard, ill, bad; *thymos*, spirit, courage.]

Dystonia. Slow, involuntary, arrhythmic muscle contractions that produce forced, distorted postures. Dystonia may occur as a separate disease entity, or it may be the symptom of another disease (e.g., Parkinson's disease). Levodopa may induce dystonia. [Gr. *dys-*, hard, ill, bad; *tonos*, tension.]

Dystrophy. Degeneration with loss of function. [Gr. *dys-*, hard, ill, bad; *trophé*, from *trephein*, to nourish.]

E

Ecchymosis. A purple-blue patch caused by absorption of blood into the skin. [Gr. *ekchymosis*, ecchymosis, from *ek*, out; *chymos*, juice.]

Echographia. Pathological copying of written words and phrases. [Gr. *echo*, echo; from échos, sound; *graphien*, to write.]

Echoic memory. *See* Memory.

Echolalia. Involuntary repetition of another person's speech. Echolalia may be present in transcortical aphasia and autism, and it may be associated with frontal lobe disorders. [Gr. *echo*, an echo; from *échos*, sound; *lalia*, from *lalien*, to babble.]

Echopraxia. Pathological copying of another person's gestures and other movements. Echopraxia may be associated with frontal lobe disorders. [Gr. *echo*, *praktos*, from *prassein*, to do, practice.]

ECoG. Electrocorticography; electrocorticogram. *See* Electroencephalogram.

Ecological validity. The degree to which a measure predicts behavior in everyday situations; a form of external validity. [Gr. *oíkos*, house; *logos*, discourse.]

Ecphory. The process by which retrieval cues interact with stored information during the reconstruction of information into memory. [Gr. *ekphorie*, from *ek*, out of, outside of; *phoros*, bearing.]

ECS. Electrocerebral silence (*see* Isoelectric EEG); electroconvulsive shock (therapy).

ECT. *See* Electroconvulsive therapy.

ED. Effective dose.

Edema, cerebral. Excessive water accumulation resulting in tissue swelling and increased intracranial pressure. Vasogenic edema is excessive water accumulation in the extracellular space. Cytotoxic edema results from impaired neural and glial membranes allowing water to diffuse into cells. [Gr. *oidema*, a swelling, tumor, from *oidein*, to swell.]

EENT. Ears, eyes, nose, and throat.

Effective visual field. Portion of the visual field in which letter recognition is possible.

Efferent. Neural conduction away from central nervous system. [L. *efferens*, from *effero*, to bring out.]

Elaboration. Memory process in which the products of initial encoding are enriched by further processing.

Electrical stimulation mapping. Technique for identifying cortical sensory, motor, and language areas by applying electrical current directly to the exposed brain. Sensation or movement is elicited by stimulating cortical regions. During stimulation of language areas, there may be cessation of recitation, or phonemic and semantic paraphasias. Stimulation mapping may be conducted either intraoperatively following craniotomy or extraoperatively with subdural electrode strips or subdural grid electrodes.

Electrocerebral silence. *See* Isoelectric.

Electroconvulsive therapy (ECT). Form of treatment for depression, schizophrenia (especially catatonia), and bipolar disorder in which an electrical current is passed through

59

the brain to produce a generalized seizure. The patient is sedated and paralyzed to avoid injury associated with the convulsion. The current may be applied either bilaterally or unilaterally. Because unilateral ECT produces less cognitive impairment (e.g., confusion, retrograde and anterograde memory impairment) and is generally equivalent in efficacy to bilateral ECT, unilateral ECT is the approach of choice for most patients. Similarly, nondominant hemisphere ECT is more common than dominant hemisphere ECT because of its more favorable cognitive side effect profile, although some evidence suggests that language dominant stimulation is more therapeutic. The mechanism of action remains unknown, except that the production of a generalized seizure appears to be critical. Also called electroconvulsive shock therapy (ECS).

Electrodermal response (EDR). *See* Galvanic skin response.

Electroencephalogram (EEG). Brain waves recorded with scalp or depth electrodes. An EEG is used for the diagnosis of epilepsy, herpes simplex encephalitis, toxic and metabolic encephalopathies, and dementia. It is also used to evaluate coma and brain death. By convention, brain wave activity recorded directly from the cortical surfaces at the time of surgery is called an electrocorticogram (ECoG); recordings made from subdural strips and from depth electrodes are generally called EEG. [Gr. *enkephalos*, brain; *gramma*, a writing.]

Electrolyte imbalance. A condition of disturbed electrolytes (e.g., sodium, potassium, chloride) commonly produced by extreme dietary insufficiency or dehydration gastrointestinal abnormalities (e.g., vomiting, diarrhea). It may give rise to an acute confusional state. The elderly are particularly at risk for developing confusional states following electrolyte imbalance, which may dramatically alter mental status if mild cognitive decline associated with early dementia is already present.

ELISA. Enzyme-linked immunosorbent assay, a test that permits the rapid and sensitive detection of antibodies in CSF or blood. It is used as a rapid diagnostic technique for infectious agents that cannot be readily cultured (e.g., AIDS, Lyme disease, cytomegalovirus, cryptococcus).

Eloquent cortex. Cortical regions that, if included in surgical resection, will produce significant functional impairment. Eloquent cortex includes language areas and primary motor and sensory regions.

Embedded Figures Tests. Tests that require the subject to locate a simple geometric figure within a more complex design containing the simple figure and then to trace the shape of the simpler figure. Test variations include identifying either a single figure or several figures within the larger design.

Embolism. Sudden blocking of an artery by a thrombus fragment or any other intra-arterial or intracardiac material that has been brought to the blockage site by blood flow. The most common embolic source is the heart, and some believe that embolism is the most common cause of transient ischemic attacks and cerebral infarction. Emboli tend to lodge at bifurcations, branchings, and curvatures such as the bifurcations of the common carotid artery, internal carotid artery, and middle cerebral artery. Because the basilar artery is larger than each vertebral artery, emboli entering the basilar artery tend to be carried to the top and lodge where the artery forks to form the posterior cerebral arteries. [L. *embolus*, a stopper.]

Embolization. Interventional neuroradiologic method of using metal pellets, thrombogenic coils, balloons, or quick-acting glues to close vessels feeding an arteriovenous malformation (AVM). The is done to reduce the size of large AVMs before surgical resection. The procedure is also used to treat aneurysms that are not surgically accessible and carotid cavernous fistulas. Embolization of an artery may also be performed when uncontrolled bleeding follows a head or neck injury.

EMG. Electromyogram or electromyography.

Emotional lability. Abnormal variability in emotional expression characterized by repetitive and abrupt shifts in affect. Emotional or affective lability is common in mania and delirium and after damage to the orbitofrontal portions of the frontal lobes.

Empty speech. Fluent speech that is lacking in information content because of marked word-finding difficulties. Empty speech is characteristic of anomic (nominal) aphasia.

Empyema. Encapsulated pus in a body cavity or space (e.g., epidural or subdural). [Gr. *empyema*, suppuration, from *en*, in; *pyon*, pus.]

Encapsulated. Enclosed in a sheath or capsule.

Encephalitis. Brain inflammation from infection, usually of viral origin. The most common viral encephalitis is herpes simplex encephalitis, which damages the inferior surface of the frontal lobe and temporal lobe.

Encephalocele. Congenital anomaly involving a skull defect and herniation of cerebral tissue through the defect. [Gr. *enkephalos*, brain; *kele*, hernia.]

Encephalomalacia. Morbid softness of the brain that is usually caused by vascular insufficiency or trauma. Although "encephalomalacia" refers to infarcted brain tissue, it is sometimes used in radiological contexts to designate volume loss. [Gr. *enkephalos*, brain; *malakos*, soft.]

Encephalopathy. Nonspecific diffuse brain impairment, usually resulting from a systemic condition. It is behaviorally characterized as a confusional state. [Gr. *enkephalos*, brain; *pathos*, suffering.]

Encoding. Process by which the cognitive system builds up a stimulus representation into memory. For example, the translation of auditory input into a meaningful stimulus, such as a word or a recognized sound (bell, thunder), is encoding.

Encoding specificity principle. Principle that the retrieval of an event is a function of the overlap between the context of the learning and that of the retrieval. Thus, memory is facilitated when information available at encoding is present during retrieval.

Endarterectomy. A surgical revascularization procedure in which the carotid artery is opened and plaque removed. Endarterectomy decreases the risk of ischemic stroke in patients with significant stenosis, although its role in patients with modest stenosis is debated. [Gr. *endon*, within; arteria, artery; *ektome*, a cutting out.]

Endorphins. Compounds synthesized in the brain that bind with the same receptors as opiates. Endorphins are found primarily in the pituitary, but lesser amounts are present in the hypothalamus and other brain regions and are involved in the processing of pain perceptions. Endorphin is derived from "endogenous opiates."

ENG. Electronystagmography.

Entorhinal cortex. Anterior portion of the parahippocampal gyrus on the medial surface of the temporal lobe. It is a relay between association cortex and the hippocampus and is involved in odor processing and memory. This site is specifically affected in Alzheimer's disease.

Environmental dependency syndrome. A syndrome characterized by imitation and *utilization behavior* due to excessive responsiveness to environmental stimuli. The associated lesions are generally bilateral orbital frontal lobe.

EOMI. Abbreviation for extra-ocular movements intact (up, down, medial, and lateral movements), indicating that third (oculomotor), fourth (trochlear), and sixth (abducens) cranial nerves are functioning normally.

Ependyma. Epithelial lining of the brain ventricles and of the central canal of the spinal cord. [Gr. *ependyma*, an upper garment, from *epidyein*; *epi*, upon; *endyein*, to put on.]

Ependymoma. A glioma derived from relatively undifferentiated ependymal cells, most often from the central canal of the spinal cord. Most ependymomas are slow growing and benign, but malignant varieties occur.

Epicritic. The discrete quality of somatosensory stimulation (e.g., topographical localization of subtle touch and temperature stimuli). Epicritic sensation includes light or localized touch, light pressure, and sharp pain. The term "epicritic" was introduced by Henry Head in 1905 (British neurologist, 1861–1940). [Gr. *epikrisis*, determination, from *epicrinein*, to judge.] (Head, H., Rivers, W.H.R., and Sherren, J. 1905. The afferent nervous systems from a new aspect. *Brain* 29:99–115.)

Epidural hematoma. Extradural hematoma following trauma in which blood pools between the dura and calvaria. This commonly results from a skull fracture when a major meningeal artery is breached by a bony groove.

Epigastric. Pertaining to the region above the stomach. [Gr. *epi*, above; *gaster*, stomach.]

Epilepsy. Chronic brain disorder characterized by recurrent seizures. Epilepsy is often operationally defined by the occurrence of at least two spontaneous, unprovoked seizures. Isolated seizures may be associated with acute brain changes and do not necessarily represent a syndrome of epilepsy. *See* Seizures. [Gr. *epilepsia*, seizure; from *epi*, upon; *lepsis*, to seize, receive.]

- **Centrencephalic epilepsy**. A term derived from the hypothesis that generalized epilepsy is triggered by a subcortical pacemaker. The cortical etiology of generalized seizures is now well documented, however, and the term centrencephalic is used only in historical contexts.

- **Psychomotor epilepsy**. Epilepsy associated with temporal lobe seizures; it is named psychomotor because of prominent ictal motor automatisms (e.g., lipsmacking). The term is no longer in wide use, having been replaced by complex partial epilepsy (or complex partial seizures).

- **Reflex epilepsy**. Epilepsy associated with seizures that are precipitated by specific environmental or internal stimulation (e.g., flashing lights).

- **Rolandic epilepsy**. Benign focal motor epilepsy during childhood that is associated with central-temporal EEG spikes.

Epilepsy surgery. Neurosurgical treatment for epilepsy patients whose seizures are poorly controlled with antiepileptic drugs. Ablative procedures, such as anterior temporal lobectomy, involve the resection of epileptogenic brain areas with the goal of eliminating seizures. Palliative treatments, such as corpus callosotomy, are intended to decrease seizure severity.

Epinephrine. A neurotransmitter secreted by the adrenal gland that is associated with *sympathetic nervous system* activity.

Episodic dyscontrol syndrome. A condition associated with intermittent explosive behavior as a reaction to frustration characterized by a loss of self-control and striking out in rage that is disproportionate to the stimulus; this syndrome was first described by Bach-y-Rita (1971). As a psychiatric disorder, its existence is controversial because it is often used in the context of criminal defense proceedings. Patients are typically diagnosed using DSM-IV criteria as having intermittent explosive disorder, which excludes patients with known neurologic factors such as traumatic brain injury. Neurologic patients with dyscontrol episodes may have lesions in ventromedial structures including portions of frontal cortex, hypothalamus, septal nuclei, and amygdala. (Bach-y-Rita, G., Lion, J. R., Gliment, C. E., and Ervin 1971. Episodic dyscontrol: A study of 130 violent patients. *Am. J. Psychiatry* 127:1473–1478.)

Episodic memory. *See* Memory.

Equipotentiality. Theory of Karl Spencer Lashley (American psychologist, 1890–1958) that posits that memory impairment does not depend on the localization of a lesion but on the amount of tissue damaged. Any part of the cortex is equally able to perform tasks.

Lashley's experiments with rats led him to conclude that although sensory and motor functions were to some degree localized, memory traces were not confined to well-defined cortical circuits. Rather, they were either diffusely represented throughout the cortex or passed to subcortical centers. Because memory was diffusely represented, he considered human amnesia to result from an inability to activate memory traces, not a loss of the memory engram. A related though not identical hypothesis of Lashley is that of *mass action*, which proposes that that the entire cortex participates in every function. (Lashley, K.S. 1929. *Brain Mechanisms and Intelligence*. Chicago: University of Chicago Press.)

Errorless learning. Learning that takes place when virtually all errors are prevented during the training process. It may be more efficient than trial-and-error learning for neurologically impaired persons, especially those with severe anterograde amnesia.

Errors of action. Forms of functional breakdown in the perception-action cycle, particularly misuse of objects and sequencing deficits. It overlaps with behaviors classically attributed to apraxias, agnosias, and severe attentional disturbance.

Erythemia. An inflammatory redness of the skin or mucous tissue. [Gr. *erythema*, flush.]

Essential tremor. A benign resting tremor that is often present in the hands, head, or voice. Essential tremor often runs in families and is also known as familial tremor. It is not symptomatic of Parkinson's disease and is often treated successfully with beta-blockers.

ET. Endotracheal tube.

État lacunaire. Multiple small infarcts and loss of brain substance associated with chronic hypertension. [F. *état*, state; L. *lacuna*, hole, gap, pit.]

ETOH. Ethanol, or ethyl alcohol.

Event-related potential (ERP). *See* Evoked potentials.

Evoked potentials. Electrophysiologic responses representing summated, discrete electrical brain discharges that are elicited by a sensory stimulus or other event along the ascending pathways to the cerebral cortex. The evoked potential is time locked to the stimuli. Although the magnitude of the response is generally smaller than that of the ongoing EEG, the background EEG occurs randomly with respect to the stimuli and is averaged out over repeated trials. Evoked potentials are often divided into two broad categories: (*1*) exogenous sensory potentials, which are modality-specific responses reflecting the processing of the sensory information in afferent pathways up to the cortical sensory area, and (*2*) endogenous potentials, which are not specific to a sensory modality and reflect the task in which the subject is engaged. Endogenous evoked potentials are also called event-related potentials (ERP).

- **Auditory evoked potentials**. Specific auditory-evoked potentials range from brainstem auditory evoked responses (BAERs), which reflects the integrity of the brainstem auditory pathway and occur in the first 10 milliseconds post-stimulation, to long-latency evoked potentials (e.g., P3, or P300), which are generated in the neocortex and reflect cognitive processing speed.

- **Motor evoked potentials**. Electrophysiologic activity recorded in relation to a motor response. This includes activity preceding the movement (e.g., Bereitschaftspotential, or BP) or closely following it (e.g., primary motor potentials). This term is also used to refer to the EMG potential generated in the muscle during movement.

- **Somatosensory evoked potentials**. Evoked potentials recorded in response to somatosensory stimulation such as brief electric shocks to either the arm or leg. Somatosensory evoked potentials are used to assess the integrity of sensory function.

- **Visual evoked potentials**. Evoked potentials recorded in response to visual stimulation, usually in the form of strobe light flashes or alternating checkerboards. Visual-evoked potentials are used to assess the integrity of visual function, and they may be useful in evaluating multiple sclerosis or other diseases involving the optic tracts. Long-latency visual evoked potentials (e.g., P3, or P300) are generated in the neocortex and reflect cognitive processing speed.

Executive function. Cognitive abilities necessary for complex goal-directed behavior and adaptation to a range of environmental changes and demands. Executive function includes the ability to plan and anticipate outcomes (cognitive flexibility) and to direct attentional resources to meet the demands of nonroutine events. Many conceptualizations of executive function also include self-monitoring and self-awareness since these are necessary for behavioral flexibility and "appropriateness." Because of individual variability and changing task demands required to demonstrate executive functions, they are often difficult to assess with standardized measures. Cerebral localization also remains elusive and controversial. Regions of the prefrontal cortex may play a special role in recruiting other brain areas in a series of distributed networks that handle different components of executive functions, depending on the processing demands of the specific task.

Exner's area. (Siegmund Exner, Austrian physiologist; 1846–1926). Area in the posterior portion of the second frontal convolution postulated by Exner to be a center for "motor graphic images" essential for writing. Pathologic correlations, however, have not supported this hypothesis (Brodmann area 46).

Exomethesthesia. A rare form of allesthesia in which somatosensory stimulus location is identified off the body and in external space. [Gr. *ek*, outside of; *metechein*, to share in; *aisthesis*, sensation, from *aisthanesthai*, to perceive.]

Expectancy wave. *See* Contingent negative variation.

Explicit memory. *See* Memory.

Exploratory factor analysis. Multivariate statistical technique used to describe the relations among a set of observed measures in terms of their relations with a smaller set of common underlying variables referred to as factors. The factors are typically unobserved but are assumed to account fully for the covariation between the measured variables. In exploratory factor analysis, the search for underlying dimensions is loosely controlled by the investigator by setting criteria for the number of dimensions to be identified and the properties of those dimensions.

Expressive aphasia. *See* Aphasia syndromes.

Extensor. Muscle that, when contracted, causes a limb extension or straightening. Opposite of flexor.

External validity. Degree to which results from a particular test or measure can be generalized to situations or related to information beyond the test itself. This may be suggested by the degree to which a measure is correlated with scores from another test of the same or a similar characteristic, or with some independent criterion. *See* Ecological validity and *compare with* Internal consistency.

Extinction. **1.** The failure to detect a stimulus contralateral to a lesion during simultaneous bilateral stimulation. Single unilateral stimuli to the affected side, however, are perceived. **2.** In learning theory, the process by which the organism stops emitting a learned response after the response is no longer reinforced. [L. *exstinguere*, to put out, destroy.]

- **Motor extinction**. Contralateral limb akinesia that increases when patients must simultaneously use their extremities ipsilateral to the lesion.
- **Sensory extinction**. This was first described in the tactile modality. Visual and auditory extinction occurs, but it is rare in the auditory modality because of the large number of bilateral auditory projections. This phenomenon is commonly seen during resolution of hemispatial inattention associated with right cerebral injuries, although it occasionally may be associated with left hemisphere injury.

Extinction burst. A dramatic increase in response frequency following the withdrawal of a re-
inforcer. It is followed by either a rate decrease or cessation (extinction) if the behavior
remains unreinforced.

Extracorticospinal system. *See* Extrapyramidal motor system.

Extrapyramidal motor system. A functional, not anatomical, unit consisting of physiologically
similar but spatially distributed structures, including the basal ganglia (caudate, putamen, and globus pallidus), subthalamic nucleus, substantia nigra, and their connections
to each other and to the thalamus. In contrast to the *pyramidal motor system*, which consists
of *upper* and *lower motor neurons* that guide purposeful and voluntary movement, the extrapyramidal system modulates movements and maintains muscle tone and posture. Extrapyramidal system dysfunction results in involuntary movement disorders.

Extrapyramidal syndrome (EPS). A syndrome of *akinesia, rigidity, tremor, akathisia,* and *bucco-
lingual dyskinesia* (i.e., choreoathetoid movements of the mouth, jaw, and tongue) resulting from extrapyramidal side effects of neuroleptic medications. Extrapyramidal syndrome differs from tardive disorders, such as tardive dyskinesia, tardive dystonia, and
tardive akathisia, in the duration of neuroleptic treatment. In EPS, the movement abnormalities develop acutely, whereas in the tardive disorders, they appear after long-term
pharmacotherapy. *See* Tardive dyskinesia; Neuroleptic malignant syndrome.

Extubation. Removal of an endotracheal or tracheostomy tube apparatus.

F

F scale. MMPI scale designed to measure symptom exaggeration. It consists of items that were empirically selected because they were infrequently endorsed by the general population. Thus, when such items are endorsed, there is a suggestion that the patients may be responding carelessly or randomly, or exaggerating their deficit. Elevations may be seen on the F scale, however, due to cultural background, severe psychiatric disturbance, or poor reading ability.

Face-Hand Test. 1. Technique used to demonstrate psychogenic hemiparesis. While supine, the patient's paretic arm is raised over the face and is dropped by the examiner. Patients with psychogenic hemiparesis typically avoid hitting their face, demonstrating preserved muscle strength. **2.** Method of double simultaneous stimulation designed to assess tactile extinction. Both hands, a face and hand, or both cheeks are touched simultaneously.

Facial Recognition Test. Test of visual perception containing photographs of unfamiliar persons. Each set consists of photographs of the same person taken from different angles or under different lighting conditions. This test has demonstrated sensitivity to right hemisphere lesions, particularly more posterior right hemisphere lesions. (Benton, A.L., Sivan, A.B., Hamsher, KdeS., Varney, N.R., and Spreen, O. 1994. *Contributions to Neuropsychological Assessment. A Clinical Manual*, 2nd ed. New York: Oxford University Press.)

Factitious disorder. Intentional production of physical or psychological symptoms in which the motivation is to adopt the sick role. The motivation to portray symptoms is related to internal needs rather than the external gain characteristic of malingering. *See* Münchausen's syndrome. [L. *facticius*, artificial.]

Factor analysis. Statistical technique that explains the correlations between a set of observed variables with a second smaller set that are only indirectly observable (i.e., latent variables). Different factors may be obtained when the number of test scores is changed or when the scores are derived from different clinical populations.

Failure to thrive. A syndrome of infants or children in which growth is significantly below expectations for their age and sex. Deficits in cognitive, social, and emotional functions develop later. Malnutrition is the critical biologic factor in most cases.

False negative. Error that occurs when a test incorrectly indicates the absence of a particular trait or condition when that trait or condition actually exists. Also called type II error or beta error.

False positive. Error that occurs when a test incorrectly indicates the presence of a trait or condition when none genuinely exists. Also called a type I error or alpha error.

Falx cerebri. Dural sheet separating the two cerebral hemispheres. [L. *falx*, a sickle; *cerebrum*, brain.]

Familial tremor. *See* Essential tremor.

Famous Faces Test. A measure of remote memory that assesses the ability to recognize photographs of individuals who achieved fame in each of six decades from the 1920s to the 1970s. In addition to standard face recognition, photographs taken when these individuals were young are paired with photographs of the same people, who have remained famous, when they are old (e.g., Charlie Chaplin). (Albert, M.S., Butters, N., and Levin, J. 1979. Temporal gradients in the retrograde amnesia of patients with alcoholic Korsakoff's disease. *Arch. Neurol.* 36:211–216.)

Fantastic confabulation. Confabulation based on fictitious events that could not possibly have happened to the individual.

FAS Test. *See* Controlled Oral Word Association.

Fasciculation. Involuntary muscle twitching that is typically a sign of muscle denervation.

Fasciculus. A nerve fiber bundle. [L., diminutive of *fascis*, bundle.]

FBS. Fasting blood sugar.

Featural analysis. Perceptual process whereby a percept is constructed by analysis of the individual features.

Febrile seizure. *See* Seizure.

Fenestrated. Having openings. [L. *fenestra*, a window.]

Festinating gait. *See* Propulsive gait.

Fetal alcohol syndrome (FAS). A syndrome present in many children born to alcoholic mothers that result from exposure of the fetus to ethanol during the first trimester. Fetal alcohol syndrome is characterized by microcephaly, impaired coordination, decreased birth size, and facial abnormalities, with a high frequency of mental retardation.

FFM. Fine finger movement.

Fibromyalgia syndrome. A chronic disorder characterized by widespread musculoskeletal pain, fatigue, and multiple tender points. Fibromyalgia may be associated with sleep disturbances, morning stiffness, irritable bowel syndrome, anxiety, and other symptoms. There is a large degree of diagnostic overlap with chronic fatigue syndrome. [L. *fibra*, fiber; Gr. *myo, mys*, muscle; *-algia*, pain.]

Fifteen Item Test. *See* Rey 3 x 5 Memory Test.

Figural fluency. A family of tests developed as nonverbal analogues to *verbal fluency* tests (e.g., Controlled Oral Word Association) in which geometric designs or figures are generated within a specified period, usually 1–3 minutes. Jones-Gotman and Milner produced the first formal figural fluency measure, Design Fluency, in which nonsense figures are generated. Regard and Strauss developed the Five-Point Test in which 5-dot matrices are presented and the subject produces different shapes by connecting different dot arrangements within the rectangle. The Ruff Figure Fluency Test is a modification of the Five-Point Test that contains distractors, or variations, of the dot matrix pattern. Glosser and Goodglass's Graphic Pattern Generation consists of four different 5-dot matrices; subjects are instructed to draw different patterns by connecting the dots using four lines only. [L. *figura*, a form, shape, figure; *fluere*, to flow.] (Glosser, G. and Goodglass, H. 1990. Disorders in executive control functions among aphasic and other brain-damaged patients. *J. Clin. Exp. Neuropsychol.* 12:485–501; Jones-Gotman, M. and Milner, B. 1977. Design fluency: The invention of nonsense drawings after focal cortical lesions. *Neuropsychologia* 15:653–674; Regard, M., Strauss, E., and Knapp, P. 1982. Children's production of verbal and non-verbal fluency tasks. *Percept. Motor Skills* 55:839–844; Ruff, R. 1988. *Ruff Figural Fluency Test*. San Diego: Neuropsychological Resources.)

Finger agnosia. *See* Agnosia.

Finger Localization Test. A measure of finger identification and finger naming in which naming the finger touched is not required. Three conditions are tested, and the patient identifies the fingers touched by either naming them, pointing to the finger on an outline of a hand, or indicating the number associated with the finger (1–5). (Benton, A.L., Sivan, A.B., Hamsher, KdeS., Varney, N.R., and Spreen, O. 1994. *Contributions to Neuropsychological Assessment. A Clinical Manual*, 2nd ed. New York: Oxford University Press.)

Finger tapping. A measure of fine motor speed in which the index finger is tapped as quickly as possible against a response key that is attached either to a mechanical counter or, with some newer devices, to an electronic counter. Five trials of 10 seconds each that do not deviate by more than 10% are usually obtained for each hand; however, variability exists in test administration from 3 to 10 trials. Part of the Halstead-Reitan Neuropsychological Battery. Also called the finger oscillation test.

Finger-nose-finger test. A measure of *dysmetria* associated with cerebellar dysfunction that is similar to the finger-to-nose test but requires the additional movement of touching the examiner's finger.

Fingertip Number Writing Perception. A test of *graphesthesia* from the Reitan-Kløve Sensory Perceptual Exam in which the numbers 3, 4, 5, and 6 are written on the subject's fingertips with a pencil in a predetermined order. The numbers are written upside down out the patient's view. For children under 9 years of age, the stimuli are X's and O's. Part of the Halstead-Reitan Neuropsychological Battery.

Finger-to-nose test. Test of cerebellar function in which subjects are asked first to extend one arm and then to put the forefinger quickly and precisely on the tip of the nose. In cases of impairment, the finger will not touch the nose on the first attempt (*dysmetria*). Instead, the limb tends to overshoot the nose (*hypermetria*). Then, in a series of closer and closer approaches, the forefinger comes to rest on the tip of the nose. This series of oscillations is traditionally called *intention tremor*.

Fissure. *See* Sulcus.

Fist-edge-palm test. A motor sequencing test that assesses motor programming ability; developed by Aleksandr R. Luria (Soviet neuropsychologist, 1902–1977). A sequence of three hand positions is repeated, and persons failing this task tend to omit the "edge" portion of the sequence.

Fistula. An abnormal communication passage from normally separated regions. [L. *fistuala*, a pipe, tube.]

5-HT. *See* Serotonin.

Flaccid. Paralysis characterized by a loss of muscle tone.

Flapping tremor. *See* Asterixis.

Flexor. Muscle that causes a limb to bend or flex when contracted. Opposite of extensor.

Floccillation. *See* Carphologia.

Floor effect. Performance that is below the level of performance measured by the lowest possible score of a test. Thus, decreased level of performance cannot be reflected accurately by lowered test scores, and differences between low-functioning subjects may be masked on measures where there is a floor effect. *See* Ceiling effect.

Fluency. Aspects of spoken speech that are related to (*1*) how easily utterances are articulated, (*2*) production of at least 50 words per minute, and (*3*) utilization of sentence structure.

Fluent aphasia. *See* Aphasia syndromes.

Fluent speech. Easily articulated verbal output that is normal in quantity (100–200 words/minute), phrase length (5–8 words/phrase), and prosody. In aphasia, fluent speech includes the above, along with decreased information content and paraphasias.

Fluid intelligence. The potential to adapt to new situations and form new ideas that depends on the ability to perceive relationships and correlations. In contrast with crystallized intelligence, fluid intelligence is relatively independent of cultural and formal educational background. The division of general intellectual skill (G) into fluid (Gf) and crystallized (Gc) intelligence was made by Cattell (1963). Fluid intelligence is thought to increase through childhood and into the late teens and begins to decline in the early twenties. Tasks of Gf require reasoning, abstraction, and concept formation. (Cattell, R.B. 1963. Theory of fluid and crystallized intelligence: A critical experiment. *J. Educat. Psychol.* 54:1–22.)

Flynn effect. The tendency for standardized test scores of a population to rise over time. The magnitude of gain is related to the number of years since test standardization. (Flynn, J.R. 1984. The mean IQ of Americans: massive gains 1932 to 1978. *Psychol. Bull.* 95:29–51.)

Focal retrograde amnesia. Severe and lasting retrograde amnesia which, unlike most cases of retrograde amnesia, occurs with relatively preserved new learning ability. (Kapur, N. 1993. Focal retrograde amnesia in neurological disease: A critical review. *Cortex* 29:217–234.)

Folate. A B-complex vitamin.

Folstein Mini-Mental Status Examination (MMSE). A mental status questionnaire that assesses simple memory, orientation, visual-spatial copying, and language. The MMSE is useful as a screening test for Alzheimer's disease, but it is less sensitive to subcortical dementias or dementia secondary to ischemic vascular disease. *See* Dementia rating scales and mental status questionnaires. (Folstein, M.F., Folstein, S.E., and McHugh, P.R. 1975. Mini-Mental State: A practical method for grading the cognitive state of outpatients for the clinician. *J. Psychiatr. Res.* 12:189–198.)

Foramen magnum. The opening in the base of the skull (occipital bone) where the brainstem becomes the spinal cord. [L. *foramen,* a hole; *magnum,* great.]

Foramen of Magendie. (François Magendie, French physiologist, 1783–1855) The opening between the fourth ventricle and the subarachnoid space.

Foramen of Monro. (Alexander Monro, Jr., Scottish anatomist, 1733–1817). The intraventricular foramen on both the left and right side that connects the third ventricle in the diencephalon to the lateral ventricles.

Foramina of Luschka. (Herbert Luschka, German anatomist, 1820–1875). Two lateral connections (openings) between the fourth ventricle and the subarachnoid space.

Forced-choice. A testing method that requires subjects to respond in a multiple-choice format. If they are unable to recognize spontaneously that one of the answers is correct, they are asked to select an answer. This has application in *symptom validity testing* because precise response probabilities can be calculated, and in clinical situations where memory can be demonstrated without awareness.

Forebrain. The *prosencephalon,* consisting of the telencephalon and diencephalon.

Foreign accent syndrome. Altered prosody associated with small infarction of the sensorimotor cortex. Speaking rhythm and cadence are affected, and patients are often described as having a Scandinavian, Swiss, or French accent. In Japanese patients, the accent is characterized as Korean. Alteration in linguistic function is unnecessary, but foreign accent syndrome may be seen in the context of mild language impairment.

Forgetting. The loss of information over time. Forgetting is often reported in neuropsychological assessment as the difference between an immediate and delayed recall (usually 20–30 minutes), expressed as a percentage of the amount of material remembered during immediate recall [(immediate recall – delayed recall)/immediate recall].

Fornix. The efferent tract of hippocampus and subiculum arching over the thalamus to synapse on structures in the rostral telencephalon and diencephalon. Approximately one-half of the fibers in the fornix, which originate in the subiculum, terminate in the mammillary body. [L. *fornix,* an arch, vault.]

Fovea. Region of the retina in which the center of gaze is projected. The fovea has the greatest visual acuity and the greatest innervation of retinal neurons. [L. *fovia,* a pit.]

Fragile X syndrome. Chromosomal abnormality associated with mental retardation and physical abnormality. This syndrome named for the characteristic fragile site, a nonstaining gap at a specific chromosome location, on the long arm of the X chromosome. The clinical picture in the male is of a long face, somewhat prominent chin, large, floppy ears, and macro-orchidism without any obvious evidence of endocrine dysfunction. Neurologic involvement is highlighted by retarded language development, hyperactivity, and delayed motor development. Many patients with Fragile X syndrome have either autism or autistic features, such as poor eye contact, fascination with spinning objects, or impaired social skills.

Fragment completion. Memory task in which the patient is shown a complete stimulus and then asked to identify that stimulus in a fragmented form.

Free radicals. Cytotoxic substances characterized by unpaired electrons in outer orbits. They are particularly toxic to neural tissue and are thought to cause secondary brain damage when released by trauma (e.g., traumatic brain injury).

Free recall. Memory retrieval without the benefit of external cues or prompts. Free recall measures the ability to reproduce spontaneously information that was presented previously.

Freedom from Distractibility Index. A measure of attention, concentration, and, to a lesser degree, numerical ability calculated from the Arithmetic and Digit Span subtests of the Wechsler Intelligence Scale for Children-III (WISC-III). This index is analogous to the Working Memory Index of the Wechsler Adult Intelligence Scale-III (WAIS-III).

Freezing. A temporary inability to move, associated with Parkinson's disease. Freezing is more common in doorways, exits, and where there is a change in floor pattern.

Frenchay Aphasia Screening Test. A screening test of acquired language impairment. It is not designed to differentiate among aphasia subtypes. Four language areas are assessed: Comprehension, Expression, Reading, and Writing. (Enderby, P., Wood, V., and Wade, D. 1987. *Frenchay Aphasia Screening Test*. Manual. Windsor, Berkshire, England: NFER-Nelson.)

Frenchay Dysarthria Assessment. Test of speech impairment resulting from either central or peripheral nervous system injuries. Eleven areas are assessed: Reflex (coughing and swallowing), Respiration, Lips, Jaw, Palate, Laryngeal, Tongue, Intelligibility, Rate, Sensation, and Influencing Factors (sight, teeth, language, mood, and posture). Responses are rated on a nine-point scale. (Enderby, P.M. 1983. *Frenchay Dysarthria Assessment*. San Diego: College Hill Press.)

Friedreich's ataxia. (Nikolaus Friedreich, German neurologist, 1825–1882). Hereditary progressive gait ataxia. The ataxia may affect speech, but cognition is unaffected. Emotional lability may be present. Also called hereditary spinal ataxia.

Frontal gait. *See* Apraxia (gait apraxia).

Frontal lobe. Brain area anterior to the central sulcus and superior to the Sylvian fissure. It is divided anatomically into motor, premotor, and prefrontal areas. The gyrus in the posterior frontal lobe containing pyramidal cells that provide the primary outflow for voluntary motor function (Brodmann's area 4) is called the motor area. It is the part of the cerebral cortex that, upon application of brief electrical stimulation, shows the lowest threshold and shortest latency producing movement. It is also called the precentral gyrus since it is immediately anterior to the central sulcus.

The premotor area is anterior to the precentral gyrus. It consists of motor association cortex and is involved with volitional muscle activity of the contralateral side (Brodmann's areas 6 and 8). The supplementary motor area (SMA) is located in the medial premotor cortex. Anterior to the premotor area is the prefrontal cortex. It is the largest of these three frontal regions and consists of a significant portion of the lateral and medial frontal cortex, and the entire orbital frontal cortex. Because lesions of these frontal lobe regions often result in recognizable and distinct frontal lobe syndromes, the entire frontal lobe is often regionalized into lateral (dorsolateral), mesial, and orbital frontal areas.

- **Dorsolateral frontal syndrome (executive dysfunction syndrome)**. A syndrome consisting of difficulty generating hypotheses and flexibly maintaining or shifting sets on tasks such as the Wisconsin Card Sorting Test, reduced verbal or design fluency, poor organizational strategies for learning, poor constructional strategies for copying complex designs, and motor programming deficits. Motor programming difficulty may include poor alternating and reciprocal motor task performance (Luria's *m*'s and *n*'s) or poor performance on sequential motor tests (e.g., Luria's fist-edge-palm).

- **Mesial frontal/anterior cingulate syndrome**. A syndrome characterized by reduced spontaneous activity that ranges from *akinetic mutism* to transient abulic hypokinesia (hypokinesia from "loss of will"). Patients are typically apathetic, do not speak spontaneously, will answer questions in monosyllables, if at all, move little, eat and drink only if fed, show little or no emotion, and may be incontinent. The most severe forms of the syndrome are caused by bilateral lesions of the anterior cingulate gyrus (Brodmann's area 24) whereas unilateral medial frontal lesions of the supplementary motor area are more likely to result in transient symptoms. If able to cooperate with neuropsychological testing, the patients may perform normally on most tasks including the Wisconsin Card Sorting Test, but often they show a failure of response inhibition on go/no-go tasks.
- **Orbital frontal syndrome**. A syndrome characterized by prominent personality changes, which may include emotional lability, impulsivity, irritability, becoming more outspoken and less worried, and occasionally showing imitation and utilization behaviors (enslavement to environmental cues). Orbital-frontal syndrome is caused by lesions of the orbital region (undersurface) of the frontal lobes. This area is also called the limbic frontal lobe because of its extensive connectivity to limbic structures such as the amygdala, and it may often be disrupted following severe closed head injuries. *See* Phineas Gage.

Frontal release signs. Pathologic reflexes originally described in association with lesions of the frontal lobes but which are more commonly associated with diffuse cerebral impairment. The frontal release signs include *grasp, snout, rooting,* and *palmomental* and *glabellar reflexes.*

FTA-ABS test. Fluorescent treponemal antibody-absorption. The FTA-ABS test is a sensitive and specific serologic test for syphilis and is generally performed only after a positive Veneral Disease Research Laboratory (VDRL) or rapid plasma reagin agglutination (RPR) test result.

Fugue. A form of psychogenic amnesia in which the patient wanders and may assume a new identity. [L. *fugare,* to cause to flee, chase.]

Fuld Object-Memory Evaluation. A memory test designed for elderly patients. Ten small objects (e.g., scissors) hidden in a bag are individually identified by touch. The object is then removed from the bag and identified visually to increase the likelihood of object encoding. A generative verbal fluency task is administered followed by free recall and recall followed by selective reminding. This is repeated for five trials. A 15-minute delayed recall is obtained then followed by a 3-choice recognition for objects not recalled. (Fuld, P.A. 1982. *Fuld Object-Memory Evaluation.* Chicago: The Stoelting Co.)

Full Scale IQ (FSIQ). Measure of general cognitive and intellectual functioning. On tests such as the Wechsler Intelligence Scales (WIS), Full Scale IQ is a composite score derived from all subtest scores on both the Verbal and Performance scales. Although the IQ (intelligence quotient) was originally the quotient of mental age/chronological age, standardized scores have replaced ratio calculations because they provide more stable estimates. IQs have a mean score of 100. A specific IQ value obtained on one test, however, is not necessarily equivalent to the same IQ value on a different test. For example, the WAIS-III yields a FSIQ that is on average 3 IQ points lower than the WAIS-R, which in turn yields FSIQs that average 8 IQ points less than the WAIS. Thus, using different tests, or even different versions of the same test, might suggest a decline in FSIQ if the specific test version is not considered. The IQ scores, while correlated with academic and occupational achievement, do not measure the full range of functions that are related to success (e.g., drive, social competence, creativity). *See* Intelligence quotient.

Function words (closed class words). Words primarily conveying grammatical information. Examples of function words include articles, auxiliary words, conjunctions, inflections, and pronouns. Because of the finite number of function words in any language, they are also called closed class words. Also called functors.

Functional adequacy. Conceptualization of brain function that proposes that the residual function of the tissue to be resected during anterior temporal lobectomy determines the degree of pre- to postsurgery memory change. Patients demonstrating the greatest degree of memory decline following surgery are those in whom a hippocampus with a larger degree of functional capability is resected. *See* Functional reserve.

Functional amnesia. *See* Amnestic syndrome.

Functional Assessment Measure (FAM). *See* Functional Independent Measure.

Functional disorder. A disorder without a known structural etiology, often used to refer to a psychiatric or psychological disorder (i.e., one that impairs function). In neurology, a functional disorder refers to an apparent neurologic disorder in which the etiology is psychiatric in origin and without physiological or structural cause.

Functional Independence Measure (FIM). Ordinal scale of competence and need for assistance in self-care, physical mobility, and other functional skills; it is widely used to assess progress in rehabilitation. The Functional Assessment Measure (FAM) is used as an adjunct to the FIM to assess more subtle cognitive and psychosocial disabilities and is not used independently. The total scale when both components are used is known as FIM + FAM. 1993. *Guide for the Uniform Data Set for Medical Rehabilitation* [Adult FIM], Version 4.0. Manual. Buffalo NY: UB Foundation Activities; Hall, K.M. 1992. Overview of functional assessment scales in brain injury rehabilitation. *NeuroRehabilitation* 2:98–113.)

Functional magnetic resonance imaging (fMRI). A noninvasive technique employing rapid MRI acquisition parameters that is sensitive to blood flow changes accompanying motor, sensory, and cognitive processing. Areas of activation are superimposed onto structural MR images to identify areas associated with blood flow changes. Like neuropsychological testing, fMRI is an activation procedure and requires patient cooperation to obtain valid results. The fMRI reflects the relative difference in blood flow between activation and control conditions, so the characteristics of the control task contribute to the validity of the final activation results.

Functional reorganization. The theory that intact portions of the nervous system reorganize their inputs/outputs after injury, eventually "taking over" lost functions subserved by damaged tissue. Its existence has been supported by neuroimaging and electrophysiology studies following focal injuries.

Functional reserve. Conceptualization of brain function that proposes that the functional capacity of the temporal lobe contralateral to surgery determines the degree of pre- to postsurgery memory change after anterior temporal lobectomy. Thus, patients who experience the greatest decline in memory are those with little functional reserve associated with the remaining temporal lobe. *See* functional adequacy.

Functor. *See* Function word.

Fundus. The portion of an organ that is furthest away from its opening. The fundus of the eye contains the optic disk, optic nerve, and blood vessels. [L. *fundus*, bottom.]

Fungus. A general term used for the diverse morphological forms of yeasts and molds. Fungal infections are treated with antifungal agents. [L. *fungus*, a mushroom.]

FUO. Fever of unknown origin.

Fusiform gyrus. Spindle-shaped gyrus on the inferior surface of the temporal lobe between the inferior temporal gyrus and the parahippocampal gyrus. This area often includes a basal temporal language region that has been identified by electrical stimulation mapping. Resection of the basal language area during anterior temporal lobectomy, however, is not necessarily associated with postoperative language decline. [L. *fusus*, a spindle; *forma*, form; *gyrus*, convolution; Gr. *gyros*, circle.]

G

Gage, Phineas. A patient who sustained a frontal lobe injury in 1848 while laying railroad tracks. The injury was caused by Gage's accidental dropping of his tamping iron on a rock and igniting blasting powder. This thrust the iron through the left side of his jaw, passing through the brain and exiting just left of the midline of the frontal skull. Although he recovered physically, Gage (1823–1860) became a well-known patient because his responsible personality shifted toward poor judgement and impulsiveness, thus demonstrating the importance of frontal lobe function in humans. *See* frontal lobe syndromes.

Gait apraxia. *See* Apraxia.

Galvanic skin response (GSR). (Luigi Galvani, Italian physician and physiologist, 1737–1798). Activity of the sweat glands that is accompanied by changes in voltage and resistance of the skin; this occurs in response to both physical and psychological stimuli. The GSR is often used to record levels of arousal and emotion. Following the 1967 recommendation of the Society for Psychophysiological Research, the term GSR is less frequently used. Instead, skin conductance response (SCR), skin resistance response (SRR), and skin potential response (SPR) are used to indicate phasic activity in the relevant context. Galvanic skin response is named for galvanic electricity, a unidirectional electric current derived from a chemical source.

Galveston Orientation and Amnesia Test (GOAT). A modified mental status examination designed to assess the duration of disorientation, or *post-traumatic amnesia*, following traumatic brain injury. It is designed for repeated assessment and can be administered daily. In addition to assessing orientation (e.g., person, place, and time), the patient is asked to recall the last event before the accident that caused the injury and the first memory after the accident. It is scored on a 0–100 point scale. (Levin, H.S., O'Donnell, V.M., and Grossman, R.G. 1979. The Galveston Orientation and Amnesia Test: A practical scale to assess cognition after head injury. *J. Nervous Mental Dis.* 167:675–684.)

Gamma knife. *See* Stereotaxic radiosurgery.

Gamma-aminobutyric acid (GABA). The major inhibitory neurotransmitter of presynaptic transmission of the nervous system. Benzodiazepines and barbiturates bind to the postsynaptic GABA receptor and some antiepileptic drugs exert their effects through the GABA system.

Ganglion. Collection of nerve cell bodies outside the central nervous system. The basal ganglia is the exception to this general definition.

Ganser syndrome. (Sigbert J.M. Ganser, German psychiatrist, 1853–1931). A factitious disorder in which patients pretend to lose their minds or become insane. Symptoms may include amnesia, disturbance of consciousness, unusual behavioral acts, or hallucinations. Responses are often characterized by senseless or approximate answers to questions.

Gatekeeper. In the U.S., a person or policy that controls access to health care service.

Gates-MacGinitie Reading Tests. A series of norm-referenced tests to assess general reading ability. Nine levels of the test exist for administration to students in kindergarten through twelfth grade. (MacGinitie, W.H. and MacGinitie, R.K. 1989. *Gates-MacGinitie Reading Tests: Manual for Scoring and Interpretation.* Chicago: The Riverside Publishing Company.)

Gaussian distribution. (Carl Friedrich Gauss, German mathematician, 1777–1855). *See* normal distribution.

Gaze palsy. Paralysis of gaze. A lateral gaze palsy, in which the eyes typically deviate toward the side of the cerebral lesion, is associated with acute lesions and is more common and more severe after right than left cerebral injury. A vertical gaze palsy in which the eyes are unable to move vertically is associated with progressive supranuclear palsy (PSP) or damage to the tegmentum. [palsy: a contraction of paralysis, from Gr. *paralyein*, to loosen, dissolve, weaken.]

Gegenhalten. Fluctuating resistance to passive stretching of the muscles in which patients seem unable to relax on command. When muscles are passively stretched, the patient's inability to cooperate interferes. Gegenhalten is seen in frontal lobe disease or diffuse cerebral degeneration. Also called paratonia. [G. *Gegenhalten*, counterholding, holding against.]

Gelastic seizure. *See* Seizure.

General Neuropsychological Deficit Scale. *See* Neuropsychological Deficit Scale.

General paresis. Dementia associated with *neurosyphilis*. This term is no longer in widespread use.

Generalized seizure. *See* Seizure.

Generalized tonic-clonic (GTC) seizure. *See* Seizure.

Geriatric Depression Scale. A 30–item yes/no questionnaire designed to assess depression and dysphoria in the elderly. The test questions are read to the patient, which assists patients with visual problems or dementia. (Brink, T.L., Yesavage, J.A., Owen, L., Heersema, P.H., Adey, M., and Rose, T.L. 1982. Screening tests for geriatric depression. *Clin. Gerontol.* 1:37–43.)

Gerstmann syndrome. (Josef Gerstmann, Austrian neurologist, 1887–1969). Syndrome comprising right-left disorientation, *acalculia*, *agraphia*, and defective *finger localization* and identification. Whether these signs represent a single, true neuropsychological disability (a disturbance of the body schema) or a group of common of manifestations of left parietal damage is debated. Originally attributed to a lesion in the left angular gyrus.

Gesell Developmental Schedules. (Arnold Gesell, American psychologist and pediatrician, 1880–1961). Empirically derived measures of infant and early childhood development that can be administered to children between 4 weeks and 6 years of age. These measures are behavioral observations in the areas of motor, adaptive, language, and personal social functions. (Gesell, A. 1956. *Developmental Schedules*. New York: The Psychological Corporation.)

Gilles de la Tourette's syndrome. (Georges Gilles de la Tourette, French physician, 1857–1904). Rare disorder characterized by vocal and multiple motor tics of childhood onset. The vocal tics consist of sniffling or throat clearing, but they may progress to louder noises, such as grunting, and to *coprolalia*. Although coprolalia is considered one of the prominent features, it is present only in approximately 60% of patients. Echolalia may also be present. Patients may have attention deficits without hyperactivity, although general intellectual function is typically intact. Often shortened to Tourette's syndrome.

Give-way weakness. A sign of poor effort during muscle strength testing that may be due to psychogenic illness, malingering, or pain. The patient is requested to prevent the examiner from moving the affected arm or leg during strength testing. Muscle resistance is present for a very brief period before quickly returning to a paretic posture with no resistance. Patients with neurologic injury, in contrast, display fairly uniform resistance, gradually giving way to force.

Glabellar reflex. Inability to inhibit eye-blinking when tapped above the bridge of the nose. This response normally extinguishes after a few taps. This reflex is often seen in Parkinson's disease, frontal lobe disease, or diffuse cerebral disease. In schizotypal disorders, there may be an absence of any eye-blink response. Also called Meyerson's sign.

Glasgow Coma Scale (GCS). A rating scale of responsiveness in three dimensions (best eye response, best verbal response, best motor response) used to assess level of consciousness. The sum of the three scales ranges from 3 to 15. Scores of 8 or less are indicative of coma. Although not universally accepted, in some studies of traumatic brain injury, scores of 9–12 are called moderate injuries and scores of 13–15 are called mild injuries. GCS scores have been correlated with neurobehavioral outcome following traumatic brain injury. (Teasdale, G. and Jennett, B. 1974. Assessment of coma and impaired consciousness: A practical scale. *Lancet* 2:81–84.)

Glasgow Outcome Scale (GOS). A scale designed to assess functioning after traumatic brain injury. Outcome is classified as: 1, death; 2, persistent vegetative state (absence of cortical function); 3, severe disability (conscious but disabled, dependent on others for daily support); 4, moderate disability (disabled but independent); or 5, good recovery (resumption of normal life). (Jennett, B. and Bond, M. 1975. Assessment of outcome after severe brain damage. *Lancet* 1:480–487.)

Glia. Non-neural, supportive cells of the nervous system, including astrocytes, oligodendrocytes, microglial cells, and ependymal cells of astrocytes, oligodendroglia, and microglia. [Gr. *glia*, glue.]

Glioblastoma (glioblastoma multiforme). A highly malignant primary brain tumor arising from one of the neuroglial cells, most often from astrocytes. Glioblastomas typically infiltrate in a "butterfly" pattern in which the tumor spreads from one hemisphere to the other through the corpus callosum. This allows tumor infiltration into both frontal lobes.

Glioma. A primary brain tumor arising from glial cells, most often from astrocytes. Gliomas in children are generally located in the posterior fossa and there is a good response to surgical therapy. In contrast, astrocytomas or gliomas in adults are generally highly infiltrative and malignant.

Gliosis. Overgrowth of glial fibers in response to injury or disease.

Global aphasia. *See* Aphasia syndromes.

Globus pallidus. Medial portion of the lenticular nucleus, which is part of the basal ganglia. The globus pallidus plays a prominent role in motor modulation and is the site targeted for lesioning in pallidotomy for symptomatic treatment of Parkinson's disease. [L. *globus*, a ball, sphere; *pallidus*, pale.]

Glove-and-stocking anesthesia. Impaired sensation over the periphery of all four limbs seen in polyneuropathies and somatoform disorders.

Glutamate. An amino acid that serves as an excitatory neurotransmitter. High levels of glutamate produce neuronal excitotoxicity (associated with sustained influx of sodium and calcium), which may be a contributory cause of neuronal damage in strokes, hypoxia, and traumatic brain injury.

Go/no-go tasks. Tests that assess the ability to inhibit a response after a particular response set has been established; these were developed and popularized by Aleksandr Luria (Soviet neuropsychologist, 1902–1977). These tasks share the common principle that two different stimuli are randomly presented at a rapid rate. Each stimulus requires a different response from the patient, one of which is no response. A common go/no-go test involves presenting one or two fingers, displayed as if a person were counting. When one finger is presented (go sign), the subject is to display two fingers. When two fingers are present (no-go sign), the subject is to display no fingers. Patients who have difficulty with this task may display two fingers after being presented with two fingers by the examiner.

Goldstein-Scheerer Tests of Abstract and Concrete Thinking. (Kurt Goldstein, American neurologist born in Germany, 1878–1965; Martin Scheerer, American psychologist born in
Germany, 1900–1961). A battery of five tests designed to measure concept formation.
The tests were developed in 1941 and were designed without standardization data to measure qualitative aspects of abstract intellectual function. (Goldstein, K. and Scheerer, M.
1941. Abstract and concrete behavior: An experimental study with special tests. *Psychol.
Monogr.* 53.)

Gordon Diagnostic System. A portable, microprocessor-based unit that administers a series of
game-like tasks measuring vigilance (continuous performance tasks) and impulse control
(delay task). This unit is often used in the differential diagnosis of childhood attention-
deficit/hyperactivity disorder. (Gordon, M. 1983. *The Gordon Diagnostic System.* DeWitt,
NY: Gordon Systems.)

Gorham Proverbs Test. A test of abstraction that employs proverb interpretation. In addition
to spontaneous responding, a multiple-choice format facilitates administration to patients
with nonfluent aphasia. (Gorham, D.R. 1956. *Clinical Manual for the Proverbs Test.* Missoula,
MT: Psychological Test Specialists.)

Graded Naming Test (GNT). A screening test to measure naming deficits. It consists of 30
black-and-white line drawings that are sequenced in order of difficulty, although many
items are not readily known in North America. Unlike the Boston Naming Test, no semantic of phonemic cues are provided. An appendix provides equivalent scores on the
WAIS Vocabulary test, National Adult Reading Test (NART), and the Shonell Graded
Word Reading Test. (McKenna, P. and Warrington, E.K. 1983. *Manual for the Graded Naming Test.* Windsor, Berkshire, England: NFER-Nelson Publishing Co.)

Graham-Kendall Memory for Designs Test. Test of visual memory consisting of 15 geometric
designs that vary in complexity. Designs are presented for 5 seconds and are then drawn
from memory immediately after exposure. It may be considered a test of visual attention
or visual short-term memory since it does not examine retention over longer delays (e.g.,
20–30 minutes), which is a characteristic practice of most visual spatial memory tests.
(Graham, K.F. and Kendall, B.S. 1960. Memory-for Designs Test: Revised general manual. *Percept. Motor Skills* 11:147–188 (Monogr. Suppl. 2-VII.)

Grammar. Rules governing the phonology, semantics, morphology, and syntax of a language.
Grammar is sometimes used in a more restrictive sense to refer to only the rules governing the morphology and syntax of a language exclusive of phonology and semantics.

Grand mal seizure. A generalized tonic-clonic seizure. The term is no longer in active use.
[F. *grand*, large; *mal*, sickness, from L. *malum*, an evil.]

Grapheme. A letter or letter combination that represents a specific sound or *phoneme*. [Gr.
graphe, a writing, a representation, from *graphein*, to write, draw.]

Graphesthesia. The ability to identify letters and numerals that are traced or written onto the
skin (e.g., palm, fingers). Graphesthesia was described in 1920 by Sir Henry Head
(1861–1940). (Head, H. 1920. *Studies in Neurology.* London: Oxford University Press.) [Gr.
graphe, a writing, a representation, from *graphein*, to write, draw; *aisthesis*, feeling, from
aisthanein, to feel.]

Graphomotor apraxia. *See* Apraxia.

Grasp reflex. An abnormal reflex that is elicited by stroking either the patient's palm across
its width or the fingers lengthwise. A patient with this reflex will involuntary grasp the
stimulating fingers despite repeated requests not to grasp. This reflex is called a frontal
release sign, although it more commonly associated with diffuse disease than with focal
frontal lobe damage.

Gray Oral Reading Tests. (William S. Gray, American educator, 1885–1960). A reading test of
prose passages that progressively increase in difficulty. The paragraphs are read aloud by

the subject and are followed by five comprehension questions. Reading rate, reading accuracy, and oral reading comprehension are measured. These scores are combined to make summary scores for Passage (rate and accuracy) and Total Reading Ability (Passage and Comprehension). Two alternative forms are available. (Wiederholt, J.L. and Bryant, B.R. 1992. *Gray Oral Reading Tests*, 3rd ed. Austin, TX: Pro-ed.)

Greek cross. A simple test of constructional ability in which the patient is instructed to copy a cross that contains four arms of equal size. A Greek cross is included in the Reitan-Indiana Aphasia Screening Test, with explicit instruction not to lift the pencil while copying. Russell, Neuringer, and Goldstein (1970) modified the Reitan-Indiana Aphasia Screening Test by having the cross copied twice and by including a score for spatial relations that reflects performance on both cross copies. (Russell, E.W., Neuringer, C., and Goldstein, G. 1970. *Assessment of Brain Damage: A Neuropsychological Key Approach*. New York: Wiley-Interscience, 1970.)

Grip strength. A measure of hand or grasp strength that is assessed with a dynamometer, typically measured in kilograms. Part of the Halstead-Reitan Neuropsychological Battery.

Grooved Pegboard Test. A test of fine motor speed and manipulative dexterity. The subject must fit keyhole-shaped pegs into similarly shaped holes on a square board. The pegs, which have an edge along one side, must be rotated to match the holes before they can be inserted. The scores obtained are the time required to complete the task with each hand and the number of times the pegs are dropped with each hand.

GSR. *See* Galvanic skin response.

GSW. Gunshot wound.

G-tube. Gastrostomy tube.

Guillain-Barré syndrome. An autoimmune disease of peripheral myelin associated with paresthesias in the distal extremities and leg weakness. This syndrome is the most common demyelinating disease of the peripheral nervous system.

Gyrus. Convolution of the brain surface that is caused by infolding of the cortex. [L. *gyrus*, convolution; *gyros*, circle.]

H

HA. Headache.

Hachinski ischemia scale. A scale for assessing risk factors, clinical signs, and historical variables associated with cerebrovascular disease. It is used to determine the likelihood of vascular causes as the source of cognitive impairment in dementia (e.g., multi-infarct dementia). Its sensitivity to subcortical vascular dementia has not been established. (Hachinski, V.C., Iliff, L.D., Zilhka, E., DuBoulay, G.H., McAllister, V.L., Marshall, J., Russell, R.W., and Symon, L. 1975. Cerebral blood flow in dementia. *Arch. Neurol.* 32:632–637.)

Hallervorden-Spatz syndrome (HSS). (Julius Hallervorden, East Prussian/German neurologist, 1882–1965; Hugo Spatz, German neuropathologist, 1888–1969). Rare hereditary degenerative disorder characterized by marked reduction in the myelin sheaths of the globus pallidus and substantia nigra, with accumulations of iron pigment, progressive rigidity beginning in the legs, choreoathetoid movements, dysarthria, and progressive emotional and mental deterioration. HSS is transmitted as an autosomal recessive trait. Clinical symptoms usually begin in the first or second decade and progress to death before the thirtieth year. The cognitive deficits include prominent visual-spatial impairment and generalized dementia.

Halstead Category Test. (Ward C. Halstead, American psychologist, 1908–1968). Test of abstraction containing six stimulus series in which the visual stimulus is associated with a number between 1 and 4. The task is to determine the principle used to determine the associated number (e.g., Roman numeral, spatial location) through feedback regarding response correctness; the same principle runs through the series. A pleasant bell sounds after correct responses and a harsh buzzer sounds after incorrect responses. The presence of the harsh buzzer sound is thought by some to increase the stress level, thereby increasing the likelihood of performances in the impaired range. The final subtest is a memory task consisting of items from the first six series. The original version consists of rear slide projection to a special presentation box. Both a booklet form and a computer form have been developed, although their strict equivalence to the original version has not been demonstrated. The test was originally employed as a measure of frontal lobe function, but it is sensitive to lesions regardless of their location. Developed by Halstead, this test is part of the Halstead-Reitan Neuropsychological Battery. (Halstead, W.C. 1947. *Brain and Intelligence.* Chicago: University of Chicago Press.)

Halstead Impairment Index. (Ward C. Halstead, American psychologist, 1908–1968). Summary value based on test performance with the Halstead-Reitan Neuropsychological Battery. This value is the proportion of test scores considered to be in the "brain-injured" range. Brain impairment is generally inferred with an impairment index of at least 0.5, whereas scores of 0.4 and lower are characteristic of healthy non-neurologic or nonpsychiatric patients. The criteria for impairment established by Halstead were based on a relatively young sample of 28 subjects, however, and no provision for the effects of normal aging was made. Consequently, use of the Halstead Impairment Index alone may lead to faulty inferences.

Halstead-Reitan Neuropsychological Battery (HRNB). A battery of tests first collected by Halstead and subsequently applied by Reitan to evaluate the effects of brain injury on cognitive performance. The battery of tests comprising the HRNB includes the Halstead Category Test, Tactual Performance Test, Seashore Rhythm Test, Speech Sounds Perception Test, and Finger Tapping Test. Performance on these five tests provides seven scores that make up the Halstead Impairment Index. In addition to the above tests, the Trail Making Test, Reitan-Indiana Aphasia Screening Test, Reitan-Kløve Sensory Perceptual Examination, Grip Strength, WAIS, and Minnesota Multiphasic Personality Inventory are generally administered as part of the battery, although scores do not contribute to the Halstead Impairment Index. A more recent summary score, based on a larger number of scores, is the *Neuropsychological Deficit Score*. Tests originally included by Halstead, the Critical Flicker Fusion and the Time Sense Test, were dropped by Reitan because of their poor sensitivity to brain damage. *See* Neuropsychological Deficit Score.

Hamartoma. A nodule of faulty tissue development that resembles a neoplasm but does not have an abnormal growth rate and thus does not produce pressure effects. [Gr. *hamartion*, a bodily defect, *-oma*, morbid growth, tumor.]

Hamilton Rating Scale for Depression. A measure of depression in which depressive symptoms are rated on a 3- or 5-point scale. It differs from other rating scales such as the Beck Depression Inventory in that the scale is filled out by an observer or interviewer. This test has been revised and different versions exist. (Hamilton, M. 1967. Development of a rating scale for primary depressive illness. *Br. J. Soc. Clin. Psychol.*, 6:278–296.)

Handedness. The tendency to prefer one hand over the other for performing skilled and unskilled movements. Handedness is often used as an indirect measure of cerebral language dominance since the majority of right-handed subjects with no evidence of early left hemisphere brain injury are left cerebral language dominant.

Handicap. According to the World Health Organization, a disadvantage for an individual on account of a disability that prevents the fulfillment of expected social roles.

Haptic Intelligence Scale for adult blind (HIS). A test of nonverbal intelligence that is patterned after the performance subtests from the Wechsler Intelligence Scales for blind individuals who are 16 to 64 years old. Four WIS subtests were modified: Digit Symbol (raised symbols and dots), Block Design (different textures), Object Assembly (puzzle assembled after subject is told the number of items), and Object Completion (missing part from common household objects). Two additional subtests were developed: Pattern Board, which requires the patient to reproduce a pattern in a pegboard after the pegs have been removed, and Bead Arithmetic, which requires the subject to use an abacus for number manipulation. (Shurrager, H.D. and Shurrager, P.A. 1964. *Manual for the Haptic Intelligence Scale for Adult Blind*. Chicago: Stoelting.)

HBP. High blood pressure.

HDL. High-density lipoprotein. *See* Lipoprotein.

Head injury. Nonspecific term referring to an injury to the head, such as a laceration or bruise, or to brain damage that may result from an injury to the head. When modified by the terms mild, moderate, or severe, head injury often refers to a brain injury involving a period of coma or a concussion. Closed head injuries are contrasted with open head injuries, which involve penetration of at least the skin, skull, and dura (i.e., the subdural space) and may involve penetration of the cerebral cortex, cerebellum, or brainstem.

Heavy metal poisoning. Poisoning from metals having higher atomic numbers than calcium in the periodic table of elements. *See* Lead poisoning.

Hebb's Recurring Digit Test. (Donald O. Hebb, Canadian psychologist, 1904–1985). Learning task in which a same-length digit series is presented to the patient. The length of the digit series exceeds the patient's forward digit span by one digit. Every third digit sequence is identical, and the task is to see how quickly the patient learns the repeated digit sequence. The patient is not told that some sequences are repeated. The Corsi block tapping test is based on this test. (Hebb, D.O. 1961. Distinctive features of learning in the higher animal. In: Delafresnay, J.F. (ed.), *Brain Mechanisms and Learning.* New York: Oxford University Press, pp. 37–51.)

HEENT. Head, ears, eyes, nose, and throat.

Hemangioma. A vascular malformation that resembles a neoplasm. Also called cavernous angioma.

Hematoma. A circumscribed or localized area of blood from vessel leakage or bleeding. [Gr. *haima*, blood; *tomé*, cut.)

- **Epidural hematoma**. A collection of blood between the skull and dura; typically associated with skull fractures.
- **Intracerebral hematoma**. A collection of blood within the brain; typically associated with missile wounds, depressed skull fractures, and shear injuries to deep blood vessels.
- **Subdural hematoma**. A collection of blood in the subdural space resulting from lacerated cortical blood vessels, exposing the cortex to blood product and *mass effects.* Over time (days to weeks), the hematoma enlarges and eventually compresses the cerebral hemisphere and produces symptoms. In the elderly, subdural hematomas may develop insidiously over a period of weeks after a seemingly minor fall or other trauma (chronic subdural hematoma), and patients are brought to medical attention only after developing personality and cognitive changes. Subdurals are typically treated by surgical evacuation through small twist-drill holes.

Hemiakinesia. The failure to use an extremity contralateral to a cerebral lesion that does not arise through primary motor loss. This is typically associated with right cerebral injuries as part of the *neglect syndrome.* Relatively normal motor strength is sometimes present when the patient pays attention to the extremity.

Hemialexia. A *paralexia* characterized by an inability to read in the left visual field due to corpus callosum lesions or visual neglect.

Hemianopia (hemianopsia). A loss of vision for one-half of the visual field of either one or both eyes.

Hemiballismus. *See* Ballismus.

Hemiplegia. Paralysis of one side of the body that is caused by brain injury. The degree of paralysis is often incomplete (hemiparesis), and the arm is usually weaker than the leg.

Hemispatial inattention. Hemispatial neglect. Hemispatial inattention is frequently used to describe a milder form of neglect. Also called hemi-inattention.

Hemispatial neglect. *See* Neglect.

Hemispherectomy. Surgical removal of a diseased cerebral hemisphere to control intractable epilepsy. Hemispherectomy is reserved for patients with congenital hemiplegia or chronic encephalitis that has progressed to produce hemiplegia. Hemispherectomy has provided insight into the plasticity of the right hemisphere to acquire language function following early left hemisphere injury. Originally, hemispherectomy was anatomically complete. However, functional hemispherectomy combines complete commissurotomy with incomplete removal of the hemisphere, typically sparing the frontal and occipital poles to support the remaining hemisphere. *See* Commissurotomy.

Hemispheric asymmetry. Hemispheric specialization in which one hemisphere is more greatly involved in processing certain tasks than the other cerebral hemisphere. The cognitive functions that display the greatest hemispheric asymmetry are language in the left cerebral hemisphere and visual-spatial processing in the right hemisphere. In addition, structural hemispheric asymmetries are present in some brain regions. The planum temporale of the left hemisphere, for example, is generally longer and larger than that of the right hemisphere and is thought to reflect an anatomic basis for left hemisphere language dominance.

Hemorrhage. Bleeding from either vessel leakage or vessel rupture. [Gr. *haimorrhages*, bleeding violently, from *haima*, blood; *rhegynai*, to break, burst.]

- **Cerebral hemorrhage**. Cerebral hemorrhage is frequently associated with hypertension. The effects of hemorrhage depend on the anatomic location, size, and degree of mass effect. Also called hypertensive hemorrhage, intracerebral hemorrhage (ICH), or parenchymal hemorrhage.
- **Subdural hemorrhage**. Bleeding in which the cerebral veins entering the sinuses are broken (e.g., cerebral veins entering the superior sagittal sinus). Subdural hemorrhage is typically traumatic in origin.

Hemosiderin. A protein residual of the breakdown of blood. Hemosiderin deposits may be observed anywhere that there has been prior bleeding into or around tissue. Subarachnoid hemorrhage may result in hemosiderin deposits on the brain surface and on the nerve roots. This may result in nervous system dysfunction, which is called siderosis.

Hereditary spinal ataxia. *See* Friedreich's ataxia.

Herniation, brain. Abnormal protrusion of the brain through a natural opening due to increased intracerebral pressure. Two types of brain herniation may be present: tonsilar herniation and transtentorial herniation. Tonsilar herniation is a protrusion of the cerebellar tonsils through the foramen magnum, which exerts pressure on the medulla, and is often fatal. Transtentorial herniation is the downward displacement of the medial structures (e.g., uncus) through the tentorial notch by a supratentorial mass, which in turn exerts pressure on the brainstem. Transtentorial herniation is also called uncal herniation or temporal herniation.

Herpes simplex encephalitis. Viral brain infection caused by herpes simplex virus type 1. It is the most common cause of serious nonepidemic encephalitis. The virus has a predilection for the inferior and medial surfaces of the frontal and temporal lobes. Memory impairment and complex partial seizures often occur. The course of the infection is generally 1–2 weeks. [Gr. *herpes*, a creeping, from *herpein*, to creep; *enkephalos*, brain.]

Heschl's gyrus. (Richard L. Heschl, Austrian pathologist, 1824–1881). Transverse temporal gyri on the inferior bank of the Sylvian fissure that serve as primary auditory cortex; Brodmann's areas 41 and 42.

Heterophone. A word with two alternative pronunciations (e.g., "read"). [Gr. *heteros* other; *phone*, a sound, voice.]

Heterotopia. A neuromigrational disorder in which neurons fail to migrate to expected locations. This results in displacement of gray matter into the white matter. Patients with heterotopias are frequently mentally retarded. [Gr. *heteros* other; *topos*, place.]

Heterotopic ossification. Abnormal bone growth into joint spaces of the arms and legs, causing pain and contracture; this occurs frequently after severe traumatic brain injury.

Hidden Figures Test. *See* Embedded Figures Tests.

Hindbrain. The pons, cerebellum, and medulla. The hindbrain is divided into the metencephalon (pons and cerebellum) and myelencephalon (medulla). Also called rhombencephalon.

Hippocampus. Part of the limbic system located in the medial aspects of the temporal lobe that is important in memory formation. The hippocampus produces a curved elevation in the floor of the inferior horn of the lateral ventricle. It is a common seizure focus in complex partial epilepsy (temporal lobe epilepsy). [Gr. *hippocampos*, seahorse.]

Hiscock-Hiscock Forced-Choice Recognition Task. A forced-choice digit recognition task designed to detect response exaggeration. (Hiscock, M. and Hiscock, C.K. 1989. Refining the forced-choice method for the detection of malingering. *J. Clin. Exp. Neuropsychol.* 11: 967–974.)

HIV. *See* Human immunodeficiency virus.

H.M. Initials of William Scoville's (1954) patient who became severely amnesic following bilateral temporal lobectomy control of intractable epilepsy. H.M. demonstrated the importance of the hippocampus in declarative memory function. Other patients had undergone bilateral temporal lobectomy, but surgery was performed to treat serious psychiatric disorders, which made the demonstration of amnesia more difficult. H.M. (b. 1926) was operated on in 1953. (Scoville, W. 1954. The limbic lobe in man. *J. Neurosurg.* 11:64–66.)

Hoffmann sign. (Johann Hoffmann, German neurologist, 1857–1919). A sign of hyperreflexia that may occur with *upper motor neuron* disease. It may also be present in anxious healthy individuals. It is elicited by a quick downward flexion of the end (i.e., distal phalanx) of the middle (third) or ring (fourth) finger. The response consists of a pincher flexion movement of the index finger and the thumb.

Hold vs. Don't Hold Tests. An approach to estimating the premorbid level of intellectual function as a basis for judging the relative change that results from neuropsychological impairment. Developed by Babcock (1930), hold tests are so named because they are considered relatively resistant to the effects of brain pathology. Two such "hold" tests are the Vocabulary and Picture Completion subtests from the Wechsler Intelligence Scales (WIS). Other tests, such as the Digit Symbol Substitution subtest, are thought to be sensitive to brain pathology regardless of its location; consequently they are considered "don't hold" tests. This approach is a rough approximation to estimating neuropsychological decline. (Babcock, H. 1930. An experiment in the measurement of mental deterioration. *Arch. Psychol.* 117:105.)

Holoprosencephaly. A neuromigrational disorder with craniofacial abnormalities that develops during the fifth and sixth weeks of gestation. The two cerebral hemispheres, either totally or in part, form a single telencephalic mass. Children with holoprosencephaly are typically severely retarded. [Gr. *holos*, whole; *pros*, in front; *enkepahalos*, the brain.]

Homeopathic dosage. A medication dosage that is smaller than that required to produce a therapeutic effect. [Gr. *homos*, same; *pathos*, suffering.]

Homonymous. Having the same effect on both sides. [Gr. *homonymous*, of the same name, from *onyma*, name.]

Homonymous hemianopsia. Hemianopsia affecting the analogous right or left halves of the visual fields of both eyes.

Homophone. A word having the same pronunciation as another word but a different spelling and meaning (e.g., "sale," "sail"). [Gr. *homos*, same; *phone*, a sound, voice.]

Homunculus. The representation of pre- or post-central gyrus sensory or motor functions depicted by drawing the associated parts of the body next to a coronal representation of the brain. The original homunculus was drawn by Wilder Penfield (Canadian neurosurgeon, 1891–1976) on the basis of his pioneering work in functional cortical mapping with electrical stimulation. [L. diminutive of *homo, hominis*, a man.]

Hooper Visual Organization Test (VOT). A test of visual perceptual organization containing 30 drawings of readily recognizable cut-up objects. The task is to name each object verbally if the test is individually administered, or by writing the name of the object if a group administration is used. No time limit for a response is employed. (Hooper, H.E. 1983. *Hooper Visual Organization Test*. Manual. Los Angeles: Western Psychological Services.)

Hoover's sign. (Charles F. Hoover, American physician, 1865–1927). A sign of psychogenic paresis or malingering that is tested by having a supine patient lift the nonparetic leg. Normally there is a reflexive downward movement in the other leg. The absence of the downward movement is a positive Hoover's sign.

Horner's syndrome. (Johann F. Horner, Swiss ophthalmologist, 1831–1886). Ptosis, constriction of the pupil (miosis), anhidrosis, and flushing of the affected side of the face caused by paralysis of the cervical sympathetic nerves.

HTLV. Human T-cell lymphocytotrophic virus; human T-cell lymphoma/leukemia virus.

HTLV-III. Human T-cell lymphotropic virus-type III.

HTN. *See* Hypertension.

Human immunodeficiency virus (HIV). A retrovirus that depresses cell-mediated immunity and is the etiologic agent of AIDS. HIV-related disease can affect any part of the nervous system. Subtle neuropsychological impairment may be present in some patients who are HIV positive but are otherwise neurologically asymptomatic. The virus is immunologically unstable, but it produces antibodies that can be detected by Western blot and ELISA tests.

Huntington's disease. (George Sumner Huntington, American physician, 1850–1916). An autosomal dominant disorder that produces basal ganglia lesions and is characterized by dementia, chorea, and psychiatric symptoms. On autopsy, severe atrophy is seen in the head of the caudate nucleus and, somewhat less prominently, in the putamen. Functional imaging studies have revealed prominent abnormalities in the striatum. Considering the integral connections between the prefrontal cortex and striatum, some of the neuropsychological features may be more appropriately ascribed to compromised functional or structural integrity of frontal cortical zones. Although chorea is often considered the first sign of the disease, behavior changes such as depression may precede the movement disorder by 10 years or more. This disease was previously called Huntington's chorea.

Hx. History.

Hydrocephalus. An abnormal increase in cerebrospinal fluid (CSF) within the skull that is marked by dilatation of the cerebral ventricles. Hydrocephalus commonly occurs secondary to obstruction of CSF pathways from tumors or meningeal disease. Associated features include imbalance and gait apraxia, incontinence, and a slowed rate of responsiveness. Gait impairment is usually the most prominent symptom, and it results from stretching of the corticospinal tract in the internal capsule. The CSF pressure is typically elevated but may occasionally be normal (i.e., normal pressure hydrocephalus). In infants, hydrocephalus is usually caused by cytomegalovirus or toxoplasmosis and it often produces enlargement of the skull because the sutures have not fused. [Gr. *hýdor*, water; *kephale*, head.]

- **Communicating hydrocephalus.** Hydrocephalus in which there is no obstruction in the ventricular system. Cerebrospinal fluid passes readily out of the ventricles into the spinal cord and subarachnoid space of the brain. Communicating hydrocephalus results from diseases of the subarachnoid space, such as meningitis, that clog CSF pathways at the base of the brain and trap CSF in the fourth ventricle, which causes retrograde obstruction. It can also be caused by a pathological increase in CSF production (e.g., choroid plexus papilloma). This disorder is called communicating hydrocephalus because the CSF pathways are unobstructed up to the subarachnoid space.

- **Hydrocephalus ex vacuo.** An enlargement of the cerebral ventricles due to atrophy or loss of adjacent cerebral tissues. Some degree of hydrocephalus ex vacuo is present with normal aging, but more significant ventricular enlargement is associated with diffuse brain pathology. [L. *ex vacuo*, due to emptiness.]

- **Noncommunicating hydrocephalus.** Hydrocephalus with obstruction in the ventricular system that prevents free passage of the CSF from the brain into the spinal canal. Hydrocephalus is often caused by tumors near the smaller channels of the CSF system. Also called obstructive hydrocephalus.
- **Normal pressure hydrocephalus.** A disorder of CSF dynamics that results in an enlargement of the ventricles and is characterized by normal or only intermittently elevated intracranial pressure. The enlarged ventricles are associated with inadequacy of the subarachnoid spaces. This disorder is usually seen in middle-aged and older persons.
- **Obstructive hydrocephalus.** Noncommunicating hydrocephalus.

Hydrocephalus ex vacuo. *See* Hydrocephalus.

Hyperactivity syndrome. Developmentally high activity levels in children that are characterized by disruptive behaviors including excessive motion (e.g., exploring, experimenting) and usually accompanied by distractibility and low frustration tolerance. *See* Attention-deficit/hyperactivity disorder.

Hyperacusis. Abnormal acuteness of hearing due to heightened neural irritability. Hyperacusis is often seen in Bell's palsy. [Gr. *hyper*, over, above, excessive; *akouein*, to hear.]

Hyperesthesia. Increased sensitivity to sensory stimulation such as pain or touch. [Gr. *hyper*, over, above, excessive; *aisthesis*, feeling.]

Hypergraphia. A compulsion to write excessively with copious output that is often contains minute details of personal history. Hypergraphia may be associated with temporal lobe epilepsy (TLE), although most TLE patients do not display this characteristic, or it may be associated with mania. [Gr. *hyper*, over, above, excessive; *graphein*, to write.]

Hyperkinesia/hyperkinesis. *See* Hyperactivity syndrome. [Gr. *hyper*, over, above, excessive; *kinesis*, movement.]

Hyperlexia. Above-average reading ability (decoding) in the presence of mental retardation. It often involves spared ability to read aloud without understanding word meaning. [Gr. *hyper*, over, above, excessive; *lexis*, word.]

Hypermetria. A condition in which voluntary movements overreach the intended target. [Gr. *hyper*, over, above, excessive; *métron*, measure.]

Hyperreflexia. Excessive activity of tendon reflexes associated with loss of corticospinal inhibition that suggests *upper motor neuron* disease. [Gr. *hyper*, over, above, excessive; L. *reflexus*, reflected.]

Hypertelorism. An abnormally large distance between the eyes. [Gr. *hyper*, over, above, excessive; *tele*, far off; *horizo*, to separate.]

Hypertension. Elevated arterial blood pressure. Chronic hypertension increases the likelihood of vascular disorders including small vessel infarction or hemorrhage. [Gr. *hyper*, over, above, excessive; L. *tensio*, a stretching.]

Hypertensive encephalopathy. A rapidly evolving syndrome of severe acute hypertension that is characterized by headache, nausea, and vomiting; it may progress to acute visual disturbances, seizures, stupor, and coma. These symptoms of diffuse cerebral disturbance may be accompanied by focal or lateralizing neurologic signs. Hypertensive encephalopathy is associated with cerebral edema and punctate hemorrhages rather than the infarctions and diffuse hemorrhages associated with chronic severe hypertension.

Hyperthyroidism. Excessive functional activity of the thyroid gland that is characterized by increased metabolism, goiter, and disturbances in the *autonomic nervous system* and in creatinine metabolism. Behavioral symptoms include emotional lability, anxiety, inappropriate temper outbursts, and euphoria. Also called Graves' disease.

Hypertrophy. Enlargement in tissue bulk that is not due to tumor formation. [Gr. *hyper*, over, above, excessive; *trophe*, nourishment.]

Hypesthesia. Decreased sensitivity to stimulation. [Gr. *hypo*, under; *aisthesis*, feeling.]

Hypochondriasis. Morbid anxiety and fear about serious illness. [Gr. *hypochondrion*, the soft part of the body below the cartilage and above the navel; *hypo*, under; *chondaros*, cartilage; the condition was supposed to have its origin in this region.]

Hypoglycemia. Diminished blood glucose that may lead to tremulousness, cold sweats, pilorection, hypothermia, headache, and ultimately, seizures and coma. Hypoglycemia is sometimes accompanied by confusion, hallucinations, and bizarre behavior. [Gr. *hypo*, under; *glykys*, sweet.]

Hypokinesis. Abnormally diminished motor activity often associated with Parkinson's disease. [Gr. *hypo*, under; *kinesis*, movement.]

Hypometria. Abnormally small movements often associated with Parkinson's disease. A common example of hypometria is micrographia. [Gr. *hypo*, under; *métron*, measure.]

Hypophonia. Low-volume speech due to reduced phonation intensity; whispering or weak voice. [Gr. *hypo*, under; *phanai*, to speak.]

Hypophysis. *See* Pituitary gland.

Hyporeflexia. Depressed activity in tendon reflexes associated with dysfunction of the reflex arc. Hyporeflexia suggests *lower motor neuron* disease; bilateral hyporeflexia is associated with peripheral neuropathies, and unilateral hyporeflexia is suggestive of radiculopathy. [Gr. *hypo*, under; L. *reflexus*, reflected.]

Hyposmia. Abnormally decreased sensitivity to odors. [Gr. *hypo*, under; *osmé*, sense of smell.]

Hypotelorism. Abnormal closeness of the eyes. [Gr. *hypo*, under; *tele*, far off; *horizo*, to separate.]

Hypotension. Abnormally low blood pressure. [Gr. *hypo*, under; L. *tensio*, a stretching.]

Hypothalamus. Part of the *diencephalon* that forms the floor and part of the lateral wall of the third ventricle. The nuclei of this region integrate the peripheral autonomic mechanisms, endocrine activity, and many somatic functions (e.g., general regulation of water balance, body temperature, sleep, food intake, and the development of secondary sex characteristics). One of the primary functions of the hypothalamus is control of the pituitary. [Gr. *hypo*, under; + thalamus.]

Hypothermia. Low body temperature. [Gr. *hypo*, under; *therme*, heat.]

Hypothyroidism. A decreased or absent thyroid hormone. In adults, hypothyroidism may superficially resemble dementia. Although cognitive impairment may be present, there is greater lethargy than in dementia. Ataxia, dysarthria, and nystagmus are common. Also called myxedema.

Hypotonia. Absent or decreased muscle tone.

Hypoxia. Decreased oxygen supply to tissue. The term refers to a moderate decrease in oxygen supply. Hypoxia may result from circulatory deficiency (ischemic hypoxia) or oxygen deficiency in the red blood cells (anemic hypoxia). Common causes of hypoxia are hypotensive shock, cardiac arrest, vasospasm, and cardio-thoracic surgery. Anemic hypoxia may result from carbon monoxide poisoning, cyanides, or anesthesia overdose. The greatest effects are in the hippocampus, resulting in anterograde memory impairment. Complete or nearly complete absence of oxygen is called anoxia. *See* anoxia. [Gr. *hypo*, under; + oxygen.]

Hysteria. A term previously used to refer to a number of clinical phenomena, including the overuse of repressive defenses, an overly dramatic and emotionally self-indulgent presentation (as in hysterical personality disorder), and the presentation of somatoform complaints and illness behaviors. Because of its pejorative connotation, the term has become obsolete. [Gr. *hystera*, uterus, womb.]

Hysterical amnesia. Memory loss of non-neurologic origin arising from an emotionally disturbing experience. The term is no longer in wide use; "psychogenic amnesia" is preferred.

I

IAP. Intracarotid amobarbital procedure. *See* Wada Test.

Iatrogenic effect. An unfavorable and unintended response to medical or surgical treatment that results from the treatment itself. [Gr. *iatros*, a physician, from *iasthai*, to heal, cure; *-gen*, producing.]

ICA. Internal carotid artery.

ICD. *See* International Classification of Disease.

Iconic memory. *See* Memory.

ICP. *See* Intracranial pressure.

Ictal. Referring to an ictus; a sudden event. The term is most often used with seizures but may be used with strokes or other paroxysmal attacks. [L. *ictus*, a blow, stroke, from *icere*, to strike, hit.]

ID. Infectious disease.

IDDM. Insulin-dependent diabetes mellitus.

Ideational apraxia. *See* Apraxia.

Ideograph. Form of orthography in which a character or figure symbolizes an object or idea with no direct correspondence between symbols and *phonology* (e.g., Chinese). [Gr. *idea*, a form, the look or appearance of a thing as opposed to its reality, from *idein*, to see.]

Ideomotor apraxia. *See* Apraxia.

Idioglossia. Unintelligible speech. [Gr. *idio-*, from *idios*, one's own, combining form meaning personal, distinct; *glossa*, tongue, language.]

Idiopathic. A disease process of unknown cause. [Gr. *idio-*, from *idios*, one's own, combining form meaning personal, distinct, own; *pathos*, suffering.]

IM. Internal medicine; intramuscular.

Imaginal code. Memory code derived from processing an image. *See* Dual-code theory.

IME. Independent medical examination.

Impairment. According to the World Health Organization, a loss or abnormality of structure or function at the level of tissue or organ that can lead to disability.

Imperception. Impairments in visuoperception and spatial thinking. The term imperception was introduced by J. Hughlings Jackson (British neurologist, 1835–1911.] *See* Extinction and neglect syndrome.

Implicit memory. *See* Memory (nondeclarative [implicit] memory).

Incidence. The number of new cases of a particular phenomenon within a specified period.

Incidental learning. Learning that occurs without volitional effort. It is tested with tasks in which the subject is unaware that memory recall will be assessed.

Inconsistent words. Words whose pronunciation follows grapheme-to-phoneme conversion rules but which have visual "neighbors" that follow different pronunciation conventions (e.g., "hint," "pint").

Independent variable. In an experimental design, the experimental manipulation that is employed to examine its influence on the dependent variable. In a true experimental design, subjects are randomly assigned to the experimental conditions to determine the effect of the independent variable on the dependent variable. A quasi-experimental design relies on subject variables that cannot be randomly assigned (e.g., disease state) to assess their effects on the dependent measure.

Infarction, cerebral. Area of cerebral necrosis due to vascular insufficiency. Tissue death results either from a lack of nutrients or from build-up of acid end products that reduce tissue pH. [L. *infarcire*, to stuff in.]

Inflection. In linguistics, a suffix added to a morpheme to change grammatical status (e.g., plural, past tense). Also, a change in the pitch or tone of voice that contributes to the intonational contour of a spoken utterance. [L. *inflectere*, to bend.]

Initiation deficit. The failure to act, or behavior requiring intensive cueing, despite a demonstrated ability to perform desired behavior. Patients can often describe intended actions while remaining unable to initiate them. This deficit is associated with injury to mesial frontal cortex and is seen with resolving akinetic mutism.

Inner speech. Experience of hearing one's own words without speaking.

Innervation apraxia. *See* Apraxia (limb-kinetic apraxia.)

Instrumental Activities of Daily Living. *See* Activities of Daily Living.

Insula. Cerebral cortex concealed from the surface and lying at the bottom of the Sylvian (lateral) fissure. Also called the island of Reil. [L. *insula*, an island.]

Intelligence. A multifaceted concept that refers to the ability to understand complex ideas, adapt effectively to the environment, learn from experience, engage in various forms of reasoning, and overcome obstacles by thought. Psychometric intelligence is generally described in relation to same-age peers (e.g., Wechsler Intelligence Scales, Stanford-Binet Intelligence Scale), although the term is also used to describe cognitive developmental levels (e.g., Piagetian stages).

Intelligence quotient (IQ). A summary measure of general cognitive or intellectual function. Originally, the IQ was a calculated quotient obtained by dividing the mental age (MA) by the chronological age (CA). Although Alfred Binet (1857–1911) and Théodore Simon developed the principle of "mental age," it was William Stern (1871–1938), a German psychologist, who first calculated the ratio of the two scores. The IQ is no longer a calculated quotient but a standardized summary score reflecting performance on all subtests. Most IQ scores have a mean value of 100 and a standard deviation of 15. The term IQ is often used as shorthand notation for Full Scale IQ, or FSIQ.

Intensive care unit (ICU) psychosis. The development of confusion following major surgery. It is thought to be related to extended periods in a sterile hospital room with minimal stimulation, no regular routine, pain, and frequent staff awakenings. Thus, it is considered the result of environmental factors, not the surgical procedure; the confusion rapidly clears following transfer to a regular hospital bed. It is, however, more common in patients recovering from cardio-thoracic surgery than in those recovering from other procedures.

Intention tremor. *Dysmetria* that intensifies when a voluntary, coordinated movement is attempted. This is a sign of cerebellar dysfunction. It is commonly assessed with the finger-to-nose test, or finger-nose-finger test.

Interferon. A naturally occurring protein that suppresses the immune system and is produced by exposure of cells to viruses. Interferon therapy, including such agents as beta-interferon and alpha-interferon, is often used in treating multiple sclerosis. Potential side effects include flu-like symptoms, anemia, and depression.

Interhemispheric fissure. *See* Longitudinal fissure.

Internal carotid artery. *See* Arteries, cerebral.

Internal consistency. Estimate of the *reliability* of a measure or score based on the average correlation among items within a test. This is a partial misnomer because the size of the reliability coefficient depends on both the average correlation among items (the internal consistency) and the number of items. Coefficient alpha is the basic formula for determining the reliability based on internal consistency. Internal consistency is different from item homogeneity.

International Classification of Diseases (ICD). A classification of diseases and disease syndromes that is published by the World Health Organization (WHO). Each disease is designated by a number. The present version, ICD-10, was published in 1990.

Intracarotid sodium amytal test (ISA). *See* Wada Test.

Intracerebral hemorrhage (ICH). *See* Hemorrhage (cerebral).

Intracranial pressure (ICP). The pressure within the cranial vault. Increased ICP results from increased volumes of cerebral spinal fluid (CSF), blood, or brain tissue, which may include tumors and edema. The ICP is measured by recording the pressure of the subarachnoid fluid. [L. *intra*, within, inside; Gr. *kranion*, skull.]

Inversion error. A reading error due to letter inversion (e.g., "but" for "put").

Involuntary movement. A family of movements associated with disorders of the *extrapyramidal motor system*, including *athetosis, ballismus, chorea, dyskinesia, dystonia*, tremor, and *tics*. Involuntary movements are usually not present during sleep.

Ipsilateral. Occurring on the same side, usually used in reference to a cerebral lesion and its clinical manifestations. [L. *ipse*, self or same; *latus*, side.]

IQ. *See* Intelligence quotient.

Ischemia. Lack of adequate blood flow. Cerebral ischemia may be focal when the territory of a particular vessel is affected, or it may be generalized when a heart attack is the cause. [Gr. *iskhein*, to suppress; *haima*, blood.]

Ischemic penumbra. The portion of the ischemic region surrounding the "central core" of dead tissue that is associated with decreased neuronal function and reduced energy metabolism. Early reperfusion within 6 hours of the ischemic event may lead to tissue recovery; otherwise, tissue infarction will develop. [Gr. *iskhein*, to suppress; *haima*, blood; L. *pene*, almost; *umbra*, shade.]

Ishihara Test of Color Blindness. (Shinobu Ishihara, Japanese ophthalmologist, 1879–1963). The pseudoisochromatic test plates used to assess color vision. The stimuli have numbers or figures formed by colored dots against a ground of contrasting colored dots that are distinguishable only by color. Some plates include figures that cannot be seen by those with normal color vision since the dots have an identical hue, but varying luminance. (Ishihara, S. 1982. *The Series of Plates Designed as a Test for Colour-Blindness*. Tokyo: Kanehara Shuppan.)

Island of Reil. (Johann C. Reil, German neurologist and histologist, 1759–1813). *See* Insula.

Isocortex. *See* Cortex, cerebral (neocortex).

Isoelectric. The record obtained from a pair of equipotential electrodes. This term is often applied to electrocerebral inactivity, or electrocerebral silence, that is associated with *brain death*. [Gr. *isos*, equal.]

J

Jacksonian march. (J. Hughlings Jackson, British neurologist, 1835–1911). Focal motor seizure progression that begins focally in one part of the body and then spreads systematically to adjacent areas. This progression reflects the spread of epileptic activity through the sensorimotor homunculus. A characteristic Jacksonian march will first involve the fingers, then arm, and then face.

Jakob-Creutzfeldt disease. *See* Creutzfeldt-Jakob disease.

Jamais vu. The feeling that familiar places or things are suddenly unfamiliar. This symptom is sometimes associated with a seizure aura. [F. *jamais*, never; *vu*, seen.]

Jargon. Unmonitored paraphasia containing little or no information content.

Jargon agraphia. *See* Agraphia spelling disorders.

Jargon aphasia. *See* Aphasia syndromes.

Jaw jerk. A pathologic reflex of temporal muscle contraction that is elicited by tapping downward on a partially open jaw. Also called chin reflex or masseter reflex.

Job coaching. Assistance given by a job trainer to a disabled worker who cannot independently meet competitive employment standards. In addition to training the worker and putting supports into the workplace, the coach may perform part of the job temporarily to provide a competitive work product.

Judgment of Line Orientation. A test of visual-spatial processing containing stimulus materials of two spokes of a semi-circular wheel that point in different directions. The task is to identify which lines of the entire semi-circle containing 11 lines are pointing in the same direction (i.e., have the same spatial orientation) as the stimuli. This test is a relatively pure measure of right hemisphere function. (Benton, A.L., Sivan, A.B., Hamsher, KdeS., Varney, N.R., and Spreen, O. 1994. *Contributions to Neuropsychological Assessment. A Clinical Manual*, 2nd ed. New York: Oxford University Press.)

Just-noticeable-difference (JND). The smallest increment or decrement in the value of a stimulus (e.g., weight, sound, illumination, color) that can be detected as different from the comparison stimulus.

Juvenile amaurotic idiocy. *See* Tay-Sach's disease.

K

K scale. A MMPI validity scale that measures the tendency to present oneself in a socially favorable light. K scale elevation varies with socioeconomic status. A very low K score raises the possibility of exaggerated problems, which reflects severe emotional disturbance.

Kana. The phonologic form of the Japanese alphabet, which contrasts with the pictographic writing approach, *Kanji*. Kana and Kanji may have differential sensitivity to left (Kana) and right (Kanji) hemisphere cerebral lesions, although the original finding has not always been replicated with independent attempts at validation.

Kanji. Japanese pictographic writing (ideograph) in which each character has a specific meaning. *See* Kana.

Kappa. The tenth letter of the Greek alphabet (κ). In statistics, it is a measure of reliability, reflecting agreement among raters that is adjusted for the expected level of chance agreement.

Karyotype. The chromosomal characteristics of an individual. The 46 chromosomes are usually arranged by size and according to the location of the centromere. [Gr. *karyon*, a nut (used in biology to denote a nucleus); *typos*, a blow, the mark of a blow, figure, outline, character of a disease.]

Katz Adjustment Scale-Relatives Form (KAS-R). Nonempirical scale devised to assess the personal, interpersonal, and social adjustment of psychiatric patients in the community. It has been used to describe the degree to which relatives of patients with traumatic brain injuries believe cognitive and behavioral difficulties interfere with the patient's interpersonal relationships. The scale consists of five inventories, each designed to describe the relative's perception of different aspects of the patient's life. (Katz, M.M. and Lyerly, S.B. 1963. Methods for measuring adjustment and social behavior in the community: I. Rationale, description, discriminative validity and scale development. *Psychol. Rep.* 13:503–535.)

Kaufman Assessment Battery for Children (K-ABC). Test of cognitive development and intelligence for children 2.5–12.5 years of age. It is intended, in part, to eliminate or minimize cultural differences by making extensive use of diagrammatic and pictorial material, thereby minimizing verbal requirements. Ten subtests are considered Mental Processing Subtests (Magic Window, Face Recognition, Hand Movements, Gestalt Closure, Number Recall, Triangles, Word Order, Matrix Analogies, Spatial Memory, and Photo Series). Six subtests are considered Achievement Subtests (Expressive Vocabulary, Faces and Places, Arithmetic, Riddles, Reading/Decoding, and Reading/Understanding). Four global scales are obtained: Sequential Processing, Simultaneous Processing, Achievement, and Nonverbal Function. (Kaufman, A.S. and Kaufman, N.L. 1983. *K-ABC: Kaufman Assessment Battery for Children.* Circle Pines, MN: American Guidance Service.)

Kaufman Brief Intelligence Test (K-BIT). An individually administered test suitable for individuals 4–90 years old that provides an estimate of intelligence. It consists of two subtests: Vocabulary and Matrices. The Vocabulary subtest requires that the subject name pictured objects that best fit clues (a phrase description and a partial spelling of the word, e.g., a light color; YE_L_W) and perform a confrontation naming task. The Matrices subtest is a multiple-choice task that requires the ability to solve visual analogies. Separate scores are provided for Vocabulary, Matrices, and total scale. (Kaufman, A.S. and Kaufman, N.L. 1990. *Kaufman Brief Intelligence Test.* Circle Pines, MN: American Guidance Service.)

Kayser-Fleischer ring. (Bernhard Kayser, German physician, 1869–1954; Bruno Fleischer, German ophthalmologist, 1874–1965). An abnormal, green-pigmented copper ring at the outer margin of the cornea. These are not pathognomic of Wilson's disease, but they occur in all but a small percentage of patients with the disease.

Kendrick Cognitive Tests for the Elderly. Tests designed to assist in the differential diagnosis of dementia from depression by assessing memory and speed of responding. The Object Learning Test consists of four cards with six items that are repeated. The cards are presented for increasing lengths of time and contain progressively more stimulus items. Recall is obtained after each card presentation. The Digit Copying Test contains a sheet with 100 numbers that are to be copied as quickly as possible in 2 minutes. Previously called the Kendrick Battery for the Detection of Dementia in Elderly. (Kendrick, D.C. 1985. *The Kendrick Cognitive Tests for the Elderly.* Windsor, England: NFER-Nelson Publishing Co.)

KeyMath Diagnostic Arithmetic Test. A set of measures to identify mathematical strengths and weaknesses in children from kindergarten through grade 9. There are 13 subtests grouped into three major categories: Basic Concepts (Numeration, Rational Numbers, and Geometry), Operations (Addition, Subtraction, Multiplication, Division, and Mental Computation), and Applications (Measurement, Time and Money, Estimation, Interpreting Data, and Problem Solving). (Connolly, A.J. 1991. *KeyMath Revised: A Diagnostic Inventory of Essential Mathematics.* Circle Pines, MN: American Guidance Service.)

Kindling. Experimental animal model for epilepsy and seizure expression induced by repeated electrical stimulation or by repeated administration of neurotoxic chemicals.

Kinesia paradoxica. *See* Bradykinesia.

Kinesthesia. Perception of various parameters of movement (e.g., range, extent, direction, force, momentum) generated by receptors in the muscles, tendons, and joints. [Gr. *kinesis,* movement; *æsthesis,* sensation.]

Klinefelter's syndrome. (Harry F. Klinefelter, Jr., American physician, b. 1912). A chromosomal anomaly, usually not evident before puberty, in which there is an extra X chromosome (i.e., XXY). Patients are male in development, but often they have gynecomastia and small testicles. Most patients have mild mental retardation, and many suffer psychosis. Also called XXY syndrome.

Klüver-Bucy syndrome. (Heinrich Klüver, American neuroscientist/psychologist, 1897–1979; Paul Bucy, American neurosurgeon, b. 1904). Behavioral disturbances following bilateral anterior temporal lobe ablation in monkeys that destroys important limbic structures. This syndrome is characterized by a tendency to place objects in the mouth, by a loss of normal fear, apparent *visual agnosia,* development of placidity and tameness in a previously aggressive animal, and hypersexuality.

Knee jerk. A *deep tendon reflex* in which twitch-like contractions of the quadriceps muscle are elicited by sharply tapping the patellar tendon when the leg hangs loosely, flexed at a right angle. This reflex is hyperactive, or brisk, with *upper motor neuron* disease, and hypoactive, or depressed, with *lower motor neuron* disease. Also known as patellar reflex.

Knox Cube Imitation Test. Subtest of the *Arthur Point Scale of Performance Battery* designed as a nonverbal measure of attention span. Four blocks are aligned in a row, and the examiner taps out sequences of increasing length that are imitated by the patient. Although this procedure is similar to that of the *Corsi Block Tapping Test,* it is a measure of spatial attention rather than spatial learning since there are no repeated sequences. (Stone, M.H. and Wright, B.D. 1980. *Knox's Cube Test: Junior and Senior Version.* Chicago: Stoelting Co.)

Kohs Block Design Test. This test is a forerunner to the Wechsler Block Design subtest and contains 17 block designs with four different colors (i.e., red, white, blue, and yellow), as in the Block Design subtest from the Wechsler Intelligence Scales (WIS). Also like the WIS Block Design test, the task is to construct designs that match the test booklet stimuli. Because both the total time and the number of individual moves are recorded, the notation of individual moves provides a level of analysis not directly available from the WIS Block Designs. Kohs Blocks are part of the Arthur Point Scale of Performance Tests. (Kohs, S.H. 1919. *Kohs Block Design Test.* Chicago: Stoelting Co.)

Korsakoff's psychosis/syndrome/disease. (Sergei Korsakoff [also Korsakov], Russian psychiatrist, 1853–1900). Korsakoff's psychosis is an older term for this cognitive disorder, which includes a prominent anterograde memory deficit, i.e., amnesia, a disturbance of orientation, and a susceptibility to external stimulation and suggestion, hallucination, and confabulation. It arises from vitamin B_1 (thiamin) deficiency. The onset may be acute or gradual and is usually preceded by Wernicke's encephalopathy. The severely abnormal nutrition that sometimes accompanies chronic alcoholism is a common cause. The primary neuropathology (punctate hemorrhages) involves the midline diencephalon. "Korsakoff's syndrome" or "Korsakoff's disease" are commonly used to describe the amnestic syndrome secondary to alcohol abuse and are sometimes incorrectly applied to any amnestic syndrome. *See* Wernicke-Korsakoff syndrome.

Kurtosis. A measure describing the degree to which a distribution of scores is clustered around the mean. A distribution that is more peaked than a normal distribution is leptokurtic, and a distribution of scores that is flatter is platykurtic. [Gr. *kyrtosis*, convexity, from *kyrtos*, convex.]

Kuru. A chronic, rapidly progressive, and uniformly fatal nervous system disease characterized by prominent ataxia with dementia in the late disease stages. Kuru is caused by *prion* transmission and was the first such disease found to be transmissible to subhuman primates. It is found only among the Fore people of New Guinea and was transmitted through ritual cannibalism, a practice that has stopped. Pathologically, the brain shows severe cerebellar loss, spongiform changes, and prion-amyloid plaques. [Fore language *kuru*, shivers, or trembles.]

L

L (Lie) scale. A MMPI validity scale created to measure whether patients are presenting themselves as having an unrealistic degree of personal virtue.

La belle indifference. A lack of concern for sensory and motor impairment. In contrast to *anosodiaphoria*, which reflects lack of concern for neurologic impairment, this term is commonly applied to psychogenic conditions (e.g., conversion disorder). [F. *la belle indifference*, the beautiful indifference.]

Labbé, vein of. (Leon Labbé, French surgeon, 1832–1916). A vessel that interconnects the superficial middle cerebral vein and the lateral sinus. It is often used as a brain landmark, and historically it has marked the posterior limit for left temporal lobectomies to avoid postoperative language decline. Also called the superior anastomotic vein.

Labile. Unstable, easily changed. The term is usually applied to rapid mood swings (i.e., labile mood). [L. *labilis*, liable to slip, from *labi*, to slip, fall.]

Lacuna, cerebral. A small area of cerebral ischemic infarction, generally less than 5 mm on CT and less than 1.5 cc in volume, resulting from occlusion of the small distal branches of the middle cerebral artery, posterior cerebral artery, or basilar artery. Lacunae are associated with hypertension and arteriosclerosis. [L. *lacuna*, hole, hollow pit, from *lacus*, a hollow, tank, lake.]

Landau-Kleffner syndrome. A developmental epilepsy syndrome of acquired aphasia. The child initially develops normally but then progressively loses previously acquired language, beginning with verbal expression. Nonverbal functions are relatively preserved. Paroxysmal EEG abnormalities involving the temporal or temporal-parietal-occipital regions are present. (Landau, W.M. and Kleffner, F.R. 1957. Syndrome of acquired aphasia with convulsive disorder in children. *Neurology* 7:523–530.)

Language. A communication system of symbolic expression that has an organized grammar and syntax to convey semantic content. The term language has been used differently, but without qualification, "language" generally refers to verbal symbol use. It includes verbal expression and comprehension and may be expressed through gesture (e.g., sign language) or through different modalities (i.e., Braille). Language is impaired with brain injury, as reflected by aphasia, agraphia, and alexia. "Speech," in contrast, refers to physical oral expression, does not require comprehension, and may be affected by peripheral factors unrelated to functions of the cerebral hemispheres (e.g., dysarthria from cerebellar damage).

Larynx. The organ of voice production. It is located between the pharynx and the trachea.

Lateral dominance tests. A general term for tests of hand and eye preference. Although many different versions exist, there is considerable overlap in the types of items included. Hand preference tests include hammering a nail and using scissors. Eye preference is commonly tested by demonstrating how one would look through a telescope or sight a billiard shot. Handedness is typically considered a continuous variable ranging from being exclusively right-handed, to mixed-handed, to exclusively left-handed. Handedness is often used to infer the likelihood of atypical cerebral language dominance. Commonly employed tests are the Annett Questionnaire, Harris Test of Lateral Dominance, Edinburgh Handedness Inventory, and Reitan-Kløve Lateral Dominance Examination from the Halstead-Reitan Neuropsychological Battery.

LDL. Low-density lipoprotein. *See* Lipoprotein.

L-dopa. *See* Levodopa.

Lead pipe rigidity. Rigidity commonly associated with involuntary movement disorders in which steady resistance is felt throughout the range of movement. The rigidity yields to constant pressure, giving the impression of bending a lead pipe.

Lead poisoning. Poisoning from lead ingestion that may produce acute encephalopathy or chronic effects. Lead is the most common metal neurotoxin as it is present in older plumbing and older paints. Children are at higher risk for lead poisoning because they have an immature blood-brain barrier. Moderate levels of lead poisoning in young children have been associated with learning and behavioral disorders and lowered IQ scores. Damage to the CNS primarily involves the hippocampus, although more severe lead encephalopathy may lead to edema and death. Peripheral neuropathy is common.

Learning. The process of acquiring new information into memory.

Learning and Memory Battery (LAMB). A battery of tests designed to assess verbal and nonverbal learning and to measure digit span. The tests include three verbal subtests (Paragraph, Word List, and Word Pairs), two numerical subtests (Digit Span and Supraspan Learning), and two visual subtests (Simple Figure and Complex Figure [Taylor Complex Figure]). Norms are available for ages 20 through 80 years. (Schmidt, J.P. and Tombaugh, T. 1995. *LAMB: Learning and Memory Battery*. Manual. North Tonawanda, NY: Multi-Health Systems.)

Learning curve. Graph in which a learning index is plotted as a function of trials.

Learning disorder/disability (LD). A heterogeneous group of disorders manifested by significant difficulties in the acquisition of reading, mathematics, or written expression. They are intrinsic to the individual and presumed to be due to nervous system dysfunction. Although LD may occur concomitantly with other handicapping conditions or environmental influences, it is not the direct result of those conditions or influences. A LD is operationally defined by many school systems as a discrepancy between intelligence test scores and scores on standardized achievement tests.

Leiter International Performance Scale. A test of general cognitive ability that is designed for children with hearing or language impairments, or for non-English-speaking individuals. Nonverbal instructions direct the child to match and sequence blocks with pictured stimuli. This test is appropriate for children 2–18 years of age. (Leiter, R.G. 1979. *Leiter International Performance Scale: Instruction Manual*. Chicago: Stoelting Co.)

Lemniscus. Sensory fiber bundle in the medulla and pons that relays discrete or *epicritic* functions. [L. *lemniscus*, a ribbon adorning a victor's wreath, from Gr. *lemniskos*, a fillet or band.]

Lennox-Gastaut syndrome. (William G. Lennox, American neurologist and electroencephalographer, 1884–1960; Henri Gastaut, French neurologist and electroencephalographer, 1915–1995). Childhood encephalopathy characterized by generalized seizures, diffuse slow (1–2.5 Hz) spike and wave EEG complexes, and a high incidence of mental retardation. The cognitive impairments associated with this syndrome are often worsened by multiple, high-dose antiepileptic medications needed to obtain some measure of seizure relief. Motor development is generally not as impaired as cognitive development.

Lenticulostriate arteries. *See* Arteries, cerebral.

Lentiform (lenticular) nucleus. Part of the *striatum* comprising the putamen and globus pallidus that lies lateral to the internal capsule. [L. *lenticula*, a lentil.]

Leptokurtic. *See* Kurtosis.

Leptomeninges. The *pia* and the *arachnoid*; the "delicate" meninges. [Gr. *leptos*, delicate; *meninx*, membrane.]

Leptomeningitis. Inflammation of the *pia* and *arachnoid*. *See* Meningitis.

Lesch-Nyhan disease. (Michael Lesch, American pediatrician, b. 1939; William Nyhan, American pediatrician, b. 1926). A rare metabolic disease that is inherited in an X-linked recessive pattern. Children appear normal at birth and usually develop normally until 6–9 months of age when hypotonia, followed by hypertonia, appears. Aggressiveness and compulsive actions also emerge. Compulsive self-mutilation, mainly of the lips, occurs early (during the second and third year), and *spasticity*, *choreoathetosis*, and tremor develop. Speech is delayed, and once attained, it is dysarthric. Mental retardation is moderately severe.

Lethargy. A state of being awake but drowsy, inactive, and indifferent to external stimuli.

Letter blindness (pure). A syndrome postulated, but not proven, to exist in the nineteenth and early twentieth century in which words could be read normally, even though individual letters could not be recognized. A relatively specific disturbance in letter naming has been described, however, that occurs in the context of normal oral reading. *See* Alexia.

Letter cancellation. General term for tests of *attention* and *hemispatial neglect* that require the subject to mark specific stimuli from a larger stimulus array. Multiple variations of this task exist. Rows containing letters are often presented on a sheet of paper, and the task is to cross out certain letters on the entire sheet. In some versions, the same target letter is used for the entire test, and in other versions, different target letters are crossed out in different rows. Patients with attentional deficits display inconsistent target responding throughout the test. Patients with hemispatial inattention tend to perform less well with stimuli on the side of the page corresponding to their neglect.

Letter fluency. *See* Controlled Oral Word Association.

Letter-by-letter reading. Type of acquired *alexia* in which print-to-sound conversion is assembled letter by letter. Some classify this behavior as a special form of *simultanagnosia*, although it occurs as a variant of alexia without agraphia.

Letter-Number Sequencing. In this subtest from the WAIS-III and WMS-III, letters and numbers are presented in a mixed-up order, and the task is first to say the numbers in ascending order and then to state the letters in alphabetical order. This subtest contributes to either the WAIS-III or WMS-III *Working Memory Index*. It is a measure of attention/concentration, or mental tracking.

Leukoaraiosis. Attenuation of the cerebral white matter. Leukoaraiosis is associated with multiple ischemic lesions, but it also occurs in Alzheimer's disease and during normal aging. [Gr. *leuko*, white; *araiosis*, thin.]

Leukodystrophy. Disturbance or degeneration of the white matter of the brain that is associated with metabolic defects. "Leukodystrophy" usually refers to one of several inherited disorders, including Fabry Disease and metachromatic leukodystrophy. [Gr. *leuko*, white; *dys-*, hard, ill, bad; *trophe*, nourishment.]

Leukoencephalitis. Inflammation of the white matter of the brain. *See* Encephalitis.

Leukoencephalopathy. Diseases affecting the white matter of the brain, especially the cerebral hemispheres. Progressive multifocal leukoencephalopathy is an opportunistic infection associated with AIDS, and before AIDS, it was a rare neurologic disease.

Leukomalacia. Morbid softening of white matter. Leukomalacia is commonly seen as a consequence of an anoxic episode producing periventricular leukomalacia. Periventricular leukomalacia is necrosis (and hence softening) of white matter observed adjacent to the anterior and temporal-occipital horns of the lateral ventricles and corona radiata. Leukomalacia can result from any other process that necrotizes white matter. [Gr. *leukos*, white; *malakos*, soft.]

Leukotomy. An incision of the white matter performed as a disconnection procedure. Most leukotomies involved the prefrontal or frontal lobe. This procedure was first performed in 1935 by Egas Moniz (Portuguese neurologist, 1875–1955), for which he was awarded the Nobel Prize in Physiology and Medicine. Frontal leukotomy was previously employed to treat severe psychiatric disorders before the introduction of neuroleptic medication in the 1950s (*see* Lobotomy). [Gr. *leukos*, white; *tomé*, cut, from *temnein*, to cut.]

Levodopa (l-dopa). A therapeutic agent commonly used in the symptomatic treatment of Parkinson's disease. Levodopa, however, does not cure the disease or halt disease progression. It replaces dopamine that is decreased on account of disease, and it is effective because postsynaptic dopamine receptors remain intact. Levodopa is administered instead of dopamine because dopamine does not cross the blood-brain barrier. There are significant peripheral effects of levodopa administration, however; it is typically administered in combination with agents that block levodopa's peripheral effects. [L. *lævus*, left.]

Levodopa-induced dyskinesia. *Dyskinesia* that develops following prolonged levodopa treatment of Parkinson's disease. It often improves following a decrease in medication. The use of drug holidays following significant dyskinesia development was advocated in the past, although they presently are performed very rarely because of the risk to the patient.

Lewy-body dementia. *See* Dementia.

Lexical agraphia. *See* Agraphia spelling disorders.

Lexical decision task. An experimental task in which subjects decide about specific lexical qualities of stimulus words or sounds. Examples include deciding if stimuli are real or are nonsense words or whether words belong to a specific semantic category. Lexical decision tasks have been used in the study of psycholinguistics and as cognitive activation tasks to study hemispheric specialization.

Lexicon. 1. Knowledge of the phonological representation and grammatical aspects of words. **2.** A dictionary. [Gr. *lexicos*, of or belonging to words, from *legein*, to say, speak.]

Lhermitte's sign. (Jacques Jean Lhermitte, French neurologist, 1877–1959). An electric-like sensation that extends from the neck down the body when the head is actively or passively flexed forward. The flexion stretches the cervical spinal cord and increases tension on demyelinated fibers. It is most often seen in multiple sclerosis, but it may be associated with cord degeneration, cervical cord tumors, or cervical cord injury.

Limbic encephalitis. A syndrome of progressive dementia resulting from an occult or remote neoplasm (e.g., lung carcinoma). There may also be behavioral changes associated with encephalopathy, such as *agitation, confusion*, hallucinations, or *seizures*. Inflammatory changes and loss of neurons occur primarily in the limbic cortex but usually involve other neural elements as well. [L. *limbus*, edge, border; Gr. *enkephalos*, brain.]

Limbic system. A group of brain structures that includes the hippocampus, dentate gyrus, cingulate gyrus, septal areas, amygdala, and parts of the diencephalon. These structure are associated with autonomic functions (e.g., arousal), motivation, emotion, recent memory, and olfaction. This system was named "limbic" by Pierre Paul Broca (French surgeon and anthropologist, 1824–1884) because of its location around the edge, or limbus, of the medial wall of the hemisphere (*grand lobe limbique*).

Limb-kinetic apraxia. *See* Apraxia.

Line bisection. Specialized tests to assess *hemispatial inattention*. Multiple approaches to testing line bisection ability exist, typically containing horizontal lines of different lengths and with different placements on the page. The task is to mark the center of each line.

Systematic placements to the right of the true center of each line suggest left hemispatial inattention.

Linguistic agraphia. *See* Central agraphia.

Lipid. Elements that are fat-soluble. [Gr. *lipos*, fat.]

Lipoprotein. Compound containing both lipids and proteins. Lipoproteins are classified by density according to their flotation constant—the higher the density, the lower the lipid content. High levels of low-density lipoproteins (LDL) are associated with an increased risk of coronary artery disease and stroke, whereas high levels of high-density lipoproteins (HDL) may reduce these.

Lissencephaly. A brain malformation associated with failure of the gyri to develop, resulting in a smooth cortical surface. Lissencephaly is associated with severe mental retardation. [Gr. *lissos*, smooth; *enkephalos*, brain.]

Literal agraphia. Antiquated term used by Carl Wernicke (German neurologist, 1848–1905) to describe an inability to write letters of the alphabet.

Literal alexia. *See* Alexia/dyslexia, acquired.

Literal paraphasia. *See* Paraphasia. [Gr. *para*, beside; *phrasis*, utterance.]

Liver flap. *See* Asterixis.

LLE. Left lower extremity.

Lobectomy. Surgical resection of a lobe in the brain. This term does not necessarily imply that the entire lobe is removed, but rather, a large portion of the lobe. The most frequently performed lobectomies involve the anterior temporal lobe in patients with intractable complex partial seizures. [lobe + Gr. *ektome*, an cutting out; *ek*, out; *temnein*, to cut.]

Lobotomy. Surgical destruction of tracts and cell bodies to isolate a cerebral lobe. The most common lobotomies were performed on patients with schizophrenia or other severe psychiatric disorders and involved disconnection of the prefrontal or frontal white matter from the rest of the brain. The term lobotomy is occasionally applied to epilepsy surgery when a disconnection procedure is performed (e.g., temporal lobotomy), rather than resection. *See* Leukotomy. [lobe + Gr. *-tomy*, from *temnein*, to cut.]

LOC. Loss of consciousness.

Locked-in syndrome. Complete paralysis due to bilateral lesions of motor pathways and lower cranial nerves in the pons or medulla, usually resulting from occlusion of a branch of the basilar artery. The third (oculomotor) cranial nerve is spared, and voluntary vertical eye movement is possible, which allows for communication by blinking (e.g., one blink for yes, two blinks for no). Cognitive function is unimpaired, and EEGs are normal. Also called coma vigil.

Locus ceruleus. A cluster of neurons in the dorsal pons situated on the floor of the fourth ventricle that contains over one-half of the norepinephrine (noradrenergic) neurons in the CNS. Locus ceruleus neurons are activated during states of heightened vigilance and may be more involved in *affective disorders*. [L. *locus*, place; *cæruleus*, dark blue.]

Logical Memory. A subtest from the *Wechsler Memory Scale* (WMS, WMS-R, and WMS-III) that assesses prose passage recall. In the WMS-R and WMS-III, retention over a 30-minute delay is assessed. Each version of the WMS has retained the "Anna Thompson" paragraph, although the second memory paragraph has been changed with each WMS revision. The WMS-III version of the Logical Memory subtest contains an extra learning trial (repeat paragraph administration) for one of the paragraphs. The Logical Memory subtest is often administered separately as an independent measure of verbal learning and memory.

Logogen. Hypothetical lexical unit representing the visual, phonological, and semantic characteristics of a word. "Input logogen" refers to the visual or auditory identification of words; output logogen is responsible for the production of a specific word. [Gr. *logos*, word, speech; -*genes*, from *gignesthai*, to be born, become.]

Logorrhea. Excessive and incessant agitated speech characterized by difficulty with grammar-based word elements, lack of meaningful content, and illogical sequences of clauses. Patients are frequently unaware of their impaired language (*anosognosia*) and may become angry when others do not appear to understand what they say. Logorrhea is associated with certain cases of Wernicke's aphasia during the acute disease stages. [Gr. *logos*, word, speech; *rheein*, to flow.]

Long tract signs. Neurologic abnormalities due to *upper motor neuron* lesions, such as hyperreflexia or Babinski signs.

Longitudinal fissure. Cleft that separates the left and right cerebral hemispheres. Also called the interhemispheric fissure.

Long-term memory. *See* Memory.

Long-term potentiation (LTP). An electrophysiological phenomenon of postsynaptic excitability following stimulation that may last up to several weeks and may reflect synaptic plasticity. Long-term potentiation was first demonstrated in the hippocampus and is thought to be an important process associated with learning and memory.

Loss of consciousness (LOC). Impaired responsiveness thought to reflect diffuse brain dysfunction, although focal injuries may also be associated with impaired responsiveness. The duration of LOC is often used as a measure of traumatic brain injury severity.

Lower motor neuron (LMN). Cell bodies and tracts of cranial nerves or anterior horn cells of the spinal cord that innervate muscle. LMN lesions are associated with weakness, decreased muscle tone, decreased muscle stretch reflexes (hyporeflexia), and muscle atrophy.

LP. *See* lumbar puncture.

LTD. Long-term disability.

LUE. Left upper extremity.

Lumbar puncture (LP). A technique for obtaining cerebrospinal fluid (CSF) by inserting a needle into the spinal canal between L_3 and L_4 or L_4 and L_5. In most standard LPs, approximately 5 cc's of CSF are drawn out. The CSF is analyzed for the presence of infection associated with meningitis or other inflammatory processes and for the presence of blood that may be associated with subarachnoid hemorrhage. [L. *lumbus*, loin.]

Lupus. *See* Systemic lupus erythematosus.

Luria figures. Any of several alternating patterns (e.g., *m n m n . . .*) designed by Aleksandr Luria (Soviet neuropsychologist, 1902–1977) to demonstrate the difficulty with task alternation associated with frontal lobe injury. Also called alternating sequences test.

Luria-Nebraska Neuropsychological Battery (LNNB). An adaptation of Luria's Neuropsychological Investigation (Christensen) that was modified to produce quantitative scoring. The battery contains 11 scales for neuropsychological evaluation of major content areas (Motor Functions, Tactile Functions, Rhythm, Visual Functions, Receptive Speech, Expressive Speech, Reading, Writing, Arithmetic, Memory, and Intellectual Processes. A second form the battery exists that contains a twelfth scale (Intermediate-Term Memory). In addition to the basic clinical scales, there are two sensorimotor scales (Right Hemisphere and Left Hemisphere) and a Pathognomic Scale. The LNNB was originally known as the Luria-Dakota Neuropsychological Battery during its development. A children's form of the test is available for 8- to 12-year-old patients. (Golden, C.J., Hammeke, T.A., and Purisch, A.D. 1980. *Luria-Nebraska Neuropsychological Battery.* Manual. Los Angeles: Western Psychological Services; Golden, C.J. 1987. *Luria-Nebraska Neuropsychological Battery: Children's Revision.* Los Angeles: Western Psychological Services.)

Luria's Neuropsychological Investigation. A collection of many of Aleksandr R. Luria's (Soviet neuropsychologist, 1902–1977) techniques compiled by Anne-Lisse Christensen. This is largely a qualitative-structured assessment battery. The battery assesses 10 areas of function (motor, acoustico-motor organization, higher cutaneous and kinesthetic function, higher visual function, receptive speech, expressive speech, writing and reading, arithmetical skill, mnestic processes, and intellectual function). It is designed to measure performance on the basis of Aleksandr Luria's model of three principal functional cortical units: (*1*) maintenance of cortical tone; (*2*) obtaining, processing, and storing information; (*3*) programming, regulating, and verifying mental activity. (Christensen, A.-L. 1984. *Luria's Neuropsychological Investigation.* Los Angeles: Western Psychological Services.)

Luxury perfusion. An angiographic phenomenon seen after a cerebral infarction in which there is an enhanced capillary blush and early venous filling on angiography. It is a transient phenomenon, typically present for several hours to days after the stroke.

Lyme disease. A multisystem disease caused by the spirochete *Borrelia burgdorferi* and transmitted by Ixodes ticks, typically occurring during the summer months. Approximately 10%–15% of nontreated patients develop acute nervous system involvement. The clinical triad includes lymphocytic meningitis, painful radiculoneuritis, and cranial neuritis (typically facial palsy). Patients with symptomatic systemic disease may have memory difficulty and difficulty with complex cognitive functioning. Named for Lyme, Connecticut, where the initial cases were reported.

M

MA. Mental age.

Macro Cisterna Magna. This cerebellomedullary cistern is a posterior fossa space receiving cerebrospinal fluid flowing out of the foramen of Magendie and foramen of Luschka. Although considered a normal anatomical variant, recent studies suggest that this may be a marker for neuronal and brain maldevelopment. [Gr. *makros*, long; L. *cisterna*, a reservoir for water, from Gr. *kista*, a chest, box; L. *magnus*, great.]

Macrocephaly. Large head with normal or only slightly enlarged ventricles. It may be indicative of macrocephalic idiocy or of an advancing metabolic disease that enlarges the brain, as in the later phases of Tay-Sachs disease, Alexander disease, and spongy degeneration of infancy. [Gr. *makros*, large, long; *kephalos*, head.]

Macropsia. Visual illusion that objects are becoming larger or moving closer. Macropsia may be a symptom associated with some partial seizures. [Gr. *makros*, large, long; *opsis*, sight, from *optikos*, denoting sight.]

Magnetic resonance angiography (MRA). A magnetic resonance imaging technique that permits visualization of cerebral vasculature. Unlike conventional angiography, which is an invasive procedure, MRA requires no intra-arterial catheter or contrast medium. Magnetic resonance angiography is sensitive to stenosis/occlusion of the carotid arteries. [Gr. *angeion*, case, vessel, capsule.]

Magnetic resonance imaging (MRI). A computerized imaging technique that employs strong magnetic fields and specific radio frequency pulses that excite protons to emit electromagnetic signals. The information gained from an MRI image depends on the relaxation time, or the time required for protons to return to a resting state after the magnetic pulse is turned off. Because different tissue types have differing relaxation times, pulse sequences can be designed to enhance specific aspects of the image. T1, T2, and proton density are designations for tissue-specific relaxation properties. In T1 images, white matter is brighter than gray matter. In T2 images, cerebrospinal fluid (CSF) is brighter than gray matter. Proton-density images employ a sequence that lies between that of T1 and T2, with image characteristics falling between T1 and T2 in brightness. Computed tomography (CT) is superior to MRI in terms of spatial resolution and the ability to image acute hemorrhage, but the contrast resolution of MRI is superior to that of CT. Recent advances have allowed the imaging of subtle blood flow changes in association with functional activation (*functional MRI*, or fMRI).

Magnetic resonance spectroscopy (MRS). A technique of noninvasively measuring chemical constituents of tissue or other substances. Distinct chemical resonance exists at different frequencies when placed in a magnetic field, and the separation of compounds based on these resonances allows for in vivo chemical identification.

Magnetoencephalography (MEG). A technique similar to EEG of measuring the magnetic signal of the brain. In contrast to EEG, the MEG is capable of three-dimensional localization of dipole sources, and as such, it may prove to be a useful adjunct in the evaluation of patients for epilepsy surgery.

Malignant. In medicine, a condition that is progressive or fatal. [L. *malignans*, from *malignare*, *malignari*, to do or make maliciously, from *malignus*, of an evil nature.]

Malingering. Intentionally feigning or exaggerating symptoms of illness or injury for external gain (e.g., compensation, leave from work, drugs). Malingering differs from somatoform disorders in that somatoform disorders result from psychological factors (e.g., to avoid intimacy or other emotional conflicts) or to manipulate others (e.g., to receive attention, special care, favors, service). [Fr. *malingre*, sickly, from Old Fr. *haingre*, *heingre*, thin, emaciated.]

Mammillary bodies. Paired, spherical masses located on the basal surface of the posterior hypothalamus. One of the major neocortical neural pathways from the hippocampus passes through the mammillary bodies (via the postcommissural fibers of the fornix) to the anterior nucleus of the thalamus (via the mammillothalamic tract), which in turn projects to the anterior cingulate gyrus. Damage to mammillary bodies has been implicated in the amnesia associated with Korsakoff's Syndrome.

Mania. State characterized by a pervasive and abnormally expansive mood, elation, irritability, flight of ideas, pressured speech, and increased motor activity. In addition, the term is used as a combining form to signify obsessive preoccupation with a specific phenomenon, such as dipsomania or erotomania. [Gr. *mania*, madness, from *mainesthai*, to rage.]

Manic-depressive disorder. *See* Bipolar disorder.

MAO inhibitors. *See* Monoamine oxidase inhibitors.

March à petis pas. Festinating, or progressively accelerating steps commonly seen in Parkinson's disease. The term was introduced by Joseph Jules Dejerine (French neurologist, 1849–1917). [Fr. *march à petis pas*, march of little steps.]

Marchiafava-Bignami disease. (Ettore Marchiafava, Italian pathologist, 1847–1935; Amico Bignami, Italian physician, 1862–1929). Progressive degeneration/demyelinization of the corpus callosum that is associated with cognitive deterioration, emotional disturbances, confusion, hallucinations, tremor, rigidity, and seizures. It is a rare disorder chiefly affecting middle-aged alcoholics, especially those who drink excessive amounts of red wine. The course is rapid and the disorder progresses from dementia to coma to death in a few months. The magnitude of the neurologic impairment cannot be easily explained by hemispheric disconnection.

Marching test. A paper-and-pencil test of gross motor function from the Halstead-Reitan Neuropsychological Battery for children. The task is to connect a series of circles, which themselves are connected with lines. After completing the test with each hand, the coordinated performance of both hands is obtained. The subject alternates hands after completing each step, and a different sequence of circles is used for the left and right hands.

Marcus Gunn pupil. (Robert Marcus Gunn, British ophthalmologist, 1850–1909). An afferent pupillary defect resulting from second (optic) cranial nerve damage in which the pupil paradoxically dilates when a light is shined in the eye. A Marcus Gunn pupil is associated with optic neuritis and is often seen in multiple sclerosis.

Masked face/masked facies. Expressionless facial appearance characteristic of many Parkinson's disease patients. This feature occasionally leads to a misdiagnosis of depression. The expressionless appearance is also called a reptilian stare.

Masking. The partial or complete suppression of stimulus perception due to the presentation of another stimulus. Both forward masking, which occurs when the masking stimulus is presented before the target stimulus, and backward masking, which occurs when the masking stimulus is presented after the target stimulus, have been demonstrated. Masking may be seen as part of the neglect syndrome and is termed extinction.

Mass action. Theory proposed by Karl S. Lashley (American psychologist, 1890–1958) that learning depends upon the entire cortex. Lashley based his theory on animal experiments, which demonstrated that it is the amount of tissue resected rather than its location that affects learning, a phenomenon that he called *equipotentiality*. Although Lashley's theory cannot account for the diverse nature of human cortical function, it does emphasize that brain regions do not work in isolation.

Mass effect. Impaired brain function from increased intracerebral volume associated with tumor, stroke, or any brain injury resulting in increased intracranial volume.

Massa intermedia. Interthalamic connection that crosses the third ventricle. The massa intermedia is absent in many normal brains.

Material-specific learning. The pattern of left hemisphere specialization of learning verbal material and right hemisphere specialization for nonverbal learning. The term modality-specific learning is occasionally applied to this phenomenon erroneously, although modality-specific learning refers to the acquisition of new information in different sensory modalities (e.g., auditory, visual) rather than to the verbal vs. nonverbal nature of the material.

Matrix Reasoning. A subtest from the WAIS-III used to assess pattern completion, classification, analogy reasoning, and serial reasoning. Because this subtest has no time limits, it does not penalize subjects who may have decreased response speed. It replaces Object Assembly from the WAIS-R in the calculation of the Performance IQ. Matrix Reasoning is similar to the Raven's Progressive Matrices.

Mattis Dementia Rating Scale (DRS). A scale developed for use in a geriatric population for assessing five cognitive domains that are commonly impaired in various dementias: attention, initiation/perseveration, construction, conceptual capability, and memory. Although called a rating scale, this procedure is more accurately viewed as a structured, extended mental status examination. (Mattis, S. 1988. *Dementia Rating Scale: Professional Manual*. Odessa, FL: Psychological Assessment Resources.)

Mayo Older Age Normative Study (MOANS). Normative data derived from individuals aged 55 to 97 years on a core battery of tests including the Wechsler Adult Intelligence Scale-Revised (WAIS-R), the Wechsler Memory Scale-Revised (WMS-R), and the Rey Auditory Verbal Learning Test (RAVLT). (Ivnik, R.J., Malec, J.F., Smith, G.E., Tangalos, E.G., Petersen, R.C., Kokmen, E., and Kurlan, L.T. 1992. Mayo's Older Americans Normative Studies. *Clin. Neuropsychol*. 6 [Suppl.]:1–104.)

Mazes. A measure of visual planning in which a route must be traced without entering blind alleys in increasingly complex mazes. The *Porteus Mazes* are often used to assess maze performance, and the Mazes subtest from the Wechsler Intelligence Scales for Children (WISC) is also commonly used, even in adult neuropsychological applications.

MCA. *See* Middle cerebral artery.

McCarthy Scales of Children's Abilities. A measure of general cognitive function and motor skills in children 2.5 and 8.5 years old. It consists of 18 cognitive and motor tests that yield standardized scores in five areas: Verbal, Perceptual-Performance, Quantitative, Memory, and Motor. The first three scales can be combined to yield a General Cognitive Index (GCI), roughly equivalent to a Full Scale IQ. (McCarthy, D. 1972. *Manual for the McCarthy Scales of Children's Abilities*. New York: The Psychological Corporation.)

Mean. The arithmetic average of multiple scores (i.e., the sum of the scores divided by the number of scores). It is a common measure of central tendency in a distribution.

Medial forebrain bundle. A fiber system in the lateral hypothalamus that connects the hypothalamus with the midbrain tegmentum and the limbic system. The medial forebrain bundle carries fibers from noradrenergic and serotoninergic cell groups in the brainstem to the hypothalamus and cerebral cortex, and dopaminergic fibers from the substantia nigra to the caudate nucleus and putamen.

Median. A measure of central tendency that separates the distribution of scores into two equal groups; one higher than the median value and the other lower. The median is often the preferred central tendency measure when the data distribution is highly skewed since it is not unduly sensitive to the effects of extreme scores (i.e., outliers).

Medulla. The portion of the brainstem lying between the spinal cord and pons. The area where the spinal cord becomes the medulla is usually defined at the foramen magnum. [L. *medulla*, the marrow, from *medius*, middle.]

Megalocephaly. An unusually large head or a progressive enlargement of the bones of the head, face, and neck. [Gr. *megas*, great, mighty, large; *kephalos*, head.]

Megaloencephaly. Abnormal largeness of the brain, distinct from the skull. [Gr. *megas*, great, mighty, large; *enkephalos*, brain.]

Melodic Intonation Therapy (MIT). A speech therapy technique that pairs verbal utterances with rhythm and melodic intonation (singing). It is designed to capitalize on the musical capabilities of the intact nondominant (right) hemisphere and is used with aphasic patients who are severely dysfluent.

Melokinetic apraxia. *See* Apraxia (limb-kinetic apraxia).

Memory. The acquisition and retention of information. Varieties of memory models have been developed within different disciplines, each with its own preferred terminology. Different terms are used to classify functionally similar types of memory, and the same terms are occasionally used to refer to different memory processes.

- **Anterograde memory**. The ability to learn and recall new information. This term is used to contrast with retrograde memory,
- **Autobiographical memory**. An aspect of episodic or declarative memory concerned with the recollection of personal events.
- **Declarative (explicit) memory**. Experiences, facts, or events that can be consciously recalled and could be either episodic or semantic events. It is more often the subject of clinical evaluation than nondeclarative (implicit) memory.
- **Echoic memory**. Sensory memory for auditory material that is of relatively large capacity but limited duration. The duration of echoic memory is approximately 2–3 seconds. (Darwin, C.J., Turvey, M.T., and Crowder, R.G. 1972. An auditory analogue of the Sperling partial report procedure. *Cognit. Psychol.* 3:225–267.)
- **Episodic memory**. Memory that is context specific and often autobiographical, preserving the temporal and spatial features of past events that are not necessarily of particular significance. It is the primary area of clinical investigation in patients with memory complaints. Episodic memory is a form of explicit memory and contrasts with semantic memory. The episodic vs. semantic memory distinction was introduced by Endel Tulving. (Tulving, E. 1972. Episodic and semantic memory. In: E. Tulving and W. Donaldson (eds.), *Organization of Memory*. New York: Academic Press.)
- **Explicit memory**. *See* Declarative memory (above).
- **Iconic memory (echoic storage)**. Sensory memory for visual material that is of relatively large capacity but extremely limited duration (i.e., 250–300 milliseconds). (Sperling, G. 1960. The information available in brief visual presentation. *Psychol. Monogr.* 74 [11].)
- **Immediate memory**. The capacity to maintain information in conscious awareness.
- **Implicit memory**. *See* Nondeclarative memory (below).
- **Long-term memory**. Retention of information over long intervals. The term is used to contrast with short-term memory, and no specific time interval exists to characterize at what point short-term memory stops and long-term memory starts.
- **Nondeclarative (implicit) memory**. A range of memory types in which performance is altered without conscious mediation. Examples of nondeclarative memory include

procedural memory, priming, and classical conditioning. This is operationally defined regarding change in performance such as savings or priming.

- **Primary memory**. The content of immediate consciousness. The term was introduced by William James to contrast with secondary memory.
- **Procedural memory**. A type of nondeclarative memory for skills that are not verbalized or consciously inspected (e.g., motor learning).
- **Prospective memory**. Memory for plans, appointments, and actions anticipated to occur in the future. Prospective memory includes timely completion of the activity and memory for the intention.
- **Recent memory**. The ability to form new memories. Recent memory is generally considered to begin where immediate memory ends, in terms of either the amount of information to be retained or its duration. In amnesia, there is a marked divergence between performance on span (immediate memory) versus supraspan (recent memory) tasks; the former is preserved and the latter defective. Recent memory includes information for events in the non-distant past, although the time interval that includes recent memory is not precise. Orientation to time and place are aspects of recent memory.
- **Remote memory**. Retention of information for distant events, such as those from childhood. While the observations that suggested these terms remain valid, the notion that chronology is the chief distinction separating recent from remote memory has been challenged. As with the short-term/long-term distinction, no specific time interval exists for demarcating recent from remote memory.
- **Retrograde memory**. The ability to recall information that had been previously stored or learned.
- **Secondary memory**. Recall of information that is no longer in consciousness. *Contrast with* Primary memory (above).
- **Semantic memory**. Memory that is context-free, reflecting general knowledge of symbols, concepts, and the rules for manipulating them. In contrast to episodic memory, semantic memories rarely concern specific information about situations in which they were learned. The facts that ancient Egyptians built pyramids and the hammer is used with nails are examples of semantic memory. Impairments in semantic memory generally do not occur unless there is an acute confusional state, dementia of at least moderate severity, or focal lesions affecting specific aspects of linguistic function. Both semantic and episodic memory are subsumed under declarative memory.
- **Sensory memory**. The first stage of memory processing in which a perceptual record is stored. The two types of sensory memory that have been most widely studied in experimental psychology are iconic and echoic memory, although they do not have any direct clinical application. Iconic memory is the sensory representation associated with vision. It fades rapidly, usually disappearing in 250–300 milliseconds. Echoic memory is the sensory memory associated with audition.
- **Short-term memory**. Retention of information over brief periods (e.g., seconds or minutes) to longer intervals (e.g., hours). The term "short-term (and long-term) memory," however, often leads to confusion. Although this meaning is commonly used by patients and general medical personnel (i.e., short-term memory impairment), no specific time interval for making a distinction between short- and long-term memory has gained common acceptance and meaning is inferred from its usage context. *Contrast with* Long-term memory (above).
- **Source memory**. Memory for the circumstances in which an episodic memory is formed. Source amnesia, in which lost memory of where and when an episode occurred, is often coupled with other forms of memory impairment and may be related to frontal lobe pathology.

- **Topographical memory**. Memory for spatial layout. [Gr. *topos*, a place; *graphein*, to write or draw.]
- **Working memory**. A limited capacity memory system that provides temporary storage to manipulate information for complex cognitive tasks such as learning and reasoning. The concept is similar to immediate or short-term memory, but it differs in its emphasis on functional operations and inclusion of multiple subsystems. According to Baddeley (1986), working memory has two types of components: storage (phonological loop and visuo-spatial sketch pad) and central executive functions. The **phonological loop** is a temporary storage system for acoustic and speech-based information. The **visuo-spatial sketch pad** is a similar system that allows manipulation of visual-spatial information. Both storage systems are relatively passive slave systems to the **central executive**, which is responsible for the selection, initiation, and termination of processing routines (e.g., encoding, storing, retrieving). The central executive is equivalent to the **supervisory attentional system (SAS)** described by Norman and Shallice (1980), which is a limited capacity system that formulates plans for situations that are novel, dangerous, or technically difficult, or where strong habitual responses or temptations are involved. Both the central executive system and the SAS are associated with prefrontal function. (Baddeley, A.D. 1986. *Working Memory*. Oxford: Clarendon Press; Norman, D.A. and Shallice, T. 1980. Attention to action. Willed and automatic control of behavior. University of California San Diego CHIP Report 99.)

Memory Assessment Scales (MAS). A battery of attention and memory tests. It contains 12 subtests and yields standard scores for Short-Term Memory, Verbal Memory, Visual Memory, and a Global Memory Scale. The subtests are List Learning, Prose Memory, List Recall, Verbal Span, Visual Span, Visual Recognition, Visual Reproduction, Names-Faces, Delayed List Recall, Delayed Prose Memory, and Delayed Visual Recognition. (Williams, J.M. 1991. *MAS: Memory Assessment Scales*. Professional Manual. Odessa, FL: Psychological Assessment Resources.)

Memory decay. The loss of recently learned information as a function of time. *See* Forgetting.

Memory Quotient (MQ). The summary score obtained from the original *Wechsler Memory Scale* (*WMS*), which was constructed to reflect overall memory ability. The MQ was criticized for the conceptualization of memory as a unitary phenomenon and inclusion of subtests are not part of memory per se (e.g., digit span). Revisions to the WMS have replaced the Memory Quotient with the General Memory Index.

Memory span. The amount of information that can be repeated immediately with complete accuracy. Memory span is assumed to reflect the capacity of short-term storage or working memory, and it is commonly assessed with digit span.

Meninges. The three membranes enclosing the brain and spinal cord, and lining the skull and vertebral canal. The meninges are the dura, arachnoid, and pia. [Gr. *meninx, meningos*, a membrane.]

Meningioma. A slow-growing benign tumor arising from the arachnoid. Surgical resection is a highly effective treatment because of tumor encapsulation and the absence of tumor infiltration. Meningiomas are more common along the superior sagittal sinus, sphenoid ridge, and near the optic chiasm on account of corresponding increases in cerebral vascularization.

Meningismus. Rigidity involving the back of the neck that results from inflammation of the meninges. The most common causes of meningismus are meningitis and subarachnoid hemorrhage. Also called nuchal rigidity.

Meningitis. Inflammation of the brain or spinal cord meninges.

- **Aseptic meningitis**. A nonbacterial meningitis. The etiology may be idiopathic, a known inflammatory response (e.g., chemical meningitis), or a nonbacterial infection such as viral meningitis. [Gr. *a-*, without; *sepein*, to make putrid.]

- **Bacterial meningitis**. Meningitis from bacterial causes, the most common of which are *Haemophilus influenzae, Neisseria meningitidis,* and *Streptococcus pneumoniae.* Stiffness of the neck (nuchal rigidity, meningismus) is an important clinical sign, although the diagnosis is based upon cerebrospinal fluid (CSF) examination. In contrast to viral meningitis, somnolence or mild confusion is common. Inflammation often extends beyond the subarachnoid space. Bacterial meningitis evolves rapidly, is often associated with CSF obstruction and seizures, and is treated with antibiotics.
- **Cryptococcal meningitis**. Meningitis resulting from infection from the yeast Cryptococcus. It typically is the result of an opportunistic infection associated with AIDS, and it is also present in other immunocompromised patients. The basilar meninges are a common site of involvement, leading to a clinical presentation of headache, cranial nerve involvement, and cerebrospinal fluid obstruction, which increases intracranial pressure. Cryptococcal meningitis is typically chronic, and if left untreated, leads to death.
- **Mollaret meningitis**. A recurrent aseptic meningitis of obscure origin.
- **Viral meningitis**. An infection of the meninges due to a virus. It is typically self-limited and treated symptomatically. There is usually no associated change in mental status.

Meningocele. A congenital anomaly in which the spinal meninges herniate through a spinal column defect without spinal column herniation.

Meningocephalitis. Inflammation of both the brain and the *meninges*; often viral in origin.

Meningomyelocele. A congenital anomaly in which the neural ectoderm develops into the spinal cord and its nerve roots fail to separate from the epithelium; the result is an external sac containing cerebrospinal fluid (CSF), incompletely formed meninges, and malformed spinal cord. This is the menigomyelocele, also called myelomeningocele. *See* Spina bifida; Spina bifida occulta.

Mental agraphia. Metaphorical term for the inability to put thoughts into written phrases. Taken literally, the term is misleading because there is no genuine impairment of linguistic ability.

Mental retardation (MR). Developmental cognitive impairment in which general intellectual function is generally at least two standard deviations below the mean. In addition, adaptive functioning is impaired. The DSM-IV recognizes the measurement error associated with IQ testing and defines significantly subaverage intellectual function as an IQ "of about 70 or below." Thus, a patient with an IQ greater than 70 may be diagnosed as mentally retarded if appropriate adaptive behavior skills are not present. Conversely, if appropriate levels of adaptive capacity are present, an IQ less than 70 need not signify mental retardation. Mental retardation differs from dementia in that higher levels of cognitive performance have never been attained in mental retardation.

Mental status examination. A structured observation and interview method of examining a set of characteristics related to orientation, attention and concentration, memory, language, visual-spatial skills, neglect syndrome, insight, abstraction, general cognitive function, and a psychiatric interview. Bedside mental status exams may include some or all of the above areas and are generally integrated into the full neurological or general physical exam.

Mental tracking. The ability to perform a cognitive operation while simultaneously retaining information in working memory. A common bedside test of mental tracking ability is to spell "world" backwards.

Mesencephalon. The midbrain. It contains the superior and inferior colliculi. [Gr. *mesos*, middle; *enkephalos*, brain.]

Meta analysis. The statistical analysis of results obtained from different, independent studies. This technique is designed to integrate research results and identify effect size and overall data trends.

Metabolic encephalopathy. *See* Toxic-metabolic encephalopathy.

Metachromatic leukodystrophy. A metabolic disorder characterized by myelin loss and accumulation of metachromatic lipids in the white matter. This condition has an autosomal recessive pattern of inheritance and is associated with general cognitive impairment and psychosis.

Metamemory. Knowledge about the nature and contents of one's own memory.

Metamorphopsia. Visual disorder in which the apparent shapes or sizes of objects are distorted. Perception of movement and color may be distorted also. Lesions may involve the occipital or parietal-occipital lobes; the right hemisphere is more often involved than the left hemisphere. [Gr. *metamorphosis*, transformation; *opsis*, sight.]

Metencephalon. The anterior subdivision of the hindbrain, or rhombencephalon (the posterior subdivision being the *myelencephalon*, or medulla), which contains the pons and the cerebellum. [Gr. *meta*, after; *enkephalos*, brain.]

Method of Loci. Mnemonic technique in which to-be-remembered items are visualized in separate locations within an imaginary space. [L. *loci*, plural of *locus*, place.]

Meyer's Loop. (Adolph Meyer, American psychiatrist, 1866–1950). A collection of fibers that originates in the lateral geniculate nucleus, swings in a broad arc over the temporal horn of the lateral ventricle, and loops into the temporal lobe. It forms part of the optic radiation. Lesions involving Meyer's loop produce visual loss in the upper quadrant contralateral to the lesion (superior homonymous quadrantanopsia). Occasionally called Meyer-Archambault loop (LaSalle Archambault, American neurologist, 1879–1940).

Meyerson's sign. *See* Glabellar reflex.

Microcephaly. An abnormally small head, usually associated with mental retardation. [Gr. *mikros*, small; *kephalon*, head.]

MicroCog. A computer-administered and computer-scored test to screen for cognitive impairment. The subtests are organized into five domains: Attention/Mental Control, Memory, Reasoning/Calculation, Spatial Processing, and Reaction Time. It is designed for individuals aged 18 through 89 years and includes both long (18 subtests) and short (12 subtests) forms. (Powell, D.H., Kaplan, E.F., Whitla, D., Weintraub, S., Catlin, R., and Funkenstein, H.H. 1993. *Manual for MicroCog: Assessment of Cognitive Functioning*. San Antonio: The Psychological Corporation.)

Micrographia. Small, often illegible handwriting that is usually associated with basal ganglia impairment such as Parkinson's disease. It is a form of hypometria.

Micropsia. A visual illusion that objects are becoming smaller or that objects are moving away. Micropsia may be a symptom of some partial seizures. [Gr. *mikros*, small; *opsis*, sight.]

Midbrain. *See* Mesencephalon.

Middle cerebral artery (MCA). *See* Arteries, cerebral.

Middle fossa. The cranial vault on which the temporal lobes rest. [L. *fossa*, a ditch, trench.]

Mill Hill Vocabulary Scale. An English vocabulary test that is widely used outside of North America as a measure of verbal intelligence. Different versions may be administered. The Definitions Form requires the subject to provide a definition, the Synonym Selection Form is a multiple-choice version, and the Definition and Synonym Selection Form is a combination of the two versions. It is widely used in conjunction with the Raven Progressive Matrices. (Raven, J.C., Court, J.H., and Raven, J. 1982. *Manual for Raven's Progressive Matrices and Vocabulary Scales*. London: H.K. Lewis and Co.)

Millon Clinical Multiaxial Inventory (MCMI). A questionnaire designed to assess personality function with a true/false format similar to that of the MMPI. The scales of the MCMI correspond with those of DSM-IV. Separate scales are used to distinguish Axis I from Axis II personality traits. Base-rate data, rather than normalized standard score transformations, are used to calculate and quantify scale measures. (Millon, T. 1993. *Millon Clinical Multiaxial Inventory*, 4th ed. Minneapolis: National Computer Systems.)

Mindblindness. Agnosia. This term is no longer in wide use.

Minimal brain dysfunction (MBD). A term for learning disability when there is no clear evidence of neurological disorder. The term no longer is in wide use.

Minimally conscious/minimally responsive state. The inability to interact consistently with the environment that is associated with severe brain injury even though some environmental awareness exists (e.g., selective visual tracking, intermittent nonreflexive motor activity). Awareness of the environment distinguishes minimal consciousness from a persistent vegetative state.

Mini-Mental State Examination. *See* Folstein Mini-Mental State Examination.

Minnesota Multiphasic Personality Inventory (MMPI). A widely used true/false objective measure of personality function. Ten clinical scales, which were empirically derived, are intended to detect the major forms of psychopathology. Many supplemental clinical scales are available. Separate validity scales measure the likelihood of intentionally trying to present oneself either favorably or unfavorably. The MMPI-2 is a revision of the MMPI. (Hathaway, S.R. and McKinley, J.C. 1940. A multiphasic personality schedule (Minnesota): I. Construction of the schedule. *J. Psychol. 14:73–84.*)

Mirror reading. An *implicit memory* task in which the reflected images of words are read.

Mirror tracing/mirror drawing. An *implicit memory* task in which a shape is traced or copied while viewing the shape and hand in a mirror.

Mixed aphasia. *See* Aphasia syndromes.

Mixed transcortical aphasia. *See* Aphasia syndromes.

Mnemonics. Techniques or devices for improving memory.

Mnestic. Pertaining to memory. [Gr. *mnéme*, memory.]

MOANS. *See* Mayo Older American Normative Study.

Mode. The most frequently occurring score or measurement in a distribution. It is one measure of central tendency.

Moderator variables. Variables that systematically vary with another variable that affects predictive accuracy. Thus, differential predictability occurs when the relationship between the predictor and criterion is influenced from the moderator variable, typically a classification variable.

Modified Card Sorting Test. *See* Wisconsin Card Sorting Test.

Mongolism. *See* Down syndrome.

Monoamine oxidase (MAO). A widely distributed enzyme in the body that is involved in the oxidative diminution of dopamine, serotonin, and norepinephrine.

Monoamine oxidase inhibitors (MAOIs). A class of antidepressant medications that inhibits the action of monoamine oxidase, an enzyme responsible for the breakdown of biogenic amines (e.g., norepinephrine).

Mood. A prevailing and sustained subjective emotional state or experience (e.g., anger, elation, or depression).

Mood disorders. Disorders in which mood disturbance is the predominant feature. Mood disorders are classified in DSM-IV as either depressive, bipolar, or etiologically based (i.e., they are due to a general medical condition or are substance induced).

Morbidity. Any deviation from psychological or physiological well-being.

Morpheme. The smallest unit of meaning in a language. Morphemes include words as well as meaningful prefixes, suffixes, and affixes (e.g., "boys" represents two morphemes, boy and -s). [Gr. *morphé*, shape, form; *mórphema*, element of form.]

Mortality. A fatal outcome.

Motor aphasia. *See* Aphasia syndromes.

Motor aprosodia. *See* Aprosodia.

Motor area/motor cortex. *See* Frontal lobe.

Motor impersistence. The inability to maintain a posture despite having the ability to form that posture. Motor impersistence is often viewed as a form of apraxia, and it is frequently associated with generalized cognitive impairment. Common approaches to testing motor impersistence include keeping the eyes closed, keeping the tongue protruded, or keeping the mouth open. A formal test of motor impersistence has been developed in the Benton Neuropsychology Laboratory. (Benton, A.L., Sivan, A.B., Hamsher, K.deS., Varney, N.R., and Spreen, O. 1994. *Contributions to Neuropsychological Assessment. A Clinical Manual.* 2nd ed. New York: Oxford University Press.)

Motor neglect. The failure to respond to a stimulus even though the subject is aware the stimulus and of the appropriate response. The failure to respond cannot be due simply to weakness. Types of motor neglect include akinesia, motor extinction, hypokinesia, and motor impersistence.

Motor neuron disease. *See* Amyotrophic lateral sclerosis (ALS).

Motor overflow. *See* Synkinesia.

Motor-Free Visual Perception Test (MVPT). A multiple-choice test of visual perception that avoids motor involvement. The MVPT measures five types of visual-perceptual abilities: spatial relationships, visual discrimination, figure-ground, visual closure, and visual memory. (Colarusso, R.R. and Hammill, D.D. 1972. *Motor-Free Visual Perception Test.* Novato, CA: Academic Therapy Publications.)

Movement disorders. Disorders resulting from impairment of the *extrapyramidal motor system.* Tremor, ballismus, dystonia, chorea, dyskinesia, and tics may be present but disappear during sleep. They are distinct from disorders of voluntary movement, which result from impairment to the pyramidal motor system consisting of upper and lower motor neurons.

MPTP. N-methyl, 4-phenyl-1, 2,3,6-tetrahydropyridine. A neurotoxin that induces parkinsonism and is used as an animal model for Parkinson's disease. Its discovery revived interest in the environmental toxin hypothesis of Parkinson's disease etiology.

MRI. *See* Magnetic resonance imaging.

MS. Multiple sclerosis.

MTD. Maximum tolerated dosage. The MTD is used for describing medications that may have side effects at higher therapeutic levels.

Multidimensional scaling. Multivariate technique to assess the scaling of a stimulus. Subjects are instructed to respond in terms of similarities and differences among the stimuli (i.e., whether stimulus A is more similar to stimulus B or stimulus C).

Multi-infarct dementia. *See* Dementia.

Multilingual Aphasia Examination (MAE). Language battery used to assess receptive, expressive, and repetition skills. Tests included are Visual Naming, Sentence Repetition, Controlled Oral Word Association, Token Test, Aural Comprehension of Words and Phrases, and Reading Comprehension of Words and Phrases. In addition, there is a spelling subtest with three response modes: oral, written, and block spelling (i.e., use of plastic letters). This test was developed in the Benton Neuropsychology Laboratory. (Benton, A. and Hamsher, K. deS. 1989. *Multilingual Aphasia Examination.* Iowa City: AJA Associates.)

Multiple correlation. Correlation coefficient that expresses the relationship between the criterion scores and an additive combination of predictor scores. A multiple correlation coefficient is indicated by a capital R.

Multiple sclerosis (MS). Demyelinating disease characterized by multi-focal chronic inflammatory lesions in the white matter. The lesions are described as being disseminated in time and place (i.e., they occur at intervals separated by at least 1 month and involving different parts of the CNS). Multiple sclerosis is an autoimmune disease that occurs roughly twice as frequently in females as in males. Cognitive and mood disorders are common, and some MS patients occasionally develop dementia.

Multiple subpial transection (MST). An epilepsy surgery technique for brain areas involving language or primary sensorimotor function (eloquent cortex). It employs a series of shallow cuts in the gray matter to disconnect the horizontal white fibers to reduce seizure propagation. This preserves the columnar arrangement of cells for functional processing. However, MST is not without morbidity, and it is generally better tolerated in motor than in language areas.

Multi-system atrophy (MSA). A *Parkinson Plus syndrome* characterized by autonomic insufficiency with degeneration of the basal ganglia, cerebellum, spinal cord, and peripheral sympathetic ganglia.

Multivariate analysis of variance (MANOVA). An extension of traditional analysis of variance (ANOVA) to situations involving two or more dependent variables. Dependent variables are combined to form linear discriminant functions that maximally separate the groups in multivariate space. A MANOVA approach may be used for repeated-measures designs, thereby eliminating the need for an adjustment in degrees of freedom (e.g., Geisser-Greenhouse) that is often required with the univariate approach to repeated-measures analysis.

Münchausen's syndrome. A factitious disorder in which patients display habitual presentation for hospital treatment of an apparent acute illness. The patient gives a plausible and often dramatic medical and social history, all of which is false. It differs from malingering and somatoform disorders in that the apparent incentive is to play the role of a hospitalized patient; this disorder is not due to clear psychological factors or external incentives (i.e., factitious disorder). *See* Factitious disorder.

Münchausen's syndrome by proxy. The repeated fabrication of an individual's disease symptoms by his or her primary caretaker (e.g., false reports of "seizures" in a child) to gain medical attention. *See* Factitious disorder.

Muscular dystrophy. *See* Duchenne muscular dystrophy.

Mutism. Absence of speech. Mutism may occur as an initial, transient response to anterior left hemisphere lesions that resolve into a Broca's aphasia, or it may occur with certain other cerebral lesions (e.g., insula) or as symptoms of a conversion disorder, depression, or other psychiatric illness. When it is associated with nonlanguage lesions, patients should not be diagnosed as aphasic. [L. *mutus*, speechless.]

MVA. Motor vehicle accident.

Myalgia. Muscle pain. [Gr. *mys, myo,* muscle; *algos,* pain.]

Myasthenia gravis. An autoimmune neuromuscular disorder associated with decreased synaptic acetylcholine receptors at the neuromuscular junction. It is characterized initially by drooping of the eyelids, double vision, and impairment of speech and swallowing. Myasthenia is treated chronically with anticholinesterase inhibitors to increase neuromuscular transmission and by resection of the thymus (thymectomy), which has an unknown mechanism of action. [Gr. *mys,* muscle; *asthenia,* weakness; L. *gravis,* heavy, weighty.]

Myelencephalon. Medulla. [Gr. *myelos,* marrow; *enkaphalos,* brain, from *en,* in; *kephale,* head.]

Myelin. A lipid that forms a sheath around many axons and acts as an electrical insulator. Myelin speeds neuronal transmission by allowing for a discontinuous and rapid conduction of the cell depolarization, which jumps between the nodes of Ranvier (i.e., saltatory conduction). Myelin damage slows nerve conduction, and demyelination is characteristic of multiple sclerosis and Guillain-Barré syndrome. Myelin is produced by oligodendroglia in the central nervous system and by Schwann cells in the peripheral nervous system.

Myelitis. Inflammation of the spinal cord.

Myoclonic seizures. *See* Seizures.

Myoclonus. Sharp, sudden, involuntary muscle jerks. Myoclonus is associated with various nervous system diseases, but it may also be seen in healthy individuals who are falling asleep. [Gr. *myo,* muscle, *klonus,* shake, shudder.]

Myoneuronal junction. *See* Neuromuscular junction.

Myopathy. Disorder of the muscle. [Gr. *mys, myo,* muscle; *pathos,* suffering.]

Myotonia. Increased muscular irritability and contractility with delayed muscle relaxation; a tonic spasm of muscle. [Gr. *mys, myo,* muscle; *tonos,* tension.]

Myotonic dystrophy. A slowly progressing disease characterized by muscle atrophy and general muscle weakness, decreased vision, eyelid drooping (ptosis), and slurred speech. It has an autosomal dominant pattern of inheritance with typical onset in the third decade.

Myxedema. *See* Hypothyroidism. [Gr. *myxo,* mucus; *odema,* a swelling, tumor.]

N

N.A. Initials of a patient who suffered a unilateral lesion of the dorsomedial thalamus as a result of a penetrating injury with a fencing foil; the patient displayed a significant anterograde memory deficit after the injury. (Squire, L.R. and Moore, R.Y. 1979. Dorsal thalamic lesions in a noted case of chronic memory dysfunction. *Ann. Neurol.*, 6:503–508.)

Nanocephaly. An extremely small skull or head. [Gr. *nanus*, dwarf; *kephale*, head.]

Narcolepsy. A condition of excessive sleepiness in which brief "attacks" of sleep intrude upon the waking hours. Narcolepsy is diagnosed with a multiple sleep latency test because the onset of the sleep attacks is preceded by little or no non-REM sleep. Narcolepsy is often associated with cataplexy. [Gr. *narké*, stupor; *-lepsin*, a fit, attack.]

Nasolabial fold. A crease running from the sides of the nose to the corners of the mouth. A "flattening" of the nasolabial fold may be an indicator of facial weakness.

National Adult Reading Test (NART). A reading test of irregularly spelled words that is used to estimate premorbid cognitive functioning; it was developed in England. There are several North American versions, including the American National Adult Reading Test (AMNART) and North American Adult Reading Test (NAART). [Grober, E. and Sliwinski, M. 1991. Development and validation of a model for estimating premorbid verbal intelligence in the elderly. *J. Clin. Exp. Neuropsychol.* 13:933–949; Nelson, H.E. 1982. *National Adult Reading Test (NART): Test Manual.* Windsor, England: NFER Nelson; Blair, J.R. and Spreen, O. 1989. Predicting premorbid IQ: A revision of the National Adult Reading Test. *Clin. Neuropsychol.*, 3:129–136.)

NE. Norepinephrine.

Neglect/neglect syndrome. The failure to attend or respond to visual, auditory, or tactile stimuli presented in the hemispace contralateral to a brain lesion that cannot be attributed to primary sensory or motor deficits. Components of the neglect syndrome may include *(1)* hemi-inattention (sensory neglect of stimuli contralateral to the brain lesion), *(2)* extinction to double simultaneous stimuli, *(3)* allesthesia and allokinesia, *(4)* hemi-akinesia (motor neglect), *(5)* asomatognosia (denial of body part), and *(6)* anosognosia (denial of hemiplegia or illness) or anosodiaphoria (inappropriate lack of concern over deficits). This syndrome is more likely to occur and is more severe after acute right (i.e., nonlanguage dominant) cerebral injures, but it may occasionally be seen for right-sided stimuli after left cerebral injuries. Common bedside approaches to testing for hemispatial neglect include line bisection tasks, drawing a flower, or clock drawing. Most neuropsychological tests of visual-spatial processing will reveal the presence of hemispatial neglect with proper qualitative inspection.

Neologism. *See* Paraphasia.

Neopallium. *See* Cortex, cerebral (neocortex).

Neostriatum. *See* Striatum.

NEPSY. A battery of neuropsychological tests intended for children 3–12 years of age. Areas assessed include *(1)* attention and executive function, *(2)* language and communication,

(3) sensorimotor function, *(4)* visuospatial function, and *(5)* learning and memory. NEPSY is derived from *NEuroPSYchology* (Korkman, M., Kirk, U., and Kemp, S. 1996. *NEPSY*. San Antonio: The Psychological Corporation.)

Neural tube. The embryonic tube that develops into the spinal cord and brain. The neural tube forms during the third week of embryonic development; its central canal becomes the ventricular system. An example of a neural tube defect is spina bifida (myelomeningocele).

Neuralgia. Paroxysmal pain that extends along the course of one or more nerves. [Gr. *neuron*, nerve; *algos*, pain.]

Neuritic plaques. *See* Senile plaques.

Neuritis. Nerve inflammation that is accompanied by pain and tenderness over the nerves. It may also be associated with anesthesia, paresthesias, paralysis, wasting, and reflex disappearance. [Gr. *neuron*, nerve; *-itis*, inflammation.]

Neurobehavioral Cognitive Status Examination. *See* Cognistat.

Neurobehavioral Rating Scale. A short, easily administered behavioral description scale based on information obtained from the interview and mental status examination. This scale is a modification of the Brief Psychiatric Rating Scale. (Levin, H.S., High, W.S., Goethe, K.E., Sisson, R.A, Overall, J.E., Rhoades, H.M., Eisenberg, H.M., Kalisky, Z., and Gary, H.E. 1987. The neurobehvioural rating scale: Assessment of the behavioural sequelae of head injury by the clinician. *J. Neurol. Neurosurg. Psychiatry* 50:183–193.)

Neuroblastoma. A tumor composed chiefly of neuroblasts that occurs mainly in infants and children up to 10 years of age. Most neuroblastomas arise in the autonomic nervous system or adrenal medulla.

Neurofibrillary tangles. Thickened, twisted strands of neural elements within neurons that are present in Alzheimer's disease, dementia pugilistica, and similar disorders. They are also present in small numbers in the brains of healthy-aged individuals.

Neurofibromatosis. Genetic condition characterized by developmental changes in the nervous system, muscles, bones, and skin. Acoustic neurofibromas are common in the late teens or early 20's. Also called von Recklinghausen's disease.

Neuroglia. *See* Glia.

Neuroglioma. *See* Glioma.

Neuroleptic drugs. Medications from a variety of chemical classes (e.g., phenothiazines, butyrophenones, thioxanthenes) designed to relieve psychotic symptoms. The first neuroleptic drug was chlorpromazine, which was originally designed as an antihistamine because of its chemical similarity to the antihistamine promethazine. Older neuroleptics target dopamine, and newer neuroleptics target dopamine and serotonin. Also called major tranquilizers. [Gr. *neuron*, nerve; *lepsis*, to seize, to receive.]

Neuroleptic malignant syndrome. A state of hyperthermia, muscle rigidity, and encephalopathy that occurs as an idiosyncratic reaction to neuroleptics, tricyclic antidepressants, lithium, cocaine, or amphetamines, and antiparkinsonian drug withdrawal. The mortality rate is high.

Neuroma. A tumor consisting primarily of nerve cells and nerve fibers. Also, a tumor growing from a nerve. [Gr. *neuron*, nerve; *-oma*, morbid growth, tumor.]

Neuromuscular junction. The terminal of a motor neuron innervating a skeletal muscle fiber. Acetylcholine is the major neurotransmitter of the neuromuscular junction.

Neuropathy. A broad term for functional disturbances or pathological changes in the peripheral nervous system. Neuropathy often designates nonspecific lesions in the peripheral nervous system, in contrast to inflammatory lesions, which are generally termed peripheral neuritis. [Gr. *neuron*, nerve; *pathos*, suffering.]

Neuropharmacology. The study of drugs that affect the nervous system. Substances foreign to the nervous system and endogenous substances (e.g., levodopa) are included.

Neuropsychiatric Inventory (NPI). A measure of 10 behavioral domains commonly associated with neuropsychiatric disorders. The domains are delusions, hallucinations, dysphoria, anxiety, agitation/aggression, euphoria, disinhibition, irritability/lability, apathy, and aberrant motor activity. The inventory is given to a caretaker who has daily contact with the patient, and to minimize time, a screening strategy is employed. If an abnormal behavior is reported, the domain is further explored with specific questions. (Cummings, J.L., Merga, M., Gray, K., Rosenberg-Thompson, S., Carusi, D.A., and Gornbein, J. 1994. The Neuropsychiatric Inventory: Comprehensive assessment of psychopathology in dementia. *Neurology* 44:2308–2314.)

Neuropsychological Deficit Score. A summary score of 42 measures derived from the Halstead-Reitan Neuropsychological Battery. Test performances are rated on a four-point scale, pathognomic signs are scored, IQ asymmetries are rated, and the magnitude of right-left performance differences is assessed. These scores are combined to yield a summary score of overall neuropsychological status. The scale is not designed to measure differences between right and left cerebral injuries.

Neurosensory Center Comprehensive Examination for Aphasia (NCCEA). A language battery comprising of 20 subtests of different aspects of language performance. The NCCEA assesses visual naming, description of use, tactile naming (right and left hand), sentence repetition, repetition of digits (forward and backward), word fluency, sentence construction, identification by name, Token test, oral reading (names), oral reading (sentences), reading names for meaning (pointing), reading sentences for meaning (pointing), visual-graphic naming, writing of names, writing to dictation, writing from copy, and articulation (word repetition). The test was developed in 1965, with revisions in 1969 and 1977. (Spreen, O. and Benton, A.L. 1977. *Neurosensory Center Comprehensive Examination for Aphasia.* Victoria, B.C.: University of Victoria, Psychology Laboratory.)

Neurosyphilis. Nervous system manifestations of syphilis that consist of deficits in "frontal lobe" function and typically begin with personality change and apathy. Other common deficiencies include a decrease in personal hygiene, poor judgment, mood swings, attention and memory impairment, and wandering behavior. Pathologically, there is extensive frontal lobe atrophy with meningeal thickening. Vascular lesions are often also present.

Neurotoxin. A substance that is destructive to nerve tissue.

Neurotransmitter. A chemical agent released by a neuron that crosses the synapse and alters the postsynaptic cell. Neurotransmitters have either a facilitatory or inhibitory effect on the activity of postsynaptic neurons and hence the flow of information within the nervous system.

Neurotrophic factors. Naturally occurring peptides that facilitate neuronal growth, promote survival, and enhance neuronal function (e.g., nerve growth factor, or NGF). [Gr. *neuron*, nerve; *trophe*, nourishment.]

Niacin deficiency. A vitamin deficiency syndrome consisting initially of confusion, impaired memory, apathy, and irritability. Niacin deficiency may be seen in alcoholics and others with poor diets.

Nidus. The central portion. Nidus is used to describe the point of abnormal development in arteriovenous malformations (AVMs), nerve origin or nucleus, or infection focus or target. [L. *nidus*, a nest.]

Nigrostriatal. Projecting from the substantia nigra to the corpus striatum. It is an important pathway for dopamine transmission, with decreased nigrostriatal dopamine associated with rigidity, tremor, and akinesia.

NMDA. *N*-methyl-D-aspartate. NMDA is a glutamate receptor that depolarizes neurons by opening ion channels that chiefly allow an influx of calcium. NMDA appears to have a role in varied processes including memory, embryonic neuron migration, and excitotoxic neuron death.

NMR. *See* Nuclear magnetic resonance.

Nociception. Perception of painful sensations. [L. *nocere*, to hurt, harm; *percipere*, to seize.]

Nociferous cortex. Cortex associated with an epileptogenic lesion that impairs the functioning of neuronal regions distant from the focus because of propagation of abnormal electrical discharges. [L. *nocere*, to hurt, harm; *pherein*, to carry or bear.]

Node of Ranvier. (Louis Antoine Ranvier, French pathologist, 1835–1922). Periodic constrictions in the myelin sheath covering axons. Greater axonal conduction velocity is possible because the signal jumps from node to node. *See* Saltatory conduction.

Nominal aphasia. *See* Aphasia syndromes.

Non compos mentis. Not of sound mind. The term is most often used to describe the condition of being unable to manage one's own affairs. [L. *non* not; *componere*, to put together, compose; *mentis, mens*, mind.]

Noncommunicating hydrocephalus. *See* Hydrocephalus.

Nonepileptic seizures (NES). Paroxysmal events that superficially resemble epileptic seizures but are not associated with abnormal electrographic seizure discharges. Commonly, NES are manifestations of conversion disorders/somatization, although they also may be seen with other psychiatric conditions, such as anxiety, psychoses, or attention-deficit/hyperactivity disorders. The term is usually reserved for psychologically based events and is not applied to metabolic, cardiogenic, or other events with a known physiologic mechanism outside of the brain. EEG/video monitoring of electrophysiological and behavioral manifestations is the definitive technique to diagnoses NES. Also called pseudoseizures.

Nonsense syllable. A syllable generally consisting of a consonant-vowel-consonant sequence that is not part of normal language (e.g., "cag"). Used in the study of memory.

Nonverbal learning disabilities (NVLD). Nonverbal learning disorders consisting of motor and sensory integration deficits, poor visual-spatial-organizational ability, and difficulty with novel and complex situations. Poor social perception and skills have been described.

Norepinephrine (NE). The neurotransmitter released by the adrenal gland that is present in autonomic ganglia.

Normal distribution. A bell-shaped score distribution that is symmetric around the mean. Approximately 68% of the scores fall between -1.0 and +1.0 standard deviations about the mean, approximately 95% of the scores fall between -2.0 and +2.0 standard deviations about the mean, and approximately 97.7% of the scores fall between – 3.0 and + 3.0 standard deviations. Also called bell-shaped or Gaussian distribution.

Normal pressure hydrocephalus. *See* Hydrocephalus.

North American Adult Reading Test. *See* National Adult Reading Test.

NPH. Normal pressure hydrocephalus. See Hydrocephalus.

Nuchal rigidity. *See* Meningismus. [M.L. *nucha*, from Arabic *nukha*, spinal marrow.]

Nuclear magnetic resonance (NMR). The absorption or emission of electromagnetic energy from a static magnetic field after excitation by a strong magnetic field. This term is most commonly applied to spectroscopic techniques (i.e., NMR spectroscopy), but it was formerly used to describe the technique's application in structural scans of tissue (NMR imaging). The term's use in the latter context has been superceded by MRI (magnetic resonance imaging).

Nucleus. A group of nerve cell bodies inside the nervous system; a similar collection of nerve cell bodies outside the nervous system is called a ganglion. [L., "a little nut".]

Nucleus basalis of Meynert. (Theodor H. Meynert, Austrian neurologist, 1833–1892). One of the basal forebrain nuclei that extend from the subthalamic nucleus to the floor of the third ventricle. These nuclei have extensive cholinergic projections to cortical and subcortical areas. The nucleus basalis of Meynert provides the major cholinergic innervation to the neocortex. Significant cell loss has been found in this nucleus in Alzheimer's disease. *See* Septal forebrain nuclei.

Null hypothesis. A statement that posits no difference between two or more experimental conditions or that restricts some parameter of interest (e.g., a regression coefficient, factor loading) to some a priori specified value, typically zero.

Nystagmus. Involuntary rapid eye movements that may be horizontal, vertical, rotary, or mixed. Lesions causing nystagmus are cerebellar, vestibular, or in the brainstem. [Gr. *nystagmos*, drowsiness, from *nystazein*, to doze, sleep.]

O

Obsessive-compulsive disorder (OCD). Anxiety disorder marked by recurrent uncontrollable thoughts (obsessions) and behaviors (compulsions) that interfere markedly with normal function. Obsessive-compulsive disorder has been linked to dysfunction in prefrontal cortex. Successful treatment is frequently a combination of behavior therapy and pharmacotherapy using selective serotonin reuptake inhibitors (SSRIs).

Obstructive hydrocephalus. *See* Hydrocephalus (noncommunicating).

Occipital lobe. The posterior brain region involved with vision. It is separated from the parietal lobe by the parietal-occipital sulcus on the medial surface, but no distinct sulcus separates it from the parietal lobe on the lateral surface of the brain.

Occupational therapy. The therapeutic use of work, self-care, and play activities to increase independent function, enhance development, and prevent disability. It may include adaptation of task or environment to maximize independence and enhance quality of life. Occupation refers to purposeful activity.

Oculomotor. Pertaining to eye movements. Also, the third cranial nerve.

Oculovestibular response. Automatic eye movements elicited by injecting ice water into the ear of a comatose patient, a procedure also called "caloric testing." No response predicts poor outcome.

Oklahoma Premorbid Intelligence Estimate (OPIE). A procedure to estimate premorbid IQ; it was developed on the WAIS-R standardization sample that combines demographic information (age, education, race, and occupation) with performance on the WAIS-R Vocabulary and Picture Completion subtests. The equations provide estimates of IQ without the same restriction of range that is found in purely demographically derived algorithms. (Krull, K., Scott, J., and Sherer, M. 1995. Estimation of premorbid intelligence from combined performance and demographic variables. *Clin. Neuropsychol.* 9:83–87.)

Olfactory. Relating to the sense of smell. [L. *olere*, to smell; *facere*, to make.]

Olfactory bulbs. Paired gray matter structures located at the bottom of the cranium and above the nasal cavity extending outward toward the eyes. The olfactory bulbs mediate smell and become the first (olfactory) cranial nerve. The olfactory nerve is vulnerable to shearing by the cribriform plate with head trauma.

Olfactory groove meningioma. A tumor that originates in arachnoidal cells along the cribriform plate. It may involve ipsilateral or bilateral anosmia and mental changes, including abulia, confusion, forgetfulness, and inappropriate jocularity.

Oligodendroglia. Glial cells that constitute the myelin sheath around neurons. [Gr. *oligos*, small; *dendron*, tree; *glia*, glue.]

Olivopontocerebellar degeneration. A *Parkinson Plus syndrome* characterized by cerebellar ataxia, postural instability, tremor, and dysarthria. Both inherited and sporadic forms of this disease have been reported. There is a loss of neurons in the pons and cerebellum.

On-off phenomenon. The tendency for anti-parkinsonian drug effects to suddenly wear off, leaving the patient with decreased mobility. The timing of this phenomenon can be highly unpredictable in some parkinsonian patients. Also called wearing-off phenomenon when the transition is less severe.

Open class words. *See* Content words.

Open head injury. Head injury that penetrates the skull and dura into the subdural space, if not the brain itself. Also called penetrating head injury.

Operculum. The area of the frontal, parietal, and temporal lobes covering the insula that borders on the Sylvian fissure. [L. "cover or lid."]

Opponent-process theory of color vision. Theory of color vision in which, given three pairs of color antagonists (red-green, blue-yellow, and white-black), excitation of one member of a pair inhibits the other member.

Opportunistic infection. An infection that is normally innocuous but becomes pathologic because the immune system is compromised (e.g., AIDS).

Optic agraphia. The inability to copy written or printed words while being capable of writing from dictation. Associated lesions are in the posterior language-dominant hemisphere. [Gr. *optikos*, denoting sight; *a-*, without; *graphein*, to write.]

Optic apraxia/optic ataxia. *See* Apraxia.

Optokinetic nystagmus. A normal, involuntary rhythmic eye movement that is induced by looking at moving visual stimuli. The eyes follow the moving stimulus until it can no longer be comfortably viewed, and then they move quickly in the opposite direction and fixate on a different object. It is abolished with parietal lobe lesions. The presence of optokinetic nystagmus is used to infer psychogenic blindness in patients who claim that they are unable to see. Also called opticokinetic nystagmus. [Gr. *optikos*, denoting sight; *kinesis*, movement; *nystagmos*, drowsiness.]

Oral apraxia. *See* Apraxia (buccofacial).

Organic brain syndrome (OBS). Obsolete nonspecific term referring to syndromes arising from brain disease.

- **Acute OBS.** Obsolete term for delirium or acute confusional state.
- **Chronic OBS.** Obsolete term for dementia.

Organophosphate compounds. Irreversible inhibitors of the enzyme acetylcholinesterase found in phosphoric acid insecticides and chemical warfare nerve gases. These compounds have widespread toxic effects throughout the central and peripheral nervous systems. Delayed neurologic effects, including weakness and ataxia, are seen several weeks after exposure. *Wallerian degeneration* occurs in the medulla, spinal cord, and peripheral nerves.

Orthography. The written form of language. [Gr. *orthós*, correct, straight; *graphein*, to write, draw.]

Orthostatic hypotension. A sudden decline in blood pressure that occurs after a rapid change in body position, as from lying prone to standing. [Gr. *orthós*, correct, straight; *statikos*, causing to stand; *hypo*, under, less than; L. *tesio*, tension.]

O-sign. Continuous open mouth (i.e., "o") seen in advanced cases of dementia or severe head trauma. This term is colloquial.

OT. *See* Occupational therapy.

Otitis media. A common pediatric disease involving acute or chronic inflammation of the middle ear mucosa and often followed by effusion within the middle ear. If left untreated, the associated hearing loss may lead to impairment of language acquisition.

Overcorrection. A behavior modification technique in which patients repeat a behavior, or rectify a situation, that has been adversely affected by their acting-out.

Overlapping figures. Two or more line drawings that partly overlap, used in the assessment of perceptual deficits.

Overt Aggression Scale. A checklist scale for assessment of aggressive behavior. It differentiates verbal from physical aggression, and aggression directed at self from aggression toward others. (Yudovsky, S.C., Silver, J.M., and Jackson, W. 1986. The Overt Aggression Scale for the objective rating of verbal and physical aggression. *Am. J. Psychiatry* 143: 35–39.)

P

Paced Auditory Serial Addition Test (PASAT). A test of sustained and divided auditory attention in which a series of randomized numbers is presented. The task is to add each number to the digit immediately preceding it. For the numbers 2-8-6-1-9, for example, the correct responses beginning after the number 8 are 10-14-7-10. The digits are presented at four differing rates. This test has predictive ability for return to work following traumatic brain trauma. In addition to attentional impairment, PASAT performance may be influenced by IQ, arithmetic ability, and math anxiety. (Gronwall, D.M.A. 1977. Paced auditory serial-addition task: A measure of recovery from concussion. *Percept. Motor Skills* 44: 367–373.)

Paeleostriatum. *See* Globus pallidus.

Paired associate learning. A memory task that assesses the ability to learn the relationship between paired stimuli (e.g., rich-cactus). Following presentation of the paired stimuli, memory is tested by presenting the initial item of the pair (e.g., rich) and the task is to respond with the second word (e.g., cactus). The paired stimuli may be words, designs, or other stimuli. For example, the Wechsler Memory Scale-Revised contains a subtest that pairs designs with colors.

Palatal lift. A fitted device worn against the palate to improve speech intelligibility in severely dysarthric patients.

Palilalia. Repetition of syllables, words, or phrases occurring at the end of an utterance that interrupts the flow of speech. Repetitions characteristically increase in speed but decrease in volume. Palilalia is often present in parkinsonism and is attributed to basal ganglia disease. [Gr. *palin*, again; *lalia*, voice, from *lalien*, to babble.]

Palinopsia. Visual perseveration characterized by the continuance of a visual sensation after the stimulus is no longer present. Palinopsia is seen in depressed visual fields, but it does not occur in visual fields that are completely blind. It is associated with both parietal and occipital lobe lesions. [Gr. *palin*, again; *opsis*, sight.]

Pallidotomy. An approach to surgical management of Parkinson's disease (PD) that involves lesioning the medial globus pallidus by using stereotaxically placed electrodes. The lesion disrupts the excessive excitation contributing to many parkinsonian features.

Pallidum. Globus pallidus.

Palmomental reflex. A reflex elicited by scraping the palm with a sharp object (e.g., key); this produces a reflexive contraction of the ipsilateral mental muscle in the chin. Although called a frontal lobe release sign, it is more common with diffuse brain disease than with focal frontal lobe impairment. However, because it also occurs frequently in healthy elderly subjects, the reflex has limited clinical utility. [palm + L. *mentum*, chin.]

Palsy. Partial paralysis or paresis.

Panencephalitis. Inflammation of the entire brain, resulting in both gray and white matter lesions, which are typically viral in origin. [Gr. *pan*, all, whole; *enkephalon*, brain.]

Panic attacks. Acute anxiety episodes in which individuals experience a variety of *autonomic nervous system* symptoms (e.g., pounding heart, dry mouth), with inexplicable feelings that they are about to die or lose control. The attacks may be only several minutes in duration or they may last hours. [Gr. *panikos*, of (the Greek God) Pan (who would arouse terror in lonely places).]

Pantomime Recognition Test. A test of the ability to understand meaningful, nonlingual pantomimed actions. Pretended handling of objects is presented on a videotape, and the patient is to point to the correct object. Because pantomime recognition is typically assessed in aphasic patients, both instructions and responses have minimal linguistic or praxic demands. (Benton, A.L., Sivan, A.B., Hamsher, K.deS., Varney, N.R., and Spreen, O. 1994. *Contributions to Neuropsychological Assessment. A Clinical Manual*, 2nd ed. New York: Oxford University Press.)

Papez, circuit of. (James Wenceslaus Papez, American anatomist, 1883–1958). Interrelationships among the various parts of the limbic system that were proposed by Papez (1937) as the substrate for controlling emotions and emotional expression. According to Papez, the "mechanism of emotion" is the hippocampo-mamillo-thalamo-cingulate-hippocampal circuit.

Papilla, optic. Point of entry of the optic nerve into the eye. [L. diminutive of *papula*, pimple.]

Papilledema. Blurring of the margins of the optic disk that results from increased intracranial pressure (ICP). Increased ICP is transmitted to the disk through the optic nerve. Not to be confused with papillitis.

Papillitis. Inflammation of the optic nerve where it enters the eye. It is typically caused by exacerbation of multiple sclerosis.

Paragrammatism. Inaccurate selection of function words that convey grammatical information, of grammatical forms, and of word order. Paragrammatism may be evident in spoken or written language

Paragraphia. Written spelling errors, or written word substitutions, that result from altered language function.

Paralexia. A reading error consisting of a sound or word substitution during the act of reading aloud that is characterized by miscomprehension in reading or by paraphasic oral reading.

- **Semantic paralexia**. A reading error consisting of a semantically related word substitution (e.g., "gun" for "pistol"). This error type is characteristic of deep dyslexia.
- **Visual paralexia**. A reading error in which the target word is misread and the word that is substituted shares many letters with the target word (e.g., "wife" for "life").

Parallel distributed processing (PDP). A model of neural processing that incorporates both parallel and serial processing functions. Each processing unit functions both locally and in parallel with other units. Information is assumed to be distributed throughout the brain, with memory and knowledge dependent on the pattern of unit connectivity.

Parallel tests. Tests constructed to be similar in content, high in reliability, and equivalent. Also called alternate forms.

Paralysis agitans. Latin term used by James Parkinson to describe the "shaking palsy;" Parkinson's disease. *See* Parkinson's disease. [New L. *paralysis agitans*, shaking palsy.]

Paramnesia. False memory.

Paraneoplastic syndromes. Remote disorders associated with carcinoma that do not result directly from tumor effects. In many cases involving the nervous system, the neurologic effects precede the diagnosis of cancer. The most common paraneoplastic syndrome affecting cognition is limbic encephalitis, and the primary tumor is typically lung carcinoma.

Paranoia. Abnormal thought processes characterized by the development of ambitions or suspicions into systematized delusions of persecution. [Gr. *para*, beyond; *nous*, mind.]

Paraphasia. Incorrect word selection (semantic or verbal paraphasia) or incorrect production of sounds within a word (phonemic or literal paraphasia). Paraphasia is a common feature of the speech production associated with aphasia. [Gr. *para*, beside; *phanai*, to speak.]

- **Neologism**. A paraphasic error consisting of nonsensical, unrecognizable words that have no apparent phonemic or semantic relevance to the target word (e.g., "galdop" for pencil). [Gr. *neos*, new; *logos*, word.]
- **Literal paraphasia**. *See* Phonemic paraphasia (below).
- **Phonemic paraphasia**. A production error in which a word is distorted by substituting, omitting, or adding phonemic elements, but is made with clear articulation (e.g., "perencil" for pencil). The target word is still recognizable. Also called literal paraphasia.
- **Semantic paraphasia**. A production error in which a word is substituted for the intended word (e.g., "art" for pencil). It is generally used synonymously with verbal paraphasia. In some reports, however, semantic paraphasia has been used to indicate an error that is semantically related to the target (e.g., "pen" for "pencil") and verbal paraphasia for a real-word error that is not related semantically to the target (e.g., "car" for "pencil" (above).]
- **Verbal paraphasia**. *See* Semantic paraphasia (above).

Paraplegia. Paralysis of both legs.

Parasympathetic nervous system. A component of the *autonomic nervous system* that is involved with specific visceral functions and with conservation and restoration of energy stores.

Paratonia. *See* Gegenhalten. [Gr. *para*, beside, next; *tonos*, tension.]

Parenchyma. Essential neural tissue that is supported by the connective tissue framework, or stroma. [Gr. *parenchyma*, something poured in beside; *para*, beside, next; *enchyma*, an infusion, from *enchein*, to pour in.]

Paresis. Partial or incomplete motor paralysis. The term is generally used in the context of focal deficits associated with *upper motor neuron* lesions. In the older literature it refers to neurosyphilis, in which increasing motor weakness accompanies cognitive changes. Complete paralysis is called plegia. [Gr. *paresis*, a letting go, from *parienai*, to loose, let fall.]

Paresthesia. A somatic sensation in the absence of external stimulation. Paresthesia is generally unpleasant, involving sensations of burning, pricking, tickling, or tingling, but it may include feelings of warmth or coldness (thermal paresthesia). It may also be a complex perception, such as the feeling that insects are crawling on the skin (formication paresthesia). [Gr. *para*, beside, next; *aessthesis*, sensation.]

Parietal lobe. The upper central lobe that is separated inferiorly from the temporal lobe by the Sylvian fissure, from the frontal lobe anteriorly by the central sulcus, and posteriorly from the occipital lobe by the parietal-occipital fissure. [L. *paries*, wall of a room.]

Parkinson Plus syndromes. A group of diseases exhibiting features of parkinsonism but distinct from Parkinson's disease. Parkinson Plus syndromes include progressive supranuclear palsy (PSP), cortico-basal ganglionic degeneration, multisystem atrophy, and olivopontocerebellar atrophy. Compared with patients with Parkinson's disease, those with Parkinson plus syndrome tend to have a poorer prognosis and do not respond well to dopamine replacement therapy.

Parkinson's disease (PD). (James Parkinson, British neurologist, 1755–1828). Idiopathic progressive disease of mid- to later life that is characterized by *bradykinesia, hypometria, cogwheel rigidity, resting pill-rolling tremor*, truncal and postural instability, and festinating gait. The etiology of PD is unknown. Neuropathologic changes include a loss of melanin-containing cells in the pars compacta of the substantia nigra, which projects primarily to the putamen (dopaminergic nigrostriatal pathway). The dopamine concentration in the putamen and caudate is significantly reduced. Speech difficulty may include hypokinetic dysarthria characterized by decreased speech volume, imprecise articulation, and accelerating speech rate with a tendency for words to run together. Cognitive impairment includes psychomotor slowing and executive dysfunction. For this reason, some have considered Parkinson's disease to be a subcortical dementia. Depression develops in a high percentage (25%–30%) of patients.

Parkinsonian tremor. A resting *pill-rolling tremor.* Parkinsonian tremor typically begins unilaterally and is generally less responsive to dopamine replacement therapy than other parkinsonian features.

Parkinsonism. The features of Parkinson's disease without reference to disease entity. The neurological symptom complex consists of hypokinesis, bradykinesia, tremor, and cogwheel rigidity. Parkinsonism may be idiopathic, postencephalitic, or drug induced. Causes of parkinsonism include postencephalitic parkinsonism, multi-infarct/atherosclerotic parkinsonism from putamenal or caudate infarction, carbon monoxide poisoning, toxic exposure, substance abuse, and multiple head trauma/dementia pugilistica.

Parosmia. An abnormal sense of smell. [Gr. *para*, beside; *osme*, odor, smell.]

Paroxysmal. A sudden onset of a symptoms. This term is often applied to disorders such as epilepsy in which seizures occur suddenly. [Gr. *paroxysmos*, from *paroxyno*, to sharpen, irritate, from *oxys*, sharp.]

Partial correlation. A measure of the relationship between two variables that exists after accounting for the relationships of a third measure to each of the two variables.

Partial seizure. A seizure in which the electroencephalographic abnormality involves a single brain region (e.g., medial temporal lobe) rather than the entire brain. Partial seizures may consist of simple partial seizures in which consciousness is not impaired or complex partial seizures in which there is altered consciousness. Complex partial seizures may spread to other brain regions (i.e., secondary generalization) and involve tonic-clonic activity.

Patellar reflex. *See* Knee jerk.

Pathognomonic signs. Findings that are specific for a given disease and that are not associated with other conditions.

Pathologic inertia. A lack of drive, initiative, or motivation that is associated with brain injury.

Pathologic left-handedness. Left-handedness that occurs as a result of early left hemisphere injury in a patient biologically programmed to be right-handed. The shift from right- to left-handedness is often accompanied by a shift from left to right cerebral language dominance.

PCA. *See* Posterior cerebral artery.

PCoA. *See* Posterior communicating artery.

Peabody Individualized Achievement Tests (PIAT). Academic achievement battery that includes mathematics, reading recognition, reading comprehension, spelling, and general information. The PIAT is appropriate for grades K–12. (Dunn, L.M. and Markwardt, F.C. 1970. *Peabody Individual Achievement Test Manual.* Circle Pines, MN: American Guidance Service.)

Peabody Picture Vocabulary Test (PPVT). A test of recognition vocabulary in which a line drawing associated with the stimulus vocabulary word is selected from a four-picture, multiple-choice array. The PPVT-III is appropriate for ages 2.5 through 90 + years. Two separate forms are available. (Dunn, L.M. and Dunn, L.M. 1997. *Peabody Picture Vocabulary Test,* 3d ed. Circle Pines, MN: American Guidance Service.)

Peduncles. In neuroanatomy, stalk-like connecting structures in the brain that are composed either exclusively of white matter (e.g., cerebellar peduncles) or of white and gray matter (e.g., cerebral peduncles). [L. *pedunculus*, dimimunitive of *pes*, foot.)

Penetrating head injury. *See* Open head injury.

Penn Inventory for Post-traumatic Stress Disorder. A questionnaire designed to determine the presence of post-traumatic stress disorder (PTSD). The questionnaire was modeled after the Beck Depression Inventory and the items were chosen to represent all aspects of the DSM-III-R definition of PTSD. (Hammarberg, M. 1992. Penn Inventory for Posttraumatic Stress Disorder: Psychometric properties. *Psychol. Assess.* 4:67–76.)

Percentile (percentile rank). A score indicating the percentage of scores at or below the comparison value. The score is more correctly termed centile because the distribution is divided into 100 equal subgroups.

Perceptual Organization Index. A summary measure from the Wechsler Intelligence Scale for Children-III (WISC-III) and the Wechsler Adult Intelligence Scale-III (WAIS-III) that is designed to reflect the ability to interpret and organize visual material. For both instruments, the Perceptual Organization Index is based upon performance on the Picture Completion and Block Design subtests. For the WISC-III, the index is also based upon performance on the Picture Arrangement and Object Assembly subtests; performance on the Matrix Reasoning subtest also contributes to the index for the WAIS-III.

Performance IQ (PIQ). A composite score summarizing the Performance scale subtests of the Wechsler Intelligence Scales (WIS). The PIQ is commonly viewed as a measure of nonverbal cognitive functioning, however, scores based on more homogeneous content are often used (i.e., Perceptual Organization Factor, Perceptual Organization Index) for neuropsychological rather than cognitive assessment. The WAIS-III Performance subtests are Picture Completion, Digit Symbol-Coding, Block Design, Matrix Reasoning, and Picture Arrangement. Object Assembly and Symbol Search are optional subtests. The WISC-III subtests that contribute to PIQ are Picture Completion, Coding, Picture Arrangement, Block Design, and Object Assembly. Symbol Search and Mazes are optional subtests.

Peripheral nervous system (PNS). A system of *afferent* and *efferent* nerves that connects the central nervous system with the sensory receptors, muscles, and viscera of the body. Includes the autonomic nervous system.

Periventricular white matter. White matter adjacent to the lateral ventricles. This area is a common site of small vessel disease associated with hypertension.

PERRL. Pupils equal, round, and reactive to light. This notation is often used to indicate normal third (oculomotor) cranial nerve function.

PERRLA. Pupils equal, round, reactive to light, and accommodating. This notation is commonly used to indicate normal third (oculomotor) cranial nerve function.

Perseveration. Persistence of the same response, even when it is shown to be inappropriate. It is associated with both diffuse and frontal lobe disease. Perseveration may involve motor acts, speech, or ideas. [L. *per*, very or thoroughly; *severus*, strict.]

Persistent vegetative state (PVS). Condition of profound nonresponsiveness in the wakeful state that is caused by brain damage. It is characterized by a nonfunctioning cerebral cortex, the absence of any discernible adaptive response to the external environment, akinesia, mutism, and inability to signal in any way. EEGs are isoelectric or show abnormal slowing.

Personality disorder. Enduring, inflexible, and maladaptive pattern of inner experience and behavior. It begins in teens or early adulthood and produces social and interpersonal dysfunction that is resistant to treatment. Ten specific types are recognized within three clusters: eccentric (e.g., schizoid), acting-out (e.g., antisocial, borderline), and fearful (e.g., obsessive-compulsive).

Personality Inventory for Children (PIC). An inventory that characterizes the personality of children 5½–16 years of age. It is composed of true-false questions regarding the child's behavior, disposition, interpersonal relations, and attitudes, and it is completed by a parent (preferably the mother). The PIC profiles are divided into three validity scales, one screening scale for general maladjustment, three developmental scales, and nine clinical scales. (Wirt, R.D., Lachar, D., Klinedinst, J.K., and Seat, P.D. 1984. *Multidimensional Description of Child Personality: A Manual for the Personality Inventory for Children*, Revised. Los Angeles: Western Psychological Services.)

Personality tests. A class of tests designed to examine personality; it covers emotional status and more enduring personality features. Personality tests are broadly conceptualized as either projective (e.g., Rorschach) or objective (e.g., MMPI).

PET. *See* Positron emission tomography.

Petit mal seizure. Older term for absence seizures. [Fr. *petit*, small; *mal* illness.]

Pfeiffer Short Portable Mental Status Questionnaire. A standardized mental status examination that does not contain any measurement of language or visual-spatial function. (Pfeiffer, E. 1975. SPMSQ: Short Portable Mental Status Questionnaire. *J. Am. Geriatr. Soc.* 23: 433–441.)

Phakomatosis. Inherited disorders involving organs of ectodermal origin (the nervous system, eyeball, retina, and skin). Examples include tuberous sclerosis, neurofibromatosis, and Sturge-Weber syndrome. [Gr. *phakos*, lentil, a wart-like a lentil.]

Phenothiazines. A class of antipsychotic drugs, the first of which was chlorpromazine.

Phenylketonuria (PKU). An inborn autosomal recessive error of metabolism in which phenylalanine tolerance is reduced. Without early dietary therapy restricting phenylalanine intake, mental retardation develops.

Phonagnosia. The inability to recognize familiar voices. [Gr. *phoné*, voice; *a-* without; *gnosis*, knowledge.]

Phonation. The utterance of vocal sounds.

Phoneme. A speech sound that is the basic unit of spoken language. It is the smallest unit of sound that speakers of a language distinguish as being different from another unit. [Gr. *phonema*, a sound, from *phoné*, a voice.]

Phoneme Discrimination Tests. Tests in which pairs of nonsense syllables are presented on a tape recorder, and the task is to determine whether the syllables differ in one phonemic feature or are the same.

Phonemic paraphasia. *See* Paraphasia.

Phonemics. The study of the sound system of a spoken language.

Phonetic disintegration. A pattern of articulation breakdown associated with aphasia.

Phonetics. The science of vocal sound production and perception.

Phonological agraphia. *See* Agraphia spelling disorders.

Phonological awareness. The ability to appreciate the phonological constitution of an utterance.

Phonological spelling. Spelling based on grapheme-to-phoneme conversion rules.

Phonology. The study of speech sounds of a language and the rules behind their production.

Phrenology. The belief popular in the mid-18th to mid-19th century that functional brain localization is reflected in the shape of the skull. Franz Joseph Gall (1758–1828) was a major proponent that skull features reflect cortical regions and that the cortex could be divided into functional units associated with specific behaviors and talents (e.g., he localized speech to the anterior lobes). Johann Christoph Spurzheim (1776–1832), a student of Gall, helped popularize phrenology with the public. (Gall, F.J. and Sprutzheim, J. 1810–1819. *Anatomie et Physiologie du Système Nerveux en Général, et du Cerveau en Particulier*. Paris: F. Schoell [Gall was sole author on first two volumes of set]. [Gr. *phrenos*, mind; *logos*, discourse.]

Physiatrist. A physician specializing in physical medicine and rehabilitation (PM & R) for disorders affecting the nervous system (stroke, traumatic brain injury, spinal cord injury), sports injury, orthopedic injury, and amputation.

Physical therapy (PT). Therapy designed for the evaluation and rehabilitation of mobility limitations resulting from either physical injury or somatic effects of nervous system injury.

Pia (pia mater). The portion of the meninges that is closest to the brain. The pia and arachnoid form the leptomeninges. [L. *pia*, feminine of *pius*, kind or tender; *mater*, mother; used as a metaphor for protector.]

Pick bodies. Dense intracellular structures, approximately the same size as the cell nucleus, that cause a mild increase in neuron size. Pick bodies are associated with Pick's disease and are not associated with normal aging or Alzheimer's disease.

Pick's disease. (Arnold Pick, Czech psychiatrist and neuropathologist, 1851–1924). A rare idiopathic, progressive dementia associated with severe atrophy of the frontal lobes and anterior temporal lobes. Atrophy usually involves the posterior two-thirds of the superior temporal gyrus and asymmetric atrophy is common. In contrast to Alzheimer's disease, visual spatial function may be relatively preserved since the parietal lobe is often unaffected. Memory is spared relative to Alzheimer's disease, although aphasia may be a prominent feature. Personality change is often the initial behavioral manifestation.

Pill-rolling tremor. *See* Resting tremor.

Pituitary adenoma. A benign epithelial tumor in which tumor cells arise from the pituitary. Pituitary adenomas are usually diagnosed because of hormonal irregularities, and they rarely grow sufficiently large to produce significant neuropsychological impairment. The initial symptoms associated with a pituitary adenoma, however, may be erroneously attributed to psychological causes such as depression or "old age." If undetected, pituitary adenomas may compress the optic chiasm, causing bitemporal hemianopsia or bitemporal superior quandrantanopsia.

Pituitary gland. The "master gland" of the endocrine system. The pituitary is under direct control of the hypothalamus and is continuous with it in the brain.

Pixel. The smallest discrete part of a digital image display, commonly used to describe MRI images and, in particular, areas of activation in functional MRI images. The word "pixel" is a derived from "picture element."

PKU. *See* Phenylketonuria.

Plantar. Pertaining to the sole of the foot. [L. *planta*, the sole of the foot.]

Planum temporale. Cortical area on the posterior superior surface of the superior temporal gyrus between Heschl's gyrus and the posterior margin of the Sylvian fissure. The planum temporale of the left hemisphere is generally longer and larger than that of the right hemisphere and is thought to reflect an anatomic basis for left hemisphere language dominance. This region is important for language comprehension.

Plasticity. General term applied to an alteration in structure or function brought about by development, learning and experience, or cerebral injury. In neuropsychological application, it refers to phenomena indicating recovery or reorganization of nervous system function following injury. [Gr. *plastikos*, fit for molding, from *plastos*, molded, from *plassein*, to mold.]

Platykurtic. *See* Kurtosis.

Plegia. Complete paralysis of a limb. Incomplete paralysis is called paresis. [Gr. *plege*, a stroke.]

Plumbism. Lead poisoning. [L. *plumbum*, lead.]

PM&R. Physical medicine and rehabilitation.

Pneumoencephalography. A radiological imaging technique that preceded CT and MRI and was used to outline the cerebral ventricles and subarachnoid space. It was developed by Walter Dandy in 1918 (American neurosurgeon, 1886–1946) after he observed that air introduced into the ventricular system after a missile wound resulted in a clear outline of the ventricles when X-rayed. [Gr. *pneuma*, wind, breath, spirit; *enkephalos*, brain.]

Polyglot. An individual who is fluent in more than one language. Polyglots have been of great interest in aphasiology because of the tendency for aphasic polyglots to display different patterns of language impairment and recovery for each language. [Gr. *polys*, much, many; *glotta*, tongue.]

POMS. *See* Profile of Mood States.

Pons. Part of the brainstem lying between the medulla and midbrain that forms a bridge between the right and left halves of the cerebellum. The pons consists of a large ventral portion, which is composed of descending fiber tracts, cranial nerve nuclei, and transverse fibers that project to the cerebellum to form the middle cerebellar peduncles, and a smaller part, known as the tegmentum, which contains the pontine reticular formation.

Porch Index of Communicative Abilities (PICA). A test of adult communication that contains 18 subtests for verbal, gestural, and graphic response modalities. It differs from most other tests of aphasia in that it uses a 16-point scoring system that reflects the accuracy, responsiveness, completeness, promptness, and efficiency of each response. Because of the amount of detail contained in the test, a 40-hour workshop is recommended by the test publisher. (Porch, B.E. 1981. *Porch Index of Communicative Ability: Vol. 2. Administration, Scoring, and Interpretation* (revised ed). Palo Alto, CA: Consulting Psychologists Press.)

Porteus Mazes. (Stanley Porteus, Australian psychologist, 1883–1972). A test of planning in which subjects are to solve each maze from the series without entering blind alleys. It consists of a series of mazes, each on a separate sheet. This maze series differs from the WISC mazes in that performance is not timed.

Portland Digit Recognition Test. A *symptom validity* memory test for digits with a *forced-choice* response format to detect exaggerated memory deficits. (Binder, L.M. 1993. Assessment of malingering after mild head trauma with the Portland Digit Recognition Test. *J. Clin. Exp. Neuropsychol.* 15:170–182.)

Positron emission tomography (PET). A technique of imaging local metabolic and physiological functions of the brain that is used to construct tomographic representations of functional brain areas. Positron emission tomography may be used clinically to measure metabolic or physiologic function/dysfunction in specialized applications; for example, a hypometabolic is often associated with the seizure focus in epilepsy patients. It is also a valuable research tool for investigating functional changes associated with cognitive activation tasks (e.g., language). [*positive* + elect*ron*; Gr. *tomos*, a cut section, from *temnein*, to cut.]

Post-concussion syndrome (PCS). A constellation of symptoms that is seen in a minority of patients after mild traumatic brain injury (MTBI). Most patients with MTBI do not seek medical attention, and they are presumably asymptomatic or have complaints that resolve quickly. Many MTBI patients seen in emergency care report symptoms that include dizziness, headache, poor concentration, and sensory abnormalities (e.g., photophobia). In the days after injury, insomnia, short-term memory deficits, and affective disturbance (anxiety, irritability, depression) may develop. These symptoms resolve gradually over several weeks to months for most patients. A minority of patients, however, continues to report significant difficulties in cognitive, affective, and physical function for 3 or more months following injury. Many practitioners conform to DSM-IV criteria and reserve the term PCS for patients who report persistent symptoms, although the term is also used by some to describe these symptoms at any time after injury. The reasons for the persistence of symptoms in some but not all victims of MTBI are unclear and have been vigorously debated. Premorbid factors (psychiatric disorders, substance abuse), secondary gain (e.g., litigation), and undetected anterior temporal lobe injury have been suggested.

Posterior cerebral artery (PCA). *See* Arteries, cerebral.

Posterior communicating artery (PCoA). *See* Arteries, cerebral.

Posterior fossa. The cranial vault on which the cerebellum rests. [L. *post*, after; *fossa*, ditch, trench.]

Postictal confusion. The period following a complex partial or generalized tonic-clonic seizure in which there is clouded mental status. The duration of confusion is typically related to seizure severity and great variability among patients exists. For patients with complex partial seizures, however, it is usually several minutes to one-half hour. Following a generalized tonic-clonic seizure, the duration of confusion may be hours.

Post-traumatic amnesia (PTA). A period of anterograde amnesia in which new memories cannot be consistently made and recalled that follows recovery of consciousness in head injury or other neurological trauma. The duration of PTA is often used as a predictor of the degree of recovery.

Post-traumatic stress disorder (PTSD). The development of a characteristic set of symptoms after exposure to a psychologically extreme traumatic stressor. According to DSM-IV criteria, the response to the event must involve intense fear, helplessness, or horror (or in children, disorganized or agitated behavior). Symptoms include persistent re-experiencing of the traumatic event, persistent avoidance of stimuli associated with the trauma, and persistent symptoms of increased arousal. The full symptom picture must be present for more than 1 month, and the disturbance must cause clinically significant distress or impairment of social, occupational, or other important areas of functioning. Post-traumatic stress disorder is often diagnosed with a variety of ill-defined complaints of uncertain origin, and the significance of it as a diagnosis should be interpreted accordingly.

Postural reflexes. Mechanisms that alter muscle tone in response to position change. Loss of postural reflexes is commonly present in Parkinson's disease.

Power, statistical. In statistical hypothesis testing, the sensitivity of a test to departures from the state of the world as postulated under the null hypothesis. The power of a test statistic varies as a function of the type I error rate, the degree to which the null hypothesis is incorrect, and the standard error of the test statistic, which in turn is controlled by the sample size.

Power tests. Tests in which there is no time restriction or time component.

Practice effects. Improvement in performance as a function of having previously taken the test or performed the task.

Prader-Willi syndrome. A genetic syndrome caused by chromosomal anomaly (chromosome 15) that is characterized by hypotonia, hypogonadism, hypometria, and mental retardation. Overeating and obesity appear in the preschool years. Occasionally referred to as Prader-Labhart-Willi syndrome. (Prader, A., Labhart, A., and Willi, H. 1956. Ein Syndrom von Adipositas, Kleinwuchs, Kryptorchidismus und Oligophrenie nach Myatonieartigem Zustand im Neugeborenalter. *Schweiz. Med. Wochenschrift* 86:1260–1261.)

Pragmatic language. The correct use of language within a given context or environment. Also called pragmatics.

Praxis. The ability to perform skilled movements. [Gr. *praktos*, from *prassein*, to do, practice.]

Precentral gyrus. *See* Frontal lobe.

Pre-conscious processing. Stimulus-processing that occurs before, or in the absence of, awareness.

Predictive accuracy. The probability, given a specific test result or pattern, that a particular condition exists. This contrasts with retrospective accuracy, which is the probability that, given a particular condition of interest, a specific test result or pattern of results will be obtained. Thus, the two terms differ in the direction of the inference.

Predictive validity. The ability of a test to predict a specific criterion (e.g., structural brain pathology, job performance). Also called criterion validity.

Prefrontal cortex. *See* Frontal lobe.

Premorbid estimation. Methods of estimating performance levels before injury or disease development. Several approaches exist, and they differ with respect to the degree that they rely on qualitative and quantitative estimation; each has its strengths and weaknesses. Regression-based estimation employs characteristics of the test's standardization sample, such as a subject's occupation and region of the country, to estimate performance. A commonly employed approach to regression-based estimation is known as the Barona equation (Barona, A., Reynolds, C.R., and Chastain, R. 1984. A demographically based index of pre-morbid intelligence for the WAIS-R. *J. Consult. Clin. Psychol.* 52:885–887). As is characteristic of regression estimation, however, it overestimates performance at the lower end of the distribution and underestimates levels at the high end of the distribution. Another approach is to rely on aspects of present performance that are considered to be relatively insensitive to the effects of mild to moderate brain injury, thus reflective of pre-morbid function. Reading tests for words that cannot be phonically pronounced because of phonetic irregularities are often used as correct pronunciation reflects previous word experience. Examples of this approach are the National Adult Reading Test and the reading subtests from Wide Range Achievement Test or Wechsler Individual Achievement Tests (*see* Hold vs. Don't Hold tests). This approach, however, does not capture qualities of nonverbal performance and is not appropriate for patients with language impairment. The *best performance method* uses the highest test score to indicate the level of premorbid function, although it does not account for normal variability among tests and will usually overestimate premorbid IQ. Performance on previous standardized testing (e.g., school testing, professional exams) is often considered, but these tests are often standardized on a nonrepresentative population. There may be significant individual changes in performance levels over those years associated with additional education and greater motivation. Performance levels are often informally estimated by reference to occupational status.

Premotor area. *See* Frontal lobe.

Presenile dementia. *See* Dementia.

Prestriate cortex. The visual association cortex adjacent to the primary visual (striate) cortex (Brodmann's areas 18 and 19). [L. *præ*, before, in front of; *striatus*, furrowed or striped; *cortex*, bark.]

Prevalence. The total number of cases of a particular phenomenon that develop within a given period.

Primacy effect. The tendency for words presented earlier in a series to be recalled better than words occurring later in the list when tested using a free recall task. The primacy effect may be decreased by rapid stimulus presentation or by using words with similar meanings. *See* Recency effect.

Primary acalculia. *See* Acalculia (primary).

Primary generalized seizures. Seizures simultaneously involving both hemispheres. The major types of primary generalized seizures include absence seizures, myoclonic seizures, atonic seizures, and generalized tonic-clonic seizures.

Primary memory. *See* Memory.

Primary receptor areas. The areas of the cerebral cortex that receive the thalamic projections of the primary sensory modalities such as vision, audition, and somesthesis.

Priming. A form of *nondeclarative (or implicit) memory* in which prior exposure to a stimulus exerts an effect on a subsequent stimulus detection or identification. Semantic priming is the effect in which a response to items from a particular class of words (e.g., vegetables) is facilitated by the presentation of a different item from the same semantic class. *See* Memory.

Principal components analysis. A dimension-reduction technique that is related to, but distinct from, factor analysis, in which all information from the original measures is preserved and described in terms of new variables. Thus, the first component explains more of the variability in the data than any other component and subsequent components encompass steadily decreasing amounts of information. The objective is to derive a smaller set of variables (components) that are defined as linear combinations of the original variables, but with the added properties that the components are mutually uncorrelated and that each component accounts for the maximum amount of covariation among the variables not accounted for by the preceding components.

Prion. A protein particle smaller than a virus that may infect cells and reproduce itself. Prions contain no nucleic acids but are otherwise similar to viruses; they are the etiologic agents in Creutzfeldt-Jakob disease and kuru. [proteinaceous infectious particle.]

PRN. Shorthand notation for "as needed." [L. *pro re nata*, as the occasion arises.]

Proactive inhibition (interference). Decreased learning of new information on account of the effects of previous learning. Proactive inhibition is greater for material that is semantically related. *See* Retroactive inhibition.

Probability. There are many definitions of probability, but the most commonly used definition in the behavioral sciences is that of long-range relative frequency, which is the theoretical limit of the ratio of the number of times the event of interest occurs relative to the number of opportunities for the event to occur. Conditional probability is the likelihood that an event (A) will occur given that another event (B) has already occurred, i.e., long-range relative frequency within a subset of the population of interest. For example, the unconditional probability of successful outcome from closed head injury is the long-range relative frequency of successful outcome in the population of patients suffering a closed head injury. The probability of successful outcome from closed head injury conditional on gender being male is the long-range relative frequency of successful outcome in the population of males suffering closed head injury.

Procedural discourse analysis. A technique commonly used when analyzing a person's communication abilities in which they are asked to describe the procedures associated with an act or skill. The productions can be a variety of elements (e.g., cohesion).

Procedural memory. *See* Memory.

Processing Speed Index. A formal measure from the Wechsler Adult Intelligence Scale-III (WAIS-III) and Wechsler Intelligence Scale for Children-III (WISC-III) representing performance on the Digit Symbol-Coding and Symbol Search subtests.

Prodrome. Symptoms that signal the approach of a full-blown clinical disease. [Gr. *prodromos*, a running before.]

Profile analysis. A multivariate statistical technique related to MANOVA, but which decomposes the MANOVA group hypothesis into distinct hypotheses about *(1)* group differences in profile shape, (i.e., differences in the pattern of high and low values in the group vectors of means), and *(2)* group differences in profile elevation (i.e., differences in the group means averaged across variables). In addition, profile analysis tests *(3)* a hypothesis about overall profile flatness, which concerns differences in the means of variables averaging across groups. For profile analysis to provide a meaningful decomposition of differences among groups and measures, the variables used in the analysis must be measured on comparable scales.

Profile of Mood States (POMS). A self-administered rating scale used to measure tension/anxiety, depression/dejection, anger/hostility, vigor/activity, fatigue/inertia, and confusion/bewilderment. Responses are intended to cover feelings experienced during the previous week. The POMS is widely employed, including by the World Health Organization and pharmaceutical companies, to assess aspects of function that are not generally reflected in cognitive testing. (McNair, D.M., Loor, M., and Droppleman, L.F. 1971. *Profile of Mood States*. San Diego: Educational and Industrial Testing Services.)

Progressive supranuclear palsy (PSP). An idiopathic degenerative disease of the brain characterized by dementia, parkinsonian features, and a loss of volitional eye movement, beginning with the inability to look down. Reflex eye movements such as the *doll's eye ma-*

neuver are preserved. Progressive supranuclear palsy involves loss of neurons and gliosis in the periaqueductal gray matter, superior colliculus, subthalamic nuclei, red nucleus, palladium, dentate nucleus, vestibular nuclei, and oculomotor nucleus. Onset is typically in the sixth decade and the disease progresses to death in 5–7 years. It is also known as Steele-Richardson-Olszewski syndrome; it is a Parkinson Plus syndrome.

Projective personality measures. Personality measures that contain ambiguous stimuli onto which patients "project" their experiences and personality traits. The most common projective personality measures are the Rorschach (Hermann Rorschach, Swiss psychiatrist, 1884–1922) and the Thematic Apperception Test (TAT; Henry A. Murray, American psychologist, 1893–1993).

Propositional language. Means of linguistic exchange that substitutes articulated sounds, gestures, or marks for objects, persons, and concepts so that novel relationships can be expressed. It must be learned and thus is subject to all the modifying social and cultural influences of the environment. This concept was introduced by J. Hughlings Jackson (British neurologist, 1835–1911) to distinguish mere speaking from true speech in which relationships are expressed. Also called symbolic language.

Proprioception. Knowledge about the position of one's body in space that is based on sensory information from receptors in the muscles, tendons, and viscera. [L. *proprius*, one's own; *receptus*, to receive).

Propulsive gait. Gait disturbance characterized by progressively faster and smaller steps while walking. The patient passes from a walking to a running pace and risks falling forward. This gait is often present in Parkinson's disease.

Prosencephalon. The forebrain, consisting of the diencephalon and telencephalon. [Gr. *pros*, before, in front; *enkephalon*, brain.]

Prosody. A component of speech that conveys meaning through pitch, loudness, tempo, stress, and rhythm. It may enhance the meaning of what is said, as in declarative or interrogative statements, and it is important in conveying emotional content. [Gr. *prosodia*, a song sung to music, from *pros*, to; *ode*, a song.]

Prosopagnosia. *See* Agnosia. [Gr. *prosopon*, face, mask.]

Prospective memory. *See* Memory.

Protease inhibitors. A class of drugs that slows the spread of HIV by preventing protease from making new copies of HIV. Protease inhibitors are better at decreasing HIV replication than the reverse transcriptase inhibitors, which was the first group of HIV drugs. Called proteinase inhibitors in Europe.

Prosthesis. A device used to replace a missing body part; also used to describe compensatory devices such as memory books and to-do lists (i.e., cognitive prostheses).

Pseudoachromatopsia. Performance failure on color vision tests for reasons other than poor color vision or discrimination. An example is an inability to trace the figures of the Ishihara test on account of apraxia or neglect.

Pseudobulbar palsy. Spastic weakness of the muscles of the face, pharynx, and tongue from bilateral lesions of the corticobulbar tracts. It is often accompanied by uncontrolled weeping or laughing (i.e., pseudobulbar affect).

Pseudodementia. A potentially reversible psychiatric condition that resembles dementia. It often results from depression, but it may be associated with other psychiatric disorders.

Pseudoparesis, alcoholic. An obsolete term for alcoholic dementia, so named because of its similarity in presentation to general paresis (neurosyphilis).

Pseudoseizures. *See* Nonepileptic seizures.

PSP. *See* Progressive supranuclear palsy.

Psychic blindness. *See* Cortical blindness.

Psychic paresis of gaze. *See* Balint's syndrome.

Psychoactive drugs. Drugs capable of modifying cognition, emotion, or other mental states. Also called psychotropic drugs.

Psychogenic. Having a psychological or psychiatric etiology. [Gr. *psykhe, psukhe*, soul, life; *genesis*, birth, origin.]

Psycholinguistic Assessment of Language Processing in Aphasia (PALPA). A test of adult language function for spoken and written language. Subtests are designed to assess components of language based on a cognitive neuropsychological model of language processing. (Kay, J., Lesser, R., and Coltheart, M. 1992. *Psycholinguistic Assessments of Language Processing in Aphasia (PALPA)*. Manual. Hove, East Sussex, U.K.: Lawrence Erlbaum Associates.)

Psychometrics. The measurement of psychological functions and individual behavioral differences. [Gr. *psykhe, psukhe*, soul, life; *metron*, measure.]

Psychometrist. A technician who administers psychological tests.

Psychomotor. The motor effect of cognitive or behavioral activity.

Psychomotor epilepsy. *See* Epilepsy.

Psychomotor retardation. Slowed mental and motor activity that may be a common feature of both psychiatric and neurologic illnesses.

Psychopathology. Abnormal, or pathological, mental and behavioral conditions. [Gr. *psykhe, psukhe*, soul, life; *pathos*, suffering.]

Psychopharmacology. The study of drug effects on behavior and their biochemical mechanisms of action. This includes therapeutic agents, such as antidepressants, and drugs that are abused and may produce dependence. Drugs that alter behavior are called psychoactive drugs.

Psychophysiologic disorder. A disorder with physical signs and symptoms that have a psychological origin. Typically, psychophysiologic disorders affect a single organ system innervated by the autonomic nervous system. It is also applied to common ailments presumed to be triggered by psychological stress, such as tension headaches. Also called psychosomatic disorder.

Psychosis. Altered mental state characterized by delusions, hallucinations, loosened associations, and illogical thinking that are considered cardinal features of schizophrenia. Psychotic symptoms may also be associated with neurologic etiologies, although the term psychotic is typically reserved for psychiatric symptoms without an obvious neurologic etiology. When patients develop psychotic symptoms due to neurologic causes, the specific symptoms are generally described (e.g., delusions, paranoid delusions, hallucinations) and related to the underlying neurologic condition.

Psychosomatic. *See* Psychophysiologic disorder. This term was previously applied to a broad spectrum of conditions, including somatoform disorders.

Psychostimulants. Medication with a centrally acting stimulant effect. They are used in traumatic brain injury and other conditions to increase attention and arousal. Commonly used psychostimulants include the dopaminergic agonists (e.g. amantadine, bromocriptine and levodopa/carbidopa) and methylphenidate.

Psychotropic drugs. *See* Psychoactive drugs.

PT. 1. Prothrombin time. A measure of blood coagulation. Prothrombin time is measured in individuals receiving chronic warfarin therapy to decrease the likelihood of ischemic stroke. **2.** Physical therapy or physical therapist.

Ptosis, eye. Drooping, or complete closure, of the eyelid that typically results from third nerve impairment. [Gr. *ptosis*, a fall, a falling.]

PTSD. *See* Post-traumatic stress disorder.

PTT. Partial thromboplastin time. A measure of blood coagulation. A PTT is typically obtained in individuals receiving anticoagulation therapy.

Punch drunk syndrome. *See* Dementia (dementia pugilistica).

Purdue Pegboard. A test of manual dexterity and fine motor speed in which round pegs are rapidly inserted into a vertical row of holes. Performances for the nondominant hand, dominant hand, and both hands are obtained. (Tiffin, J. 1968. *Purdue Pegboard: Examiner Manual.* Chicago: Science Research Associates.)

Pure word deafness. *See* Agnosia (auditory agnosia).

Pursuit eye movement. Slow, smooth-tracking eye movements. Pursuit eye movements contrast with saccadic eye movements.

Pursuit rotor task. Manual tracking task used in the assessment of procedural learning skills.

Pyramidal cells. The principal motor output cells of the neocortex consisting of pyramidal-shaped neurons that typically have long axons. They originate in the precentral gyrus, pass through the medullary pyramids, and descend the spinal cord as the corticospinal tract. Lesions produce spastic hemiplegia or hemiparesis. Pyramidal cells are also present in the hippocampus, and they have been demonstrated to play a role in certain types of learning.

Pyramids and Palm Trees Test. A measure of picture and word recognition that requires knowledge of item similarity, either by property or by association. The format is the same for both pictures and words: a stimulus is presented and one of two choices is made. For example, a pyramid must be matched with either a palm tree or a pine tree. (Howard, D. and Patterson, K.E. 1992. *The Pyramids and Palm Tress Test.* Bury St. Edmunds, Suffolk, England: Thames Valley Test Company.)

Q

qhs. Shorthand notation for "at nighttime." [L. *quaque hora* + sleep.]

qid. Shorthand notation for "four times a day." [L. *quater in die.*]

Q-sign. An open mouth with a deviated tongue (i.e., "Q") often seen in severe acute stroke. This term is colloquial.

Quadrantanopsia/quadrantanopia. Defective vision or blindness in one-fourth of the visual field bounded by a vertical and a horizontal radius. A superior quandrantanopsia is associated with lesions of the contralateral temporal lobe, and an inferior quandrantanopsia is associated with lesions of the contralateral parietal lobe. [L. *quandrans*, fourth part, quarter; Gr. *an-*, without; *opsis*, pertaining to sight.]

Quadriplegia. Paralysis of all four limbs. Quadriplegia results from injury to either the brainstem or the cervical spine.

Quality of life. The characterization of health concern or disease effects on patient lifestyle and daily functioning. Two approaches to quality-of-life assessment in clinical populations are used. In one method, general health problems that may be due to any disease having an effect on quality of life are assessed; in the other, disease-specific effects are investigated. In contrast to most other health measures, quality of life reflects the patient's perspective.

Quantile. The expression of a distribution as equal, ordered subgroups. Quantiles can be made by dividing the distribution into any number of equal groups. Deciles are tenths; quartiles, quarters; quintiles, fifths; terciles, thirds; and centiles (percentiles), hundredths.

Quantitative data. Data represented numerically. Quantitative data may consist of either continuous or discrete variables.

Quantitative EEG (qEEG). A method of quantifying EEG into discrete frequency bands, generally using fast Fourier analysis. This approach still remains primarily investigative, however, because of statistical considerations involved with multiple statistical analyses, issues involving the test-retest reliability of the data, and difficulty in appropriately editing out signal artifact.

Quantity-Frequency-Variability Index. A scale for quantifying alcohol intake. (Cahalan, D. and Cisin, I.H. 1968. American drinking practices: Summary of findings from a national probability sample: I: Extent of drinking by population subgroups. *Q. J. Stud. Alcohol* 29: 130–151.)

Quasi-experimental design. An experimental design in which complete randomization is not possible (e.g., subjects cannot be randomly assigned to conditions of interest, such as presence or absence of a disease state). It may also refer to designs for studying independent variables that are inherent to the individual and cannot be randomly assigned, such as sex or handedness.

R

Radiation necrosis. Cerebral infarction from occlusion of small cerebral vessels that are damaged during high-dose radiation therapy for brain tumors. Infarction does not typically appear until approximately 6–18 months after radiation therapy has been completed. In severe cases, vascular dementia may develop.

Radiculopathy. Lesion of the nerve roots. [L. *radicula*, diminutive of *radix*, root; Gr. *pathein*, *paschein*, to suffer.]

Rancho Los Amigos Scale of Cognitive Levels and Expected Behavior. A neurobehavioral rating scale that is commonly used in rehabilitation settings to characterize patient status. Eight levels of behavior are classified. Level I. The patient is unresponsive to all stimuli. Level II. The patient produces nonpurposeful, nonspecific reactions to stimuli. Response to pain may be delayed. Level III. The patient has inconsistent reactions that are directly related to the type of stimulus presented. The patient may respond to some commands and to discomfort. Level IV. The patient is disoriented and unaware of present events, and exhibits frequent bizarre and inappropriate behavior. Attention span is short and information processing capacity is limited. Level V. The patient displays random or fragmented responses when task complexity exceeds abilities. The patient appears alert, however, and will respond to simple commands. Previously learned tasks are performed, although the ability to learn new tasks is impaired. Level VI. Patient behavior is goal directed and responses are appropriate, but incorrect responses may result from impaired memory. Level VII. Patients appear oriented to their setting, but insight, judgment, and problem-solving are limited. Correct routine responses appear robot-like. Level VIII. Patients can learn new information, although they frequently display poor frustration tolerance and impaired abstraction ability. (Hagen, C. 1981. Language disorders secondary to closed head injury: diagnosis and treatment. *Topics in Language Disorders* 1:73–87.)

Range of motion (ROM). The degree to which a joint will move from being fully straightened to being completely bent. Range of motion may refer to either passive (PROM) or active (AROM) movement.

Raphé nuclei. Groups of neurons in the medial pons and medulla that are a major source of ascending serotonergic fibers.

Rapid alternating movements. A test of cerebellar function in which the palm and then the back of the hand is placed on a surface as rapidly as possible. Failure to perform smooth movements is called adiadochokinesia or dysdiadochokinesia.

Rapid eye movement (REM). Rapid scanning eye movements that occur in clusters during sleep and are associated with dreaming.

RAS. *See* Reticular activating system.

Raven's Progressive Matrices. A multiple-choice test of visual-spatial ability and reasoning that consists of a series of visual patterns and analogies. The test requires subjects to conceptualize spatial, design, and numerical relationships. The Coloured Progressive Matrices are intended for children from 5 to 11 years old, and for adults 65 years and older. The Standard Progressive Matrices are generally used for ages 8–65 years. The Advanced Progressive Matrices are intended for individuals with above-average intellectual ability. (Raven, J.C., Court, J.H., and Raven, J. 1982. *Manual for Raven's Progressive Matrices and Vocabulary Scales.* London: H.K. Lewis and Co.)

Reaction time (RT). The amount of time between a stimulus and a response. In a simple reaction time test, a single stimulus and response are used. Choice reaction time (CRT) tasks involve multiple stimuli, with response selection being dependent on the specific stimulus presented. The CRT is proportional to the number of stimuli about which decisions are made. Reaction time performance may be affected by noncognitive factors (e.g., motor deficits, peripheral neuropathy, depression).

Readiness potential. *See* Bereitschaftspotential.

Reading disabilities. *See* Dyslexia.

Receiver operating characteristic curve (ROC). A curve derived from *signal detection theory* that plots the probability of correctly detecting the presence of a signal (i.e., hits) against the probability of false alarms. Because the signal can be defined in multiple ways, this approach has been applied both to recognition memory tasks (recognizing or failing to recognize a memory stimulus) and to the relationship between neuropsychological tests and binary outcome prediction (e.g., presence or absence of a lesion).

Recency effect. The tendency to recall items from the end of a list in *free recall* task. The absence of a recency effect may indicate interference due to problems with attention and concentration.

Recent memory. *See* Memory.

Receptive aphasia. *See* Aphasia syndromes.

Recognition. Memory that is assessed by presenting material shown earlier (i.e., targets) with new items that were not previously administered (i.e., distractors or foils). The task is to identify those items presented earlier. Two primary types of recognition procedures are used. In one, both the memory targets and distractors are presented simultaneously in an array and the words recognized are selected from the entire array. In the other approach, the stimuli are presented sequentially—typically individually, in pairs, or as part of larger groups. Subjects indicate which item from the array is correct, or with single stimuli, which item was to be remembered. Subjects may be required to choose an answer, even if they do not specifically remember the target; this is called forced-choice. The forced-choice format is often used with *symptom validity testing* because precise response probabilities can be calculated. [L. *recognitio,* a recognition.]

Recognition Memory Test. A test of verbal and nonverbal memory using single words and unfamiliar male faces as stimuli. After presentation of 50 verbal or nonverbal stimuli, subjects are tested with two alternative forced-choice recognition tasks in which the target is paired with a single distractor. As with other forced-choice measures, this test may also be used in *symptom validity testing.* (Warrington, E.K. 1984. *Recognition Memory Test Manual. Windsor,* Berkshire: NFER-Nelson.)

Recurring Digit Test. *See* Hebb's Recurring Digit Test.

Recurring Figures Test. A test of visual recognition memory that contains both geometric and irregular stimuli. Each stimulus is displayed for 3 seconds. Seven additional sets containing the original designs interspersed with new designs are presented next. The patient is to indicate which designs are new and which are old (recurring). (Kimura, D. 1963. Right temporal lobe damage. *Arch. Neurol.* 8:264–271.)

Reduplicative paramnesia. A confabulation consisting of a false belief in the duplication of people or places. It may be seen during recovery from post-traumatic amnesia, when patients indicate that they are in their hometown *and* the location of their hospital simultaneously. Patients are unaware of the contradictions of their responses. The term "reduplicative paramnesia" was introduced by Arnold Pick (Czech psychiatrist and neuropathologist, 1851–1924), who considered it a sign of cerebral disease.

Reflex epilepsy. *See* Epilepsy.

Reflex sympathetic dystrophy (RSD). A syndrome of autonomic nervous system dysfunction characterized by vascular instability; it is often manifested by limb pain and swelling. It can be triggered by stroke, traumatic brain injury, peripheral nerve injury, and myocardial infarction.

Regional cerebral blood flow (rCBF). The measurement of blood flow within a given brain region, usually based on oxygen turnover rate. Areas of increased blood flow are inferred to be more active during motor and cognitive tasks, and conversely, areas of decreased blood flow are inferred to be less active. The rCBF is not a de facto index of brain metabolism, however, because blood flow and metabolism may become uncoupled (e.g., *luxury perfusion*).

Regression analysis. A method of statistical analysis in which a single outcome variable is related to one or more predictor variables by examining the tendency for scores on the outcome to move in concert with scores on the predictors. Typically, the outcome is considered to be related to the predictors in a linear manner, although curvilinear and nonlinear relations are possible. Predictors can be either categorical or continuous variables.

Regression toward the mean. The tendency for scores at the extremes of a distribution to migrate toward the mean upon repeated assessment. This finding results from the tendency for scores to fall at the tails of the distribution, in part because of chance factors that likely will not be operating again during subsequent testing.

Regularization error. A reading error regarding words with irregular pronunciation in which a common word is substituted with another word that follows regular phonemic pronunciation patterns (e.g., "buzzy" for busy, "sue" for "sew"). Commonly associated with surface alexia/dyslexia.

Rehabilitation. Activities designed to facilitate and maximize recovery of function following injury and to maximize accommodation to functional disabilities and handicaps. In rehabilitation hospitals for brain-injured patients, rehabilitation is frequently provided by a team consisting of a physiatrist, neuropsychologist, speech-language pathologist, occupational therapist, and physical therapist. [L. *rehabilitare*, to restore, from *re-*, again; *habilis*, suitable.]

Reitan-Indiana Aphasia Screening Test. Screening instrument consisting of 32 items that constitute Reitan's modification of the Halstead-Wepman Aphasia Screening Test. It briefly tests language, constructional praxis, calculation, and right-left orientation. When used as part of the Halstead-Reitan Neuropsychological Battery (HRNB), the Aphasia Screening Test is not formally scored, does not contribute to the Halstead Impairment Index, and provides only qualitative descriptions of an individual's language performance. However, 12 "pathognomic signs" are derived that contribute to the HRNB General Neuropsychological Deficit Scale. The Aphasia Screening Test was modified by Russell, Neuringer, and Goldstein (1970) to include a formal scoring system that indicates aphasia severity. In addition to the computation items in the Reitan-Indiana Aphasia Screening Test, two other subtraction items and two other multiplication items of decreasing difficulty are presented. The test contains several geometric items for the subject to copy in addition to a skeleton key; these items are not formally scored in the Russell modification to derive an aphasia score from this test. The Russell modification also includes two trials to assess spatial relations: copying the Greek cross and cross copying. (Russell, E.W., Neuringer, C., and Goldstein, G. 1970. *Assessment of Brain Damage: A Neuropsychological Key Approach*. New York: Wiley-Interscience, 1970.)

Reitan-Kløve Sensory Perceptual Examination. A structured examination of visual, auditory, and sensory function and of higher-order sensory processing. The test contains five formal subtests: the Tactile, Auditory, and Visual Imperception subtests assess perception of unilateral and bilateral sensory stimulation; Tactile Finger Recognition assesses agnosia; and Fingertip Number Writing Perception assesses graphesthesia. Both the Tactile Coin Recognition and Tactile Form Recognition subtests assess stereognosis. This examination is part of the Halstead-Reitan Neuropsychological Battery.

Release from proactive interference. Improved memory performance for stimulus words following a shift in semantic category. When stimuli are presented from the same semantic category over repeated trials, fewer and fewer words are recalled. After a shift in semantic category, performance improves because the proactive interference effect is reduced. Originally described by Wickens (1970) using the *Brown-Peterson distractor task*. (Wickens, D.D. 1970. Encoding categories of words: An empirical approach to meaning. *Psychol. Rev.* 77:67–85.)

Reliability. The degree to which scores on a test are systematic. In technical terms, this reflects the degree to which a measure is free from measurement error (or random influence). Since there are several types of measurement error, reliability should be viewed as a generic term for several features of a measure that are either necessary or useful to achieve this aim.

Reliable change index (RCI). An empirical measure derived from repeated assessments for a target population. The measure is based on the test-retest reliability, standard error of the test, and practice effects. Reliable change indexes are used to determine whether changes present on follow-up testing exceed what is considered to result from methodological aspects associated with repeat assessment. Change-score confidence intervals (e.g., 90%) are selected by the investigator.

Reliable digit span. The maximum *digit span* length that is recalled without error on both trials of standard digit span testing such as with the Wechsler Intelligence Scales (WIS). The maximum reliable span lengths for forward and backward repetition conditions are then summed to form a single measure. This approach has been shown to be sensitive to probable malingering. (Greiffenstein, M.F., Baker, W.J., and Gola, T. 1994. Validation of malingered amnesia measures with a large clinical sample. *Psychol. Assess.* 6:218–224.)

REM. *See* Rapid eye movement.

Remote memory. *See* Memory.

Reptilian stare. A colloquial expression for the masked face of Parkinson's disease in which there is a significant decrease in spontaneous eye-blinking.

Resting tremor. A rhythmic movement of the wrist, fingers, and thumb that occurs in a relaxed and supported limb and gives the appearance that the patient is rolling a small pill between the thumb and fingertip (pill-rolling tremor). It often develops first in one hand in Parkinson's disease, and it is the feature that is least responsive to levodopa therapy. Anxiety and excitement increase the tremor; it is absent during sleep.

Retention. The persistence of information over time.

Reticular activating system. A network of nerves in the upper brainstem whose function is to regulate attention and arousal. [L. *reticulatus*, made like a net, from *rete*, a net.]

Reticular formation. *See* Reticular activating system.

Retrieval deficit. The failure of free recall for information that can be remembered under different circumstances, such as with the passage of time, with cues, or with recognition testing (a form of cueing). Retrograde amnesia exemplifies a retrieval deficit because the duration of the retrograde memory deficit "shrinks" over time. Information that cannot be initially recalled following a neurologic event, yet can be recalled later, suggests that the information was appropriately stored but could not be accessed. An exaggeration of this normal tendency may be seen in states of psychopathology (e.g., anxiety) and in some forms of brain disease. *See* Storage deficit; Tip-of-the-tongue phenomenon.

Retroactive inhibition/interference. Impairment in recall of previously learned material due to the learning of new material. *See* Proactive interference.

Retrobulbar. 1. Located behind the eyeball. **2.** Located behind the medulla. [L. *retro*, backward; *bulbus*, a bulb.]

Retrograde amnesia/retrograde memory loss. Loss of memory for information or experiences that occurred before an injury or other event. In brain injury associated with retrograde memory loss, the duration of memory loss will "shrink" over time, although a permanent memory loss for the events closest in time to the injury often remains. This suggests that retrograde amnesia has two components: a retrieval deficit and a loss of previously stored information. A retrieval deficit characterizes the temporary loss of access to pretrauma experiences whereas the loss of previously stored information characterizes the permanent inability to recall information just before the accident. Although retrograde memory loss is typically associated with anterograde memory impairment, it may occur without significant impairment in the ability to acquire new memories (i.e., focal retrograde amnesia).

Retrospective accuracy. The probability that, given a particular condition of clinical interest, a specific test finding or pattern will be obtained. This contrasts with predictive accuracy, which is the probability that, given a specific test finding or pattern, a particular clinical condition exists. Thus, the two terms differ in the directionality of the inference.

Rett's disorder. (Andreas Rett, 20th century Austrian pediatrician). A progressive syndrome affecting females in which the infant develops normally until approximately 1 year of age when the course changes to one of progressive dementia, truncal ataxia, autism, microcephaly, and clumsiness of the hands. Associated with characteristic "hand washing" movements.

Reversal error. Reading error due to reversal of letters. Also called transposition or sequencing error.

Revised Wechsler Memory Scale. A modification of the original Wechsler Memory Scale by Elbert Russell that contains only the Logical Memory and Visual Reproduction subtests but also introduces a 30-minute delay. Short-term memory, delayed memory, and percent-retained scores are obtained. This modification was the first practical answer to the criticism that the WMS contained many subtests that did not measure memory formation per se and did not examine information retention over time. The Revised Wechsler Memory Scale is not the same procedure as the Wechsler Memory Scale-Revised, which is an official test revision and restandardization by the test publisher. (Russell, E.W. 1975. A multiple scoring method for the assessment of complex memory functions. *J. Consul. Clin. Psychol.* 43:800–809.)

Rey Auditory Verbal Learning Test. A serial word-learning task in which 15 words are presented over five learning trials. After the fifth presentation, a sixth trial containing 15 new words is administered. Free-recall of the second list is tested and the subject is asked to recall the initial 15-word list. A 20- to 30-minute delayed recall trial and a recognition memory trial, using either a story or word-list format, can also be given. (Rey, A. 1958. *L'examen Clinique en Psychologie*. Paris: Press Universitaire de France.)

Rey Figure Test. *See* Complex Figure Test.

Rey 3 × 5 Memory Test. A test to assess exaggeration or feigning of memory complaints. Patients are shown items with multiple redundancies and are then asked to draw the items from memory. Because of these redundancies, all but the most severely impaired patients perform the task adequately. Also called Rey 15-item test. (Rey, A. 1958. *L'examen Clinique en Psychologie*. Paris: Press Universitaire de France.)

Rey-Osterreith Complex Figure. *See* Complex Figure Test.

Rhombencephalon. The hindbrain, which consists of the *metencephalon* (pons and cerebellum) and *myelencephalon* (medulla). [Gr. *rhombos*, object that can be turned; *enkephalos*, brain.]

Ribot's law (of regression). (Théodule Ribot, French psychologist, 1839–1916). The principle that the vulnerability of memory loss to neurological insult is an inverse function of the age of those memories. Memories for experiences most recently acquired are those most vulnerable to loss following neurologic disease, resulting in a temporal memory loss gradient. *See* also Retrograde amnesia/memory loss; Retrieval deficit.

Right-left orientation tests. A family of measures designed to test right-left orientation. Culver's version (1969) requires the identification, under time constraints, of right or left hands and feet in various positions. The version developed in the Benton Neuropsychology Laboratory consists of a series of 32 commands (e.g., "show me your left ear"). (Benton, A.L., Sivan, A.B., Hamsher, K.deS., Varney, N.R., and Spreen, O. 1994. *Contributions to Neuropsychological Assessment. A Clinical Manual*, 2nd ed. New York: Oxford University Press; Culver, C.M. 1969. Test of right-left discrimination. *Percept. Motor Skills* 29: 863–867.)

Rigidity. Increased muscle resistance to passive movement.

Ring-enhancing lesion. A cerebral lesion that is seen on CT or MRI with a contrast medium as a bright circular spot surrounded by dark areas (i.e., ring). Ring-enhancing lesions are seen in toxoplasmosis, brain abscess, and metastatic carcinoma.

Rivermead Behavioural Memory Test (RBMT). A test of everyday memory functioning that, because of its low ceiling, is intended for individuals with moderate to severe memory impairment. In contrast to traditional neuropsychological assessment, many types of everyday memory are assessed. For example, the ability to associate a name with a face is tested. Other tasks include remembering a hidden belonging of one's own, remembering an appointment, and remembering to deliver a message. A separate version exists for children between 5 and 10 years of age (Rivermead Behavioural Memory Test for Children [RBMT-C]). (Wilson, B., Cockburn, J., and Baddeley, A. 1985. *The Rivermead Behavioural Memory Test*. Bury St. Edmunds, England: Thames Valley Test Co.)

RLE. Right lower extremity.

ROC curve. *See* Receiver operating characteristic curve.

Rolandic epilepsy. *See* Epilepsy.

Rolandic fissure. (Luigi Rolando, Italian anatomist, 1770–1831). The major sulcus that runs obliquely across the superior lateral surface of the cerebral hemisphere, separating the frontal lobes from the parietal lobes. It separates the primary motor and primary sensory gyri. Also called the central sulcus.

ROM. *See* Range of motion.

Rooting reflex. An abnormal reflex that is elicited by rubbing or scratching on or near the corner of the mouth. If present, there will be a puckering or pursing of the lips. This reflex is considered a frontal release sign, although it is more common with diffuse disease than with frontal lobe lesions.

Rorschach Test. (Hermann Rorschach, Swiss psychiatrist, 1884–1922). A projective test in which patients describe what they see in black and colored inkblots.

RPR. Rapid plasma reagin agglutination test; a serologic test for syphilis.

RT. *See* Reaction time.

RUE. Right upper extremity.

Rule-based reading. A phonologically based process in which words are sounded out. Reading occurs from grapheme-to-phoneme, or print-to-sound, conversion rules. *Contrast with* Analogy theory.

Rx. Prescription.

S

s̄. Shorthand notation for "without." [L. *sine*, without.]

Saccades. Rapid movements of both eyes under both voluntary and reflex control. These quick, synchronized eye movements change the point of visual fixation, as in the series of jumps associated with scanning a line of print. [Old F. *saquer, sacher*, to pull.]

Sagittal. Dividing the body (or brain) into left and right portions along the anterior-posterior plane. [L. *sagitta*, an arrow.]

Saltatory conduction. A property of neural conduction in which the impulse jumps from one *node of Ranvier* to the next, thereby increasing the speed of neural transmission. [L. *saltatorius*, pertaining to dancing, from *saltare*, to leap.]

Savings technique. An approach to assessing retention in which a task is first learned to a specific level and is later relearned to that same level of performance. Savings reflects the difference in the amount of time, or number of trials needed to learn the task to criterion between initial and subsequent task performance.

Scanning dysarthria. *See* Scanning speech.

Scanning speech. A speech disorder of cerebellar origin that is characterized by the variable intonation associated with involuntary interruption between syllables. Each syllable may be uttered with more or less force than is normal ("explosive speech"). In addition, speech is slow. Scanning speech is one of the characteristics of ataxic dysarthria.

Schema. Mental frameworks that organize the storage of knowledge. [Gr. *skema*, form.]

Schilling test. (Victor Schilling, German hematologist, 1883–1960). A test for measuring B_{12} absorption. See B_{12}.

Schizencephaly. Abnormal divisions or cavities of the brain that develop either prenatally or during early infancy. Also called schizoencephalic porencephaly. [Gr. *schizein*, to split; *enkepahlon*, brain.]

Schizoencephalic porencephaly. *See* Schizencephaly.

Schizophrenia. A group of severe and usually chronic psychiatric disorders characterized by fragmented or bizarre thought content, delusions, disruption of normal thought associations, flat or inappropriate affect, and hallucinations of all types (auditory hallucinations are the most frequent). A decrease in activity to the point of stupor may also be observed. Schizophrenic symptoms are often categorized as either positive (e.g., hallucinations, delusions, thought disorder) or negative (e.g., social withdrawal, reduced motivation or initiation behavior) symptoms. Onset is typically during adolescence or early adulthood. [Gr. *schizein*, to split; *phrenos*, mind.]

Schizotypal. A personality disorder characterized by a pattern of interpersonal and social deficits, cognitive and perceptual distortions, odd thinking and speech, social anxiety, and eccentricities of behavior. These same features are described as the residual signs of schizophrenia.

SCID. *See* Structured Clinical Interview for DSM-IV.

Scintillation. An illusion in which there are sparks, flashes of light, or glitterings in the peripheral visual fields. Scintillation is often associated with seizures or migraine. [L. *scintillare*, to sparkle.]

Sclerosis. Scarring associated with hyperplasia or glial overgrowth that may result from neural injury. The terms sclerosis and gliosis are often used interchangeably. [Gr. *sklerosis*, hardness.]

Scotoma. An area of poor vision or blindness within the visual field, generally circular or oval, that is surrounded by an area of normal or near-normal vision. [Gr. *skotos*, darkness.]

Scrapie. A transmissible degenerative disease of sheep and goats. It is caused by *prion* transmission, the same mode of transmission as in Creutzfeldt-Jakob disease.

Screen and metric. A two-step approach to evaluation designed to decrease the total number of items administered. A relatively difficult item is presented first (screen), and if it is successfully completed, the subject is considered able to pass the easier items, and they are not presented. If the screen is failed, then the metric is administered. The metric is a series of test items of increasing difficulty that is common to most assessment approaches. Screen and metric approaches are used to increase the breadth of coverage, while allowing more comprehensive examination of areas in which problems are identified, when there are constraints of time or patient cooperation.

SDAT. *See* Senile dementia of the Alzheimer type.

Seashore Rhythm Test. A test of sustained auditory attention involving the comparison and differentiation of rhythmic sequences. The test requires the subject to identify pairs of rhythmic patterns as either the same or different. Although frequently interpreted as a measure of right temporal lobe function, the test results do not appear to have localizing significance. This is a subtest of the Seashore Tests of Musical Talent; it is also part of the Halstead-Reitan Neuropsychological Battery. (Reitan, R.M. and Wolfson, D. 1989. The Seashore Rhythm Test and brain functions. *Clin. Neuropsychol.* 3:70–78.)

Second impact syndrome. A condition in which the second of two independent mild head injuries produces greater impairment than would be expected from the cumulative effects of both injuries.

Secondary generalization. The second phase of a seizure that begins as a focal or partial seizure but progresses to a generalized one. Secondary generalization does not accompany all partial seizures, and patients with complex partial epilepsy may have some seizures that generalize and others that do not generalize. *See* Complex partial seizures.

Secondary motor area. *See* Supplementary motor area.

Segmentation. A process during reading by which a string of letters is broken down into graphemic segments that are then assigned *phonology*.

Seizure. A discrete clinical attack in which there is uncontrolled, excessive, and hypersynchronous discharge of cortical neurons. Approximately one-half of seizures are associated with acute brain disorders (e.g., stroke, hypoglycemia) and do not reflect an underlying syndrome of epilepsy. There are two broad seizure categories: generalized seizures, which affect both cerebral hemispheres simultaneously, and partial seizures, in which the initial disturbance is confined to a region of a single hemisphere. *See* Epilepsy.

- **Absence seizure**. A generalized seizure characterized by 3 Hz spike and slow-wave EEG discharges that typically begin between ages 4 and 10 years. The hallmark of an absence attack is a sudden blank stare and interruption of ongoing activities. The seizure stops quickly without awareness that a seizure has occurred and without postictal confusion. Automatisms, subtle clonic limb movements, and eye blinking often occur. Absence seizures are usually outgrown and generally are not associated with cognitive impairment. Patients with absence attacks, however, may be mistakenly thought to have "attentional" problems. Previously called petit mal seizures.

- **Complex partial seizure (cps)**. A partial seizure associated with impaired consciousness or impaired responsiveness. Complex partial seizures differ from simple partial seizures in that consciousness is not impaired in simple seizures. Partial seizures begin focally but may evolve into generalized tonic-clonic seizures (secondary generalization). The most common seizure focus for complex partial seizures is the medial temporal lobe, with the next most common focus being in the frontal lobe. Complex partial seizures are often named according to their area of seizure onset (e.g., temporal lobe seizures, frontal lobe seizures).
- **Febrile seizure**. A generalized seizure associated with a rapid rise in core body temperature. The incidence of febrile seizures reaches its peak in children between 6 months and 5 years of age. While children with positive family histories of febrile seizures are at greater risk for febrile seizures themselves, a single, uncomplicated febrile seizure is generally of little consequence. Patients with complex partial seizures of temporal lobe origin and histories of febrile seizures, however, are more likely to have hippocampal atrophy and sclerosis. [L. *febris*, a fever.]
- **Gelastic seizure**. A seizure in which laughter is the primary ictal phenomenon. Gelastic seizures are associated with complex partial seizures. They have been associated with hypothalamic hamartomas. [Gr. *gelas*, laughter.]
- **Generalized seizure**. A seizure involving both hemispheres. Generalized seizures may be primary generalized seizures, in which the seizure onset arises from both hemispheres, or secondary generalized seizures, in which the seizure begins focally and then spreads to involve both hemispheres.
- **Generalized tonic-clonic (GTC) seizure**. A generalized seizure with a sudden loss of consciousness and a generalized tonic muscle contraction. This is followed by clonic jerks that increase in amplitude while decreasing in rate. Tongue biting or incontinence may occur. GTC seizures may be the primary seizure manifestation or they may occur after a partial seizure, in which case they are called secondary generalization. Lethargy and confusion are common postictally. Previously called grand mal or major motor seizures.
- **Myoclonic seizures**. Generalized seizures characterized by myoclonic jerks (i.e., sudden, brief, single or multiple shock-like muscular contractions). The arms and legs are usually affected, and the seizure may lead to a fall. [Gr. *mys*, *myo*, muscle, *klonos*, shake, shudder.]
- **Simple partial seizure**. A partial seizure in which consciousness is preserved, such as focal motor or focal sensory seizures.
- **Uncinate seizure**. A seizure originating in the uncus that is associated with hallucinations of taste and smell, commonly unpleasant smells. [L. *uncus*, hook.]

Selective reminding test. A word-list learning procedure that differs from traditional list learning tasks in that the number of words presented during each learning trial varies. The subject is prompted only with those words not recalled on the immediately preceding trial. This allows the demonstration of word recall without the need for further prompting. A word is considered to have entered long-term storage (LTS) if it is successfully recalled on two successive trials. Thus, subsequent failure to recall is operationally defined as a retrieval difficulty. Consistent long-term retrieval (CLTR) reflects the number of words summed over trials that are recalled throughout the remainder of the test without the need for further prompting. (Buschke, H. and Fuld, P.A. 1974. Evaluating storage, retention, and retrieval in disordered memory and learning. *Neurology* 24:1019–1025.)

Selective serotonin reuptake inhibitor (SSRI). A class of antidepressant medications that enhances serotonin transmission.

Self-monitoring. A process of tracking, evaluating, and correcting one's behavioral and speech output. It may be impaired with diffuse injury and focal lesions involving frontal lobe systems. Impairment can be associated with *anosognosia*.

Self-Ordered Pointing Task. A test of working memory and strategic behavior in which a set of stimulus items is arranged in different spatial locations on multiple pages, and subjects are required to point to a different item on each page. Neuroimaging studies indicate a role for the mid-dorsolateral frontal cortex in task performance. (Petrides, M. and Milner, B. 1982. Deficits on subject-ordered tasks after frontal- and temporal-lobe lesions in man. *Neuropsychologia* 20:249–262.)

Semantic. Word meanings and the rules for their use. [Gr. *semantikos*, significant meaning.]

Semantic agraphia. *See* Agraphia spelling disorders.

Semantic category fluency. A fluency task requiring the subject to give examples of a target category (e.g., animals, foods) within a limited time, usually 60 seconds. Some evidence suggests that semantic fluency is more greatly impaired than letter fluency in Alzheimer's disease. Also called category fluency, semantic fluency, or word generatively.

Semantic dementia. *See* Dementia.

Semantic fluency. *See* Semantic category fluency.

Semantic memory. *See* Memory.

Semantic paralexia. *See* Paralexia.

Semantic paraphasia. *See* Paraphasia.

Semantic priming. *See* Memory; Priming.

Semantic system. Cognitive system for the representation of meaning.

Semiology. Symptomatology. [Gr. *semeion*, sign; *logos*, study.]

Senile dementia. *See* Dementia.

Senile dementia of the Alzheimer type (SDAT). *See* Dementia.

Senile plaques. Amorphous material composed of amyloid surrounded by degenerated dendrites that is found in high concentrations in the brains of Alzheimer's disease patients. Of the neuropathologic abnormalities associated with Alzheimer's disease, the number of plaques has been the most consistent correlation with dementia severity. Also called neuritic plaques. [L. *senix*, old, an elder.]

Senility. An obsolete term refering to dementia associated with advancing age. [L. *senix*, old, an elder.]

Sensory aphasia. *See* Aphasia syndromes.

Sensory memory. *See* Memory.

Sensory neglect. *See* Neglect syndrome.

Sensory Perceptual Examination. *See* Reitan-Kløve Sensory Perceptual Examination.

Sensory suppression. *See* Double simultaneous stimulation; Neglect syndrome; Extinction.

Sentinel bleed. Leakage of small amounts of blood that may occur intermittently before a larger hemorrhage.

Septal area. Cortex and unlined septal nuclei, the latter extending to septum pellucidum beneath the genu and rostrum of the corpus callosum, on the medial side of the frontal lobe.

Septum. A thin wall or membrane that divides two chambers. [L. *sepes, saepes*, hedge.]

Septum pellucidum. A membrane that separates the frontal horns of the lateral ventricles.

Sequenced Inventory of Communication Development. A test of communication for children ranging from 4 months to 4 years of age. The Receptive Scale measures developing aspects of awareness, discrimination, and understanding; the Expressive Scale measures imitation, initiation, response, verbal output, and articulation. (Hedrick, D.L., Prather, E.M., and Tobin, A.R. 1984. *Sequenced Inventory of Communication Development,] Revised*. Seattle: University of Washington Press.)

Serial Digit Learning. A digit supraspan learning test in which either an 8- or a 9-digit sequence of numbers is to be learned over repeated trials. (Benton, A.L., Sivan, A.B., Hamsher, K.deS., Varney, N.R., and Spreen, O. (1994). *Contributions to Neuropsychological Assessment. A Clinical Manual.* 2nd ed. New York: Oxford University Press.)

Serial learning. Any learning task in which items to be learned are presented over multiple trials.

Serial position effect. The tendency to more readily recall items presented at the beginning (*primacy effect*) and toward the end (*recency effect*) in a free-recall task.

Serial recitation. *See* Serial subtraction tasks.

Serial subtraction tasks. A measure of mental tracking ability commonly employed at the bedside that involves counting backwards by specified increments. The two most common approaches are Serial Sevens (i.e., 100, 93, 86, etc.) and Serial Threes (i.e., 100, 97, 94, etc). Also called serial recitation.

Serotonin (5-HT). 5-hydroxytryptamine. A neurotransmitter/neuromodulator located primarily in the raphe nuclei of the pons and upper brainstem that is particularly involved in affective and arousal states of the brain. Although projections spread throughout the central nervous system, they are concentrated in sensory, motor, association, and limbic regions. Generally, serotonin has an inhibitory effect on sensory relay neurons and an excitatory effect on motor neurons, which in alert states enhances motor excitability or readiness and suppresses the distracting influence of sensory cues. Psychopathological conditions associated with serotonin perturbations include mood disorders, schizophrenia, and hyperaggressive states. [L. *serum*, whey, serum; Gr. *tonos*, a stretching; so named because of serotonin's vasoconstricting activity.]

Severe Impairment Battery (SIB). A battery of tests designed for the assessment of patients with moderate to severe neuropsychological impairments. The subtests include Attention, Language, Visuospatial Ability, Orientation, Memory, and Construction. (Saxton, J., McGonigle, K.L., Swihart, A.A., and Boller, F. 1993. *The Severe Impairment Battery.* Bury St. Edmunds, Suffolk, England: Thames Valley Test Co.)

Shadowing. A dichotic listening task in which the message presented to one ear is repeated by the subject while a competing message presented to the contralateral ear must be ignored.

Shear strain injury. A primary mechanism of *diffuse axonal injury* following traumatic brain injury. Axons are injured by rotational forces that produce shearing between tissues of different densities. This is prominent at the junctures between gray matter and white (myelinated) fiber tracts.

Shipley Institute of Living Scale-Revised. A measure of verbal cognitive function consisting of Vocabulary and Abstraction subtests. Vocabulary is tested in a multiple-choice format, and abstraction is tested with a series completion task (e.g., 1-2-2-2-3-2-__). The test was initially developed for application in a psychiatric setting (Hartford Institute of Living) for use with schizophrenic patients. The difference between the two subtest scores was thought to reflect the degree of psychiatric impairment since "loss of abstract attitude" was considered a feature of schizophrenia. The Shipley presently yields scores for vocabulary, abstraction, and a total score. In addition, a conceptual quotient, abstraction quotient (which is the age-adjusted Conceptual Quotient), and both WAIS and WAIS-R Full-Scale IQ estimates can be obtained. (Shipley, W.C. 1940. A self-administering scale for measuring intellectual impairment and deterioration. *J. Psychol.* 9:371–377; Zachary, R.A. 1986. *Shipley Institute of Living Scale: Revised Manual.* Los Angeles: Western Psychological Services.)

Short forms. Tests modified to require less time for administration and scoring. Although results from short forms are often treated as equivalent to those obtained with standard administration, the psychometric properties of the short forms in general are poorly understood.

Short-term memory (STM). *See* Memory.

Shunt. In the context of brain disease, a shunt refers to a plastic tube inserted surgically between a cerebral ventricle and the abdomen to divert excessive cerebrospinal fluid (CSF) of hydrocephalus away from the brain. A ventriculoperitoneal (VP) shunt is the most frequently employed shunt and diverts CSF from the frontal horn of the lateral ventricle to the peritoneum of the abdomen. The most common complication is blockage of the shunt catheter at either end (brain or abdomen), occurring in as many as 25%–30% of patients during the first year after surgery.

Sickle cell disease. A genetic disorder of hemoglobin named for the abnormal crescent shape of the red blood cell. This disease may be associated with cognitive delay, disordered consciousness, seizures, and meningitis.

Signal detection theory. A theory developed in sensory psychophysics that describes individual differences in the ability to detect the presence of a signal from background noise. It is based on perceptual sensitivity to the signal and on the amount of certainty that subjects require before they conclude that a signal has been presented (response bias). Signal detection theory incorporates the speed-accuracy tradeoff, and it generates two unique statistics: d' describes the "distance" between the noise distribution and the signal plus noise distribution, and β is the perceptual threshold above which a signal is reported. Signal detection theory has been adapted for use in characterizing response styles for recognition memory testing.

Simple partial seizure. *See* Seizure.

Simultanagnosia. *See* Agnosia.

Single photon emission computed tomography (SPECT). A functional neuroimaging technique using radioisotope tracers to assess brain perfusion. SPECT has the advantage over PET of being less expensive and more widely available. Administering the isotope during a seizure and then obtaining a SPECT scan is often used to localize seizures in epilepsy surgery candidates with a hypermetabolic state associated with the ictus.

Situs inversus. A complete reversal of cerebral laterality and specialization in which the left hemisphere is dominant for visual-spatial processing and the right hemisphere is dominant for language. [L. *situs*, site; *inversus*, inverted.]

Size constancy. A perceptual process that allows a stimulus to be perceived as approximately the same size despite variations in its proximity.

Skewness. The degree to which a measurement falls in a symmetrical (not skewed) or asymmetrical (skewed) distribution around the mean. A negatively skewed distribution has a greater number of scores at the high end of the distribution, and a positively skewed distribution has a greater number of scores at the low end of the distribution.

Sklar Aphasia Scale. A scale often used in speech rehabilitation that is designed to measure acquired language impairment with an emphasis on functional communication skill. It consists of a preliminary interview followed by assessment of auditory decoding, oral encoding, visual decoding, and graphic encoding. A checklist for language disturbance and emotional behaviors is also obtained. (Sklar, M. 1983. *Sklar Aphasia Scale: Revised 1983 Manual.* Los Angeles: Western Psychological Services.)

Sleep apnea. A breathing disorder caused by upper airway obstruction that leads to frequent nighttime awakenings and subsequent daytime sleepiness. It may be associated with daytime impairments in attention and concentration.

SMA. 1. Sequential multichannel autoanalyzer; a blood test of liver function, kidney function, metabolic function, and electrolytes. **2.** *See* Supplementary motor areas.

Smell Identification Test. A test of smell function containing "scratch & sniff" odorants. The odor is identified using a multiple-choice format (e.g., "This odor smells most like: a. chocolate, b. banana, c. onion, d. fruit punch"). Also called the University of Pennsylvania Smell Identification Test. (Doty, R.L. 1995. *The Smell Identification Test Administration Manual*, 3rd ed. Haddon Heights, NJ: Sensonics.)

Snellen chart. (Hermann Snellen, Dutch ophthalmologist, 1834–1908). A test of visual acuity that contains a chart of printed letters of differing sizes.

Snout reflex. An abnormal reflex of pursing the lips when the upper lip is tapped. Although commonly regarded as a frontal lobe release reflex, it is more common with diffuse disease than with focal frontal lobe lesion.

Social history. A description of the major social events and patterns of an individual's life. It typically includes employment history, marital and family status, or description of recreational drug, alcohol, or tobacco usage.

Soft neurologic signs. Nonspecific signs suggestive of neurologic impairment that occur frequently in the normal population, although they do occur with greater frequency in clinical populations. Soft neurologic signs may include motor overflow when performing a motor task (*synkinesia*). Soft neurologic signs also refer to mild or subtle findings in a neurologic examination, such as a mild pronator drift or mild reflex asymmetry.

Somatagnosia. *See* Asomatognosia.

Somatic. Pertaining to the body, in contrast to viscera. [Gr. *soma*, body.]

Somatization. The tendency for psychological discomfort to be expressed through bodily symptoms.

Somatoform disorders. Disorders in which physical symptoms cannot be fully explained by a medical condition and, in contrast to malingering, no secondary gain can be identified. The motivation does not appear to be a psychological need to assume the role of the patient, as occurs in factitious disorders. Somatoform disorders are thought to result from psychological factors that are not conscious or volitional.

Somatosensory area. The cortical projection area in the postcentral gyrus involved in the processing of sensory information from receptors in skin, joints, muscles, and viscera. Thus, it has a central role in the conscious perception of somatic sensation. Also called the somesthetic area.

Somesthesia. Bodily sensation of pain, temperature, touch, pressure, position and movement, and vibration. [Gr. *soma*, body; *aisthésis*, perception.]

Somesthetic area. *See* Somatosensory area.

Sound conduction error. *See* Phonetic disintegration.

Source memory. *See* Memory.

s/p. Status post; The event being described has already occurred (e.g., s/p coronary artery bypass graft).

Spacing effect. Enhanced memory for repeated items when the repetitions are separated by other events.

Span of apprehension. The amount of auditory material that can be held in immediate memory and reproduced exactly.

Spastic ataxia. The combination of spasticity and unsteadiness.

Spasticity. Increased muscle tone associated with hyperactive tendon reflexes that generally accompany *upper motor neuron* impairment. [Gr., *spastikos*, stretching or drawing.]

Spatial acalculia. *See* Acalculia.

Spatial agraphia. *See* Agraphia writing disorders.

Spatial orientation. The ability to judge the orientation of information in either two- or three-dimensional space. Spatial orientation is generally considered a primary function of the right cerebral hemisphere.

SPECT. *See* Single photon emission computed tomogram.

Speech. The process of language vocalization. Speech is not synonymous with language, which relates to symbol-based representation of language, including writing and sign language. Speech may be disrupted by brain lesions, which are generally perisylvian, and by injuries to peripheral muscles and nerves that serve articulation and vocalization. Disorders of speech articulation related to neuromuscular involvement are called dysarthria.

Speech-language pathologist. An individual who is qualified to diagnose and treat patients with a variety of speech or language impairments. Sometimes called speech therapist or speech clinician.

Speech-language pathology. The study of speech and language disorders and their treatment.

Speech pragmatics. Nonlinguistic social rules of verbal communication, including initiating and terminating speech, maintaining eye contact, and staying on topic.

Speech rate. The rate of spontaneous, conversational speech. The normal rate of speech is at least 100 words per minute. Speech rate is used in aphasia classification. A low rate of speech (e.g., 50 words per minute) is associated with anterior lesions (i.e., expressive or Broca's aphasia). *See* Fluency.

Speech-Sounds Perception Test. Multiple-choice test of spoken nonsense word perception. The target stimuli have differing beginning and ending consonant sounds with constant "ee" vowel sounds throughout. The task is to pick which of the four printed nonsense words corresponds to the spoken nonsense word. This test has frequently been interpreted to be a measure of left temporal lobe function. Reitan and Wolfson (1990), however, have demonstrated that it is more a test of attention, and it is sensitive to lesions throughout the cerebrum. Part of the Halstead-Reitan Neuropsychological Battery. (Reitan, R.M. and Wolfson, D. 1990. The significance of the Speech-Sounds Perception Test for Cerebral Functions. *Arch. Clin. Neuropsychol.* 5:2665–272.)

Speech therapy. Therapy designed to maximize recovery of speech and language in patients with acquired language impairment or to facilitate speech and language development in children with developmental speech and language disorders. Speech therapy is not limited to central disorders; it is also applied to problems such as stuttering and phonation difficulty.

Speed and Capacity of Language-Processing Test (SCOLP). A measure of language processing that consists of two subtests. The Speed of Comprehension Test contains simple true/false statements that are completed by the subject in a 2-minute period. The Spot-the-Word Vocabulary Test, which requires the subject to distinguish real words from nonwords, was designed as a measure resistant to the effect of brain injury. The discrepancy between test results is thought to reflect the degree of probable cognitive impairment. (Baddeley, A., Emslie, H., and Nimmo-Smith, I. 1992. *The Speed and Capacity of Language-Processing Test (SCOLP).* Bury St. Edmunds, Suffolk, England: Thames Valley Test Company.)

Speed tests. Timed tests in which the dependent measure is the number of items completed within the specified time limit.

Speed-accuracy tradeoff. A phenomenon associated with tests requiring response accuracy that must be performed within a limited time. By emphasizing the speed aspects of the test, performance accuracy is decreased, and maximizing accuracy decreases speed.

Spina bifida. A developmental anomaly characterized by defective closure of the bony encasement of the spinal cord, so that the cord and meninges may protrude through it. [L. *spina*, spine, prickle; *bifida*, feminine of *bifidus*, forked, from *bis*, twice; *findere*, to cleave, divide.]

Spina bifida occulta. An anomaly that develops when neural closure fails without involvement of spinal cord tissue. There is no detectable neurologic deficit.

Spinal tap. *See* Lumbar puncture.

Spinothalamic system. The ascending sensory system that carries information about diffuse touch, pain, and temperature.

Split-brain. *See* Commissurotomy.

Splitting the midline. A sign of psychogenic sensory loss in which sensory perception, typically tested with a pinprick, stops abruptly at the midline of the body. This suggests a non-neurologic etiology of the sensory loss because normal sensory fibers spread across the midline. Vibration may similarly reveal this abnormality since it spreads over bony structures and can easily be perceived on the contralateral side.

Spontaneous speech. Spoken discourse produced at the discretion of the speaker.

Standard deviation. A statistical measure of the variability or dispersion of scores around the mean. The standard deviation is the square root of the variance.

Standard error of measurement. A measure of the variability of scores obtained on a test relative to the "true scores." A small standard error of measurement indicates a reliable test.

Standard error of the mean. A measure of the degree to which a sample mean varies from sample to sample around the true mean of the entire population; the standard deviation of the sampling distribution of the sample mean. The standard error of the mean is smaller with larger sample sizes. It is typically estimated by taking the standard deviation in the sample and dividing by the square root of the sample size.

Standard score. A score transformed to reflect its distance from the mean measured in standard deviation units. This may be expressed using a variety of scales (e.g., T score, z score) and need not imply that the underlying distribution of scores is normal, although the transformation is commonly employed with normally distributed test scores.

Standardization. The process by which data from a group of individuals intended to represent the population of interest are collected and analyzed. A standardization can be conducted in groups of healthy individuals, patients with a specific neurologic disease, or other clinical populations. With adequate standardization of a test, an individual's performance can be characterized relative to individuals of similar background and characteristics. The standardization sample is frequently stratified rather than completely randomized to ensure representative sampling of important subject characteristics (e.g., age, education).

Stanford-Binet Intelligence Scale. (Alfred Binet, French psychologist, 1857–1911; Théodore Simon, French physician, 1873–1961). Aside from the Wechsler Intelligence Scales (WIS), this is the most widely used test of general intellectual functioning. The test is based on a hierarchical model of cognitive abilities, in which general reasoning factor (g) is the first level. The second level consists of crystallized abilities, fluid-analytic abilities, and short-term memory. The third level consists of verbal reasoning, quantitative reasoning, and abstract-visual reasoning. The ages at which this test can be administered range from 2 years, 0 months through age 23 years, 11 months. The Stanford-Binet test is a modification of the Binet-Simon test, which was created to screen school children at risk for learning problems. Louis Terman (1877–1956) modified the scale not only by translating it from French to English but also by adding questions and extending the age range. The test became known as the Stanford-Binet because of Terman's academic appointment at Stanford University. (Thorndike, R.L., Hagen, E.P., and Sattler, J.M. 1986. *Stanford-Binet Intelligence Scale*, 4th ed. Chicago: Riverside Publishing.)

Stanine. A score that represents where a score falls on a distribution that is divided into nine equal intervals. Stanine 1 is the lowest ninth and stanine 9 is the highest ninth of the distribution. "Stanine" is derived from "standard nine."

Stat. Immediately. [Abbrev. of L. *statim*, at once.]

Status epilepticus. A seizure lasting more the 30 minutes or repeated seizures without periods of consciousness between them. All seizure types can be associated with status epilepticus. Generalized convulsive status epilepticus is a medical emergency with a mortality rate of approximately 10% when it lasts longer than 2 hours. Patients with generalized status tend to have sequelae of hippocampal sclerosis. Nonconvulsive status epilepticus is marked by decreased alertness. Epilepsy partialis continua is a variant that is characterized by continual seizure activity without loss of consciousness.

STD. Short-term disability.

Steal phenomenon. Diversion of blood flow from vascularized tissue to tissue deprived of blood flow cue to proximal arterial obstruction or a vascular abnormality. *See* Arteriovenous malformation.

Stellate cells. Neurons with a star-shaped soma (cell body) that typically have an associative function within a particular brain region rather than an output function to other areas (i.e., *see* Pyramidal cells). [L. *stellatus*, past part. of *stellare*, to cover with stars, from *stella*, a star.]

Stereognosis. Recognition of objects by touch. Some authors have used the term to describe recognition of familiar objects by touch; this usage is common in the neurologic literature. *See* Agnosia (astereognosis). [Gr. *stereos*, solid; *gnosis*, knowledge.]

Stereograms. Meaningful visual stimuli that can be identified only with binocular vision. [Gr. *stereos*, solid; *gramma*, a writing or drawing.]

Stereotaxic guided surgery. A surgical technique in which the patient is placed in a stereotaxic apparatus before an MRI scan. This allows for greater precision in determining critical brain regions for the placement of electrodes or cannulae because the relationship between the sterotaxic frame and brain areas can be precisely determined. This procedure is commonly used for intracranial electrode implantation, as in epilepsy surgery where depth electrodes are implanted to record spontaneous discharges and ictal events; for pallidotomy to treat Parkinson's disease, in which lesions are created near the region of the internal capsule; and for the removal of diseased tissue. In addition, stereotaxic guided surgery is used in cerebral biopsies.

Stereotaxic radiosurgery. A minimally invasive technique of creating lesions with a gamma knife and modified linear accelerator. It currently is used to treat poorly accessible arteriovenous malformations (AVMs) and brain cancer, although there are many other potential applications.

Stereotypy. The persistent repetition of purposeless movements, acts, or words. [Gr. *stereos*, solid; *typos* a blow, the mark of a blow, figure, outline, character of a disease.]

Sternberg paradigm. A recognition memory task that requires people to memorize a short list of digits. Digits are then presented visually and subjects respond "yes" or "no" to indicate whether a test digit is from the memorized set. Reaction time increases with the size of the set to be memorized. (Sternberg, S. 1966. High-speed scanning in human memory. *Science* 153:652–654.)

Stimulus-boundedness. Difficulty disengaging or shifting the focus of attention from one stimulus in the perceptual field to another. Individuals showing stimulus-bound behavior seem pulled toward or "stuck" on stimuli (i.e., unable to direct their gaze away from or to stop handling test materials). Stimulus-boundedness is often attributed to frontal circuit dysfunction, but it may also be seen with diffuse brain pathology. "*Closing-in*" behavior is a related phenomenon in which an individual seems pulled toward a stimulus; for example, a design may be copied inappropriately close to or even on top of the stimulus figure.

Storage deficit. A memory deficit resulting from impaired consolidation. The classic example of a storage deficit is illustrated by patient H.M. who, after bilateral temporal lobectomy, can neither recall nor recognize material once his attention has been directed away from the task.

Stratified sample. A sample for which adequate representation of specific characteristics within the sample have been ensured by imposing certain restrictions on the composition of the sample. For example, a true random sample for studying the effects of aging requires that all subjects in the population have the same likelihood of being selected. Since there are relatively fewer elderly than younger individuals, chances are that an insufficient number of elderly subjects would be included if the examiner relied on random sampling. A stratified sample ensures adequate representation of all ages by creating independent age-groups and drawing a random sample from each age-group (stratum). [Latin *stratus*, stretched out, a layer.]

Stretch reflexes. *See* Deep tendon reflexes.

Striate cortex. The primary sensory visual cortex, Brodmann's area 17. It is named striate because of the stria (stripe) of Gennari, a thin, myelinated tract that is a prominent feature of the granular layer of the cortex and runs horizontally. Also called calcarine cortex. [L. *striatus*, furrowed; *cortex*, bark.]

Striatum. Caudate nucleus and putamen. Also called corpus striatum. [L. *striatus*, furrowed.]

Stroke (cerebral). The sudden onset of neurologic dysfunction as the result of a cerebrovascular event. Strokes are considered either ischemic, which is the most common type and includes thrombotic and embolic etiology, or hemorrhagic, in which blood leaks from a weakened vessel because of aneurysms or vascular malformations. A "progressing stroke" is one in which deficits are worsening. A stroke in the carotid distribution typically progresses for up to 18 hours, while a vertebrobasilar stroke may progress for 2–3 days. "Completed stroke" describes a stable neurologic picture without evidence of progression. Also called cerebrovascular accident (CVA). [M.E. *strook, strok,* from O.E. *strac,* a stroke, from *strican,* to strike.]

Stroma. The supportive tissue. Stroma in the central nervous system consists primarily of glia. [Gr. *stroma*, anything spread out for sitting or lying upon, mattress, bed, from *stronnynai*, to spread out.]

Stroop Color-Word Interference Test. A task consisting of color names printed in nonmatching colored ink (e.g. "RED" printed in blue ink). Reading the color names (e.g., "RED," "GREEN," "BLUE") regardless of ink color used for printing is reliably faster and more accurate than identifying the ink color while ignoring the spelled color name (i.e., the interference or inhibition condition). Many different versions of this paradigm exist for experimental and clinical purposes, most of which also measure how quickly color names can be read when they are printed in dark ink, and how quickly ink color can be identified when items contain minimal verbal content (e.g., "XXXX" printed in different colors). Various scoring schemes have been proposed, including a time difference score between the reading and "inhibition" tasks, and a ratio index of interference is commonly used. The inhibition effect is sensitive to brain damage. Diminished performance, however, has also been reported in depressed and anxious patients. (Stroop, J.R. 1935. Studies of interference in serial verbal reactions. *J. Exp. Psychol.* 18:643–662.)

Structured Clinical Interview for DSM-IV (SCID). A structured clinical interview that assesses 33 Axis-I diagnoses in adults. It does not evaluate disorders usually first evident in infancy, childhood, and adolescence, organic mental disorders, dissociative disorders, sexual disorders, sleep disorders, factitious disorders, or impulse control disorders. Specialized editions and modules have been developed for specific disorders (e.g., dissociative disorders, panic disorder, and post-traumatic stress disorder) and particular patient populations (e.g., veterans, human immunodeficiency virus infection, and nonpsychiatric patients). The SCID-II is a companion instrument that assesses personality disorders (Axis II).

Stupor. An unconscious state from which the patient can be partially aroused but cannot reach a fully wakeful state of awareness.

Subacute. Between acute and chronic. Denotes a disease course of moderate duration.

Subacute spongiform encephalopathy (SSE). *See* Creutzfeldt-Jakob disease.

Subarachnoid hemorrhage (SAH). Leakage of blood into the subarachnoid space from trauma or a vascular malformation. Traumatic SAH results from laceration of cerebral vessels that bleed into the subarachnoid space after head injury. Nontraumatic SAH most often results from ruptured aneurysms. Death is common because as little as 100 ml of blood can produce coma due to increased intracranial volume. However, a small SAH (e.g., sentinel bleeds) may have relatively minor clinical correlates and may be disregarded as simply a headache by the patient. Nontraumatic SAH is typically associated with meningismus (nuchal rigidity). Susarachnoid hemorrhage often occurs during exertion such as during exercise or during sex. [L. *sub*, under, below; Gr. *arachne*, spider, cobweb; *eidos*, resemblance; *haimorrhages*, bleeding violently: *haima*, blood; *rhegynai*, to break, burst.]

Subclinical. The presence of a disease without associated symptoms.

Subcortical. Brain regions that lie below the cortex. Among the prominent subcortical areas are the thalamus and basal ganglia.

Subcortical aphasia. *See* Aphasia.

Subcortical dementia. *See* Dementia.

Subcortical lesions. Deep lesions affecting noncortical areas. A common cause of subcortical lesions is lacunar infarction from arterial hypertension. Lacunar infarctions result from occlusion of small arteries (i.e., perforators) of the lenticulostriate branches of the middle cerebral artery, thalamic perforants of the posterior cerebral artery, and the paramedian branches of the basilar artery.

Subdural hematoma. *See* Hematoma (subdural).

Subdural hemorrhage. *See* Hemorrhage (subdural).

Subiculum. A medial temporal lobe structure between the parahippocampal gyrus and Ammon's horn. [L. *subic-, subex*, underlayer, support.]

Subject variable. Classification variable reflecting some aspect of life experiences. Subject variables are not easily manipulated and are employed in correlational and experimental designs involving covariates. The majority of clinical neuropsychological research employs subject variables.

Substantia nigra. Large midbrain nucleus that is often considered part of the basal ganglia and is associated with motor function. Many cells in the substantia nigra contain dopamine and melanin, a byproduct of dopamine metabolism. Severe cell loss in this area occurs in Parkinson's disease. [L., *substantia*, substance; *nigra*, from *niger*, black substance.]

Subtest scatter. Test performance variability of an individual's scores across subtests. This is a consideration when comparing Wechsler subtests. High Wechsler subtest scatter is often interpreted as reflecting some abnormality, whether neurologic or psychiatric. However, subtest variability is characteristic of many normally functioning people and is not necessarily indicative of pathology.

Sulcus. A groove or fissure of the brain that defines a gyrus. Major fissures demarcate lobes of the brain. [L. *sulcus*, furrow, ditch; pl. *sulci*.]

Sundowning. Increased confusion during the late afternoon and early evening hours (i.e., when the sun goes down) that is often present in patients with dementia or acute confusional states.

Sunset gaze sign. An inability to look up. The pupils appear to be "setting" in the lower lid. This sign may accompany increased intracranial pressure.

Superior anastomotic vein. *See* Labbé, vein of.

Supervisory attentional system (SAS). A theoretical system of nonroutine attentional control. The SAS is putatively localized in the frontal cortex and represents an attempt to anchor Aleksandr Luria's (Soviet neuropsychologist, 1902–1977) theory of frontal-executive functions within a cognitive science framework. *See* Memory (working memory).

Supine. The position of lying down with face upward. [L. *supinus*, backward, lying on one's back.]

Supplementary motor area. The area anterior to the primary motor cortex that is important in temporal organization of movements, especially in sequential performance of multiple movements. It is important in the initiation of voluntary movements. It is located at the anterior portion of Brodmann area 6 on the medial surface.

Supported employment. Subcompetitive employment model in which disabled persons are supported by *job coaching* or by specialized training and supervision in an enclave (group employment setting or "crew"). In some such models, performance of one competitive job is provided by two subcompetitive workers, or by one disabled worker and one part-time job coach.

Suprasella cyst. *See* Craniopharyngioma.

Supratentorial. Above the tentorium, which is the dural covering the cerebellum. The term is used to describe the cerebral hemispheres, and it is used colloquially to describe a functional deficit (i.e., a deficit in "one's head").

Surface agraphia. *See* Agraphia spelling disorders.

Surface structure. The specific linguistic form of an utterance. *See* Deep structure.

Sx. Shorthand notation for "symptom."

Sylvian fissure. (Franciscus Sylvius, Dutch anatomist, 1614–1672). The major sulcus beginning at the base of the brain on the lateral aspect of the anterior perforated substance, extending laterally between the temporal lobe and frontal lobe, and turning posteriorly between the temporal lobe and parietal lobe. It divides into posterior, ascending, and anterior branches. Also called the lateral fissure. [L. *fissura*, a cleft, from *findere*, to cleave, split.]

Symbol Digit Modalities Test (SDMT). A test of graphomotor speed that is similar to the Digit Symbol—Coding test from the Wechsler Intelligence Scales (WIS). Single digits are uniquely paired with simple visual symbols as part of an answer key. The test contains symbols with blank boxes, and the task is to fill in the number corresponding to the symbols as quickly as possible. This contrasts with the Digit Symbol—Coding test, in which numbers are the printed stimuli and the subject writes the corresponding symbol. The SDMT enables the patient to respond with the more familiar act of number writing; it also allows for a spoken response trial. A written form of this test permits group administration. (Smith, A. 1991. *Symbol Digit Modalities Test.* Los Angeles: Western Psychological Services.)

Symbolic language. *See* Propositional language.

Sympathetic nervous system. *See* Autonomic nervous system.

Symptom validity testing. Any approach designed to assess deficit exaggeration of a purported symptom. Common techniques include multiple-choice formats in which subjects are told to provide an answer, even if they are unsure of a response. This allows response probabilities to be calculated to determine if the incorrect choice is being selected more often than by chance, which suggests that the correct response is being avoided. Other approaches to symptom validity testing include examination of primacy and recency memory effects, comparison of word span and digit span, and priming effects.

Synapse. The functional contact point between neural processes or between a neuron and a receptor (muscle or gland). The electrical action potential elicits the release of chemical neurotransmitters into the synaptic cleft, which alters the post-synaptic neuron's likelihood of firing. Synapses can be either inhibitory or excitatory/facilitory. [Gr. *syn-*, together; *haptein*, to clasp.]

Syncope. A temporary loss of consciousness; fainting. Syncope may be related to reduced cardiac output, temporary reduction of blood flow to the brain, a decrease in an essential blood component, or other factors. It may also be related to psychological factors, including anxiety. [Gr. *synkope*, swoon, cut short, from *synkoptein*, chop up, cut off.]

Syndrome. Signs and symptoms that often occur together and that suggest a common etiology, prognosis, and treatment. [Gr. *syndrome*, a running together, a concurrence (of symptoms); *syn-*, together; *dromos*, race, or running.]

Synesthesia. Multisensory perception from single sensory stimulation. This gives rise to the sensation of "hearing" colors and "seeing" sounds, which has been reported with the use of hallucinogens. In his book *Mind of a Mnemonist*, Aleksander Luria (1968) described how a patient's synesthetic associations with sound were cues that greatly aided the patient's recall; for example, "He remarked to Vygotsky 'What a crumbly, yellow voice you have'." [Gr. *syn-*, together; *aessthesis*, sensation.]

Synkinesia. Involuntary movement of a muscle group during the execution of voluntary movement that involves a different muscle group. This may be seen with athetosis, in which distant muscles contract, or with diffuse brain damage in which there is movement of the contralateral hand during fine-motor movement. Also called motor overflow. [Gr. *syn-*, together; *kinésis*, movement.]

Syntax. The rules of language structure governing the assembly of words into sentences. Syntax represents the variety of relationships among words (i.e., word order) that help convey information in a coherent and meaningful manner. [Gr. *syntaxis*, put together, arrange in order; *syn-*, together; *taxis*, order, arrangement.]

Systemic lupus erythematosus (SLE). A generalized collagen vascular disease characterized by skin eruptions, neurological manifestations, lymphadenopathy, fever, and other constitutional symptoms. The neurologic features of SLE are sometimes referred to as the 3 S's- *strokes*, *seizures*, and *psychosis*. [L. *lupus*, wolf; Gr. *erythema*, a redness of the skin.]

T

T score. A standard score that as been transformed to fit a normal curve distribution with a mean of 50 and a standard deviation of 10 points. A T score of 60, for example, indicates performance that is one standard deviation above the mean and corresponds to performance at the 84th centile. T scores are used by various psychological tests such as the MMPI, and in the normative tables for an expanded Halstead-Reitan Neuropsychological Battery. (Heaton, R.K., Grant, I., and Matthews, C.G. 1991. *Comprehensive Norms for an Expanded Halstead-Reitan Battery: Demographic Corrections, Research Findings, and Clinical Applications.* Odessa, FL: Psychological Assessment Resources.)

Tachistoscope. An apparatus that allows brief presentation of visual stimuli. Stimulus duration can be on the order of milliseconds. [Gr. *tachistos*, superlative of *tachys*, swift; *scopein*, to see.]

Tactile agnosia. *See* Agnosia.

Tactile Finger Recognition. *See* Reitan-Kløve Sensory Perceptual Examination.

Tactile Form Perception. A test of *stereognosis* in which geometric figures made of fine-grade sandpaper are identified tactually. The stimuli are presented out of the subject's sight and the task is to explore each stimulus with the hand and to identify it by matching it with a visual stimulus. (Benton, A.L., Sivan, A.B., Hamsher, K.deS., Varney, N.R., and Spreen, O. 1994. *Contributions to Neuropsychological Assessment. A Clinical Manual,* 2nd ed. New York: Oxford University Press.)

Tactile Form Recognition. *See* Reitan-Kløve Sensory Perceptual Examination.

Tactual Performance Test (TPT). A test of tactile perception, motor coordination, tactile exploration, and memory. The task is to explore wooden shapes (e.g., star, triangle) while blindfolded and to place them into a formboard. Trials are given for the dominant hand, nondominant hand, and both hands together, and there is a memory trial for location and number of shapes correctly drawn. This test is a modification of the Seguin formboard and is part of the Halstead-Reitan Neuropsychological Battery. [L. *tactus*, pl. of *tangere*, to touch.]

Talairach space. A technique of displaying individual MRIs with standardized coordinates to facilitate comparison across individuals and for stereotaxic localization. Three reference lines are employed. The CA-PA line passes through the superior edge of the anterior commissure and the inferior edge of the posterior commissure. The VCA line is a vertical line traversing the posterior margin of the anterior commissure. The third reference line is the sagittal plane. (Talairach, J. and Tournoux, P. 1988. *Co-Planar Stereotaxic Atlas of the Human Brain.* New York: Thieme Medical Publishers.)

Tangentiality. Discourse that is characterized by wandering speech that never returns to the original subject matter.

Tardive dyskinesia (TD). A nonreversible involuntary movement disorder resulting from dopamine hypersensitivity after long-term *neuroleptic* therapy. Prominent dyskinesias involve the tongue, jaw, and facial expressions. Risk of TD increases with age and medication dosage. [OF. *tardif*, tardy, from L. *tardus*, slow; Gr. *dys-*, ill, bad; *kinesis*, movement, motion.]

Target Test. A test of visual spatial attention from the Halstead-Reitan Neuropsychological Battery for children. A sequence is tapped out on a large stimulus figure containing nine black dots, and after a 3-second delay, the sequence is drawn on the answer sheet.

Task analysis. A rehabilitation procedure in which the physical, cognitive, and social demands of a complex task are analyzed to identify the source of breakdown to target intervention.

Taylor Complex Figure. *See* Complex Figure Test.

Tay-Sachs disease. (Warren Tay, British ophthalmologist, surgeon, pediatrician, and dermatologist, 1843–1927; Bernard Sachs, American neurologist, 1858–1944). An autosomal recessive genetic disorder that affects primarily Jewish children of Eastern European (Ashkenazi) descent. It is initially characterized by poor visual fixation and an increased startle response shortly after birth, followed by delayed psychomotor development and motor regression. Death usually occurs between age 3 and 5 years.

TBI. *See* Traumatic brain injury.

Telegrammatism. *See* Agrammatism.

Telegraphic speech. *See* Agrammatism.

Telencephalon. Cerebral hemispheres of the brain. The telencephalon is the anterior of the two divisions of the prosencephalon. [Gr. *telos*, end; *enkephalos*, brain.]

Temporal context. Contextual knowledge that allows events to be discriminated in time.

Temporal gradient. The greater likelihood of memory loss for events closer in time to the occurrence of the neurological insult or development of neurologic disease. It is also present in normal aging. *See* Ribot's law.

Temporal herniation. *See* Herniation, brain.

Temporal lobe. The lower lateral lobe of the cerebral hemisphere, lying below the Sylvian (lateral) fissure and merging posteriorly with the occipital lobe. The temporal lobes contain the hippocampus, an important structures for making new memories. [L. *temporalis*, from *tempus*, time.]

TENS. Transelectrical nerve stimulation; an approach to pain treatment in which electrical stimulation is applied to the nerve to decrease its sensitivity.

Tentorium. The portion of the dura covering the posterior fossa. The tentorium is attached to the falx and separates the cerebellum from the occipital and temporal lobes. Colloquially referred to as the tent. [L. *tentorium*, a tent.]

Ten-twenty system. A standardized system of scalp electrode placement. Electrode placements are determined by measuring the head from external landmarks and placing the electrodes at sites that are 10% or 20% of the distance between landmarks.

Tesla. (Nikola Tesla, Yugoslavian-born American physicist, 1856–1943). The standard unit of magnetic flux density.

Test of Everyday Attention (TEA). A measure of selective attention, sustained attention, attentional switching, and divided attention that employs material and tasks that are routinely encountered in real-life settings. Examples of the tests include Map Search, Elevator Counting, Telephone Search, and Lottery, which involves listening for the "winning number" while writing down two letters preceding and numbers ending in given digits. (Robertson, I.H., Ward, T., Ridgeway, V., and Nimmo-Smith, I. 1994. *Test of Everyday Attention*. Bury St. Edmunds, Suffolk, England: Thames Valley Test Co.)

Test of Memory and Learning (TOMAL). A test of memory for children and adolescents between 5 and 19 years of age. It consists of 10 core and 4 supplemental subtests, and yields composite scores for Verbal Memory, Nonverbal Memory, Composite Memory, Delayed Recall, Learning Index, Attention and Concentration, Sequential Memory, Free Recall, and Associative Recall. (Reynolds, C.R. and Bigler, F D. 1994. *Test of Memory and Learning*. Austin, TX: POR-ED.)

Test of Memory Malingering (TOMM). A forced-choice recognition test that includes two learning trials and a retention trial. Explicit feedback on response correctness is given for each item. The TOMM is similar in composition to the Warrington Recognition Memory Test. (Tombaugh, T.N. 1996. *Test of Memory Malingering*. Tonowanda: New York: Multi-Health Systems.)

Thalamic syndrome. A combination of superficial persistent hemianesthesia, mild hemiplegia, mild hemiataxia, variable astereognosis, severe and persistent pains in the hemiplegic side, and choreo-athetoid movements in the limbs of the paralyzed side. Also called Dejerine-Roussy syndrome.

Thalamotomy. Surgical treatment of Parkinson's disease (PD) that involves lesioning the thalamus with stereotaxically placed electrodes. The lesion disrupts the excessive excitation that contributes to many parkinsonian features.

Thalamus. Sensory-relay nuclei located in the diencephalon within each cerebral hemisphere. The thalamus forms part of the lateral wall of the third ventricle and is the main relay center for sensory impulses and cerebellar and basal ganglia projections to the cerebral cortex. In addition to sensory deficits, lesions involving the thalamus may produce aphasia, executive dysfunction, or memory impairment [Gr. *thalamos*, an inner room or inner chamber.]

Thematic Apperception Test (TAT). A projective technique using pictures designed to elicit thought content, emotions, and conflicts. Subjects are asked to tell stories about each picture; the stories are to have a beginning describing what led up to the scene, a middle describing the scene, and an end describing the outcome. A variety of scoring methods, including quantitative and nonquantitative systems and rating scales, have been developed. (Murray, H.A. 1938. *Explorations in personality*. New York: Oxford University Press.) [F. *aperception*, perception, from L. *ad*, to + *percipere*, to perceive.]

Thiamine. *See* B$_1$.

Three words-three shapes test. A bedside memory task in which 6 stimuli are first copied, then immediately recalled. Subjects are not forewarned that memory will be tested. If the subject is unable to recall at least 5 items, a 30-second exposure of the 6 stimuli is provided, following by another immediate recall test. This is repeated for up to 5 trials or until 5/6 items are recalled. Delayed free recall after 5, 15, and 30 minutes is obtained, and 30-minute delayed recognition is tested if the subject does not reproduce all 6 items during the 30-minute delayed-recall condition. (Mesulam, M.-M. 1985. *Principles of Behavioral Neurology*. Philadelphia: F.A. Davis.)

Three-Dimensional Block Construction. A test of visual constructional ability in which three-dimensional block models are assembled. Three-dimensional construction tasks are thought to be more sensitive to mild right hemisphere impairment than two-dimensional block tasks. (Benton, A.L., Sivan, A.B., Hamsher, K.deS., Varney, N.R., and Spreen, O. 1994. *Contributions to Neuropsychological Assessment. A Clinical Manual*. 2nd ed. New York: Oxford University Press.)

Thrombolytic therapy. Acute treatment of ischemic stroke that uses agents to dissolve clots obstructing flow through the cerebral arteries. Thrombolytic therapy can decrease neurological impairment if it is initiated within the first few hours after stroke. *See* Ischemic penumbra. [Gr. *thrombos*, particle, lump, small mass; *lysis*, a loosening.]

Thrombosis, cerebral. Occlusion of a cerebral blood vessel by a thrombus (solidified blood within a vessel) that usually occurs at the site of a pre-existing arterial stenosis.

Thrombus. Solidified blood within a vessel. [Gr. *thrombos*, particle, lump, small mass.]

Thurstone Word Fluency. A test of written fluency from Thurstone's Primary Mental Abilities test that is similar to oral tests of verbal fluency (e.g., Controlled Oral Word Association). The test is to write as many words that begin with the letter "s" as possible during a 5-minute span, and as many words as possible that begin with "c" in four minutes. (Thurstone, L.L. and Thurstone, T.G. 1962. *Primary Mental Abilities* (Revised). Chicago: Science Research Associates.)

TIA. *See* Transient ischemic attacks.

Tic. An involuntary, stereotyped movement resembling a purposeful movement because it is coordinated and involves muscles that are normally synergistic. Tics usually involve the face and shoulders.

tid. Shorthand notation for "three times a day." [L. *ter in die.*]

Time-out. Behavior modification technique in which patients are removed temporarily from sources of reinforcement to decrease an undesired behavior.

Tinnitus. Ringing in the ears. [L. *tinnitus*, a jingling.]

Tip-of-the-tongue-phenomenon. The inability to retrieve a word despite knowledge of its meaning and *phonology*.

Todd's paralysis. (Robert B. Todd, British physician, 1809–1860). Temporary postepileptic hemiplegia or monoplegia after a seizure stops that usually lasts only a few minutes but may persist for 48 hours. A previous focal deficit may worsen or a new deficit may appear. The functional impairment depends on the area of cortex in which the seizure occurred.

Token economy. A behavior modification technique in which material rewards, or tokens representing them, are provided for desired behaviors and withdrawn for undesired behaviors.

Token Test. A test of auditory comprehension involving commands of graded length and complexity that are to be executed with tokens varying in color, shape, and size. The Token Test is too difficult for many aphasic patients, but it is sensitive to mild or latent comprehension disturbance. Many versions of this test exist. (De Renzi, E. and Vignolo, L. 1962. The Token Test: A sensitive test to detect receptive disturbances in aphasics. *Brain*, 85:665–678.)

Tonic-clonic seizure. *See* Seizure (generalized tonic-clonic seizure).

Topectomy. A surgical resection of a small area of cortex. [Gr. *topos*, a place; *-tomy*, from *temnein*, to cut.]

Top-of-the-basilar syndrome. A condition from emboli that pass through the termination of the basilar artery and occlude the thalamoperforant arteries. It consists of visual, oculomotor, and behavioral abnormalities without significant motor dysfunction. Memory impairment is common with infarction of the medial thalamus, although it is not as dense as that associated with hippocampal infarction. (Caplan, L.R. 1980. "Top of the basilar" syndrome. *Neurology* 30:72–79.)

Topographical amnesia. Specific loss of memory for places.

Topographical disorientation. The inability to find one's way about, as in following mental or paper maps.

Topographical memory. *See* Memory.

Tourette syndrome. *See* Gilles de la Tourette's syndrome.

Tower of London/Hanoi/Toronto. Problem-solving tasks used to assess frontal lobe dysfunction and residual learning capability. Although these versions differ with respect to complexity, they all involve moving different colored rings (or beads) from their positions on vertical sticks to other specific locations in the fewest number of moves. (Shallice, T. 1982. Specific impairments of planning. *Phil. Trans. R. Soc. Lond.* 298: 199–209.)

Toxic-metabolic encephalopathy. A condition associated with systemic disorders of metabolism or intoxication that is commonly characterized by altered mental status. It is one of the most common causes of confusional states in the elderly. A fluctuating course is common, and symptoms are usually worse in the evening (i.e., sundowning).

Toxoplasmosis. An opportunistic infection with the parasite *Toxoplasm gondii*. It may be congenital or acquired (e.g., through contract with cat feces), but its most common presentation is with AIDS. A CT image usually generally shows the ring-enhancing lesion associated with brain abscesses. Neuropsychological deficits may occasionally include language impairment, but confusion associated with a generalized subacute encephalopathy is more common.

Tracheostomy/tracheotomy. An opening of the neck to allow placement of a tube through the trachea to establish a direct airway for artificial ventilation.

Trail Making Test. A test of visual scanning speed developed in 1944 by the U.S. Army that has two parts. Part A consists of 25 circles numbered from 1 to 25 that are distributed on a piece of paper. The task is to "connect the dots" as quickly as possible. Part B consists of 25 circles with the numbers 1 to 13 and letters A to L. The task is connect the circles alternating between numbers and letters in sequence. The scores are the number of seconds required to finish each part, although the number of errors is often recorded. A children's version of the test contains the first 15 stimuli (circles) from the standard form. Other variants of the test include an oral version and a color form (*Army Individual Test Battery. Manual of Directions and Scorings*. Washington, D.C.: U.S. War Department, Adjutant General's Office; Armitage, S. G. 1946. An analysis of certain psychological tests for the evaluation of brain injury. *Psychol. Monogr.* 60:[277].)

Transcortical motor aphasia. *See* Aphasia syndromes.

Transcortical sensory aphasia. *See* Aphasia syndromes.

Transient global amnesia (TGA). A sudden, acute amnesia that is typically benign and resolves within 24 hours. The etiology of TGA is debated, but it appears to involve subcortical structures with postulated mechanisms of ischemia or partial seizures and spreading depression. During TGA, patients are disoriented and unable to form new memories, although they can carry out complex activities, such as driving a car. Initially, the patient is also unaware of the memory deficits. A dense retrograde amnesia is present for recently experienced information and it may extend backward several months. As the TGA recedes, the retrograde amnesia shrinks. Transient global amnesia is often precipitated by events associated with sudden body changes such as a cold shower, sexual intercourse, or a strong emotional experience.

Transient ischemic attack (TIA). A sudden onset of focal cerebral neurological dysfunction (e.g., hemiplegia) attributable to blood vessel disease which resolves in less than 24 hours. Most carotid TIAs last 3–5 minutes and most vertebrobasilar TIAs last 10–12 minutes. Transient ischemic attacks indicate atherosclerotic cerebrovascular disease, and approximately 5% of this population will develop a stroke within a year without treatment. The main treatments are endarterectomy and antiplatelet therapy.

Transitional living. A program of supervised living and structured activity for brain-injured persons that also provides retraining in independent living skills.

Transtentorial herniation. *See* Herniation, brain.

Traumatic brain injury (TBI). Brain injury caused by an external mechanical force such as a blow to the head, concussive forces, acceleration-deceleration forces, or projectile missile (e.g., bullet). The primary causes of TBI are motor vehicle accidents, falls, and interpersonal violence. Severity of injury can be assessed with a Glasgow Coma Scale score or by measuring the duration of loss of consciousness (coma, LOC), with each measure adding increased prognostic value. [Gr. *trauma*, wound, hurt.]

- **Mild TBI**. A TBI with a Glasgow Coma Scale of 13–15, loss of consciousness of up to 20 minutes, post-traumatic amnesia of up to 24 hours, no focal neurologic deficits, and no focal radiologic evidence of injury. Mild TBI accounts for approximately 80% of nonfatal TBI. *See* also Post-concussion syndrome.
- **Minor head injury**. *See* Mild TBI (above).
- **Moderate TBI**. A TBI with a Glasgow Coma Scale of 9–12.
- **Severe TBI**. A TBI with a Glasgow Coma Scale of 3–8.

Tricyclic medications. A class of antidepressant medications so named because of their chemical structure. Tricyclics are generally better tolerated than monoamine oxidase (MAO) inhibitors and do not require special diets. Frequently used tricyclic medications are imipramine, amitriptyline, nortriptyline, and doxepin. Clomipramine is a tricyclic medication used to treat obsessive-compulsive disorder

Trisomy. A genetic abnormality in which there are three rather than the standard pair of chromosomes. [L. *tres* or Gr. *tris*, three; Gr. *soma*, body.]

Trisomy 21. *See* Down syndrome.

Truncal ataxia. *See* Ataxia.

Tuberous sclerosis. A congenital disorder in which there are sclerotic masses in the cerebral cortex, adenoma sebaceum, tumors in organs, mental retardation, and epilepsy. It follows an autosomal dominant pattern of inheritance with variable penetrance and expression. [L. *tuberosus*, knobby; *sklerosis*, hardness.]

Turner's syndrome. (Henry Hubert Turner, American endocrinologist). A chromosomal condition causing short stature and infertility in females that results from the complete or partial absence of one of the two X chromosomes (XO sex chromosome constitution). Patients with Turner's syndrome typically have normal IQ levels. Also called XO syndrome.

Twenty-One Item Test. A symptom validity test used to identify nonoptimal effort. After presentation of a list of 21 nouns, the patient is asked to recall the list. Immediately after the free-recall trial, the patient is given two alternative forced-choice recognition tasks. (Iverson, G.L., Franzen, M.D., and McCracken, L.M. 1991. Evaluation of an objective assessment technique for the detection of malingered memory deficits. *Law Hum. Behav.* 15: 667–676.)

Twilight state. Transient impaired consciousness in which the patient may perform certain acts involuntarily without subsequent memory for those acts. A twilight state may be seen during recovery from general anesthesia. [M.E. *twi-*, two, double, twice + light; "the light between".]

Twist-drill hole. A small hole of several millimeters made into the skull with a drill, generally to place intracranial electrodes or to obtain a biopsy. It may also be used to drain a subdural hematoma.

Two-Point Discrimination. A discrimination task in which the examiner uses calipers to measure two-point discrimination thresholds.

Two-route model. A theory of language processing that postulates two separate means for successful production. In reading, words can be either sounded out or "sight read" for meaning; in writing, words can be either spelled phonetically or written from a memorized vocabulary.

Tx. Shorthand notation for treatment, or therapy.

Type I error. A hypothesis-testing error made by rejecting the null hypothesis when it is true. Also called alpha error.

Type II error. A hypothesis-testing error made by failing to reject the null hypothesis when it is false. Also called beta error.

U

U fibers. Short cortical fibers that connect adjacent cortical gyri.

UBO. Unidentified bright object. This term is applied to hyperintense white matter foci from T_2-weighted MRIs. The cause of the abnormal signals cannot be determined with certainty, and they may reflect a variety of conditions, such as white matter pallor, ischemia, infarction, or plaques. The clinical correlates and relationships to cognitive function are variable.

Ultrasound. A technique using Doppler technology that, in neurology, reveals the degree of vessel stenosis and thus helps identify the of cerebrovascular disease.

Uncal herniation. *See* Herniation, brain.

Uncinate seizure. *See* Seizure.

Uncus. The medially curved, anterior end of the parahippocampal gyrus located near the temporal pole. The uncus is a landmark for the lateral olfactory area. [L. *uncus*, a hook.]

Unilateral neglect. The tendency to ignore information presented in the hemispace contralateral to a cerebral lesion. This condition is usually but not always associated with right hemisphere lesions. *See* Neglect syndrome.

Upper motor neurons. The primary motor output pathway that originates in the precentral gyrus, passes through the medullary pyramids, and descends the spinal cord as the corticospinal tract. Upper motor neurons synapse with lower motor neurons in the spinal cord, which carry motor information to the periphery. Upper motor neuron lesions result in spastic hemiplegia or hemiparesis.

Utilization behavior. The propensity to grasp and use objects that are within reach regardless of whether they are related to the present task. When presented with an item, a patient appears compelled to use it for its normal purpose as if enslaved to environmental cues. A patient may start cutting paper when given a pair of scissors, for example, or hammering when presented with a hammer. It is associated with bilateral frontal lobe lesions, especially inferior frontal lesions. It has been postulated to result from disinhibition or loss of modulation of a "natural" tendency, stimulated by parietal lobe systems, to explore and manipulate the physical environment. It is a characteristic of *environmental dependency syndrome*.

V

Vagus nerve stimulation. A technique for decreasing seizure frequency in patients with medically refractory epilepsy. A pacemaker-like device is attached to the tenth (vagus) cranial nerve to deliver electrical pulses.

Validity. The degree to which a measure can be used to support a specific inference. Validity is not a property of a test but of the inferences that the test is designed to produce. Multiple types of validity exist, although the most common include construct validity, content validity, and criterion validity. [L. *validitas*, from *validus*, strong.]

Variance. Measure of the degree to which scores deviate from the mean. The variance is the expected value of the squared difference between observations and the mean of the distribution in the population. In the sample, an unbiased estimate of the population variance is obtained by computing the sum of squared deviations around the sample mean and dividing this sum by $n - 1$, where n is the number of observations. [L. *variare*, to change.]

Vascular dementia. *See* Dementia (vascular).

Vasculitis. Inflammation of a vessel.

VDRL. Venereal Disease Research Laboratories; refers to the laboratory where a serology test for syphilis was developed.

Vegetative state. *See* Persistent vegetative state.

Ventricles, cerebral. Cavities of the brain filled with cerebral spinal fluid that form a continuous space. The largest ventricles are the paired lateral ventricles in the cerebral hemispheres, which can be subdivided into the anterior horn in the frontal lobe, the posterior horn in the occipital lobe, and the inferior horn that extends into the temporal lobe. The third ventricle is located in the midline between the two halves of the diencephalon and connects to the fourth ventricle at the top of the mesencephalon via the cerebral aqueduct. The ventricular system and the subarachnoid space are continuous. [L. *ventriculus*, diminutive of *venter*, stomach or belly.]

Ventriculomegaly. Enlarged ventricles. [Gr. *megalo-*, from *megas*, large, great.]

Ventriculostomy. Operation for the treatment of hydrocephalus to establish free communication between the floor of the third ventricle and the underlying interpeduncular cistern.

Verbal agraphia. *See* Agraphia spelling disorders.

Verbal aphasia. Expressive or Broca's aphasia. [Late L. *verbalis*, pertaining to a word, from *verbum*, a word.]

Verbal code. The linguistic representation of a word. *See* Imaginal code, dual code theory. [Late L. *verbalis*, pertaining to a word, from *verbum*, a word.]

Verbal Comprehension Index. A score derived from selected verbal subtests of the Wechsler Intelligence Scales (WIS) that reflects verbal knowledge and comprehension—knowledge obtained partially from formal education—and reflects the application of verbal skills to novel situations. The WAIS-III subtests contributing to this index are Vocabulary,

Similarities, and Information. The WISC-III index is based on the same three subtests as above plus performance on the Comprehension subtest.

Verbal fluency tests. Generative fluency tasks in which as many words as possible are generated within a specified time, typically 60 seconds. Letter fluency tasks involve the generation of words that begin with a particular letter of the alphabet. Semantic fluency is similar, although words that belong to a particular semantic category (e.g., fruits, animals) are generated. Some evidence exists that Alzheimer's disease may be associated with greater impairment of semantic fluency than letter fluency. *See* Controlled Oral Word Association; Semantic category fluency.

Verbal IQ. A score derived from the scaled scores of the Wechsler Intelligence Scales (WIS) that is indicative of overall verbal intellectual functioning. The Verbal subtests for the WAIS-III are Vocabulary, Similarities, Information, Comprehension, Arithmetic, Digit Span, and Letter-Number Sequencing. The first four subtests (Vocabulary through Comprehension) may be used to calculate a Verbal Comprehension Index, and the last subtests (Arithmetic, Digit Span, Letter-Number Sequencing) may be used to calculate a Working Memory Index. The Verbal subtests from the WISC-III include Vocabulary, Similarities, Information, Comprehension, Arithmetic, and Digit Span (optional subtest).

Verbal learning. Acquisition and retention of stimuli that are verbal or linguistic in nature. The stimuli may be presented in any sensory modality. This term is often equated with left hemisphere function, and left mesial temporal lobe function in particular, but lesions throughout the cerebral hemispheres impair verbal learning as do and psychiatric/psychological disturbances. The term is used to contrast with nonverbal or visual-spatial memory.

Verbal paraphasia. *See* Paraphasia.

Vertigo. The illusion of motion involving either the environment or self. [L. *vertigo* (*vertigin-*), action of whirling, from *vertere*, to turn.]

Victoria Symptom Validity Test. A modification of the *Hiscock-Hiscock Forced Choice Recognition Task* designed for the assessment of memory deficit exaggeration. It employs forced-choice recognition of 5-digit sequences that are presented on a computer. The test includes both easy and hard items. (Slick, D., Hopp, G., and Strauss, E. 1997. *Victoria Symptom Validity Test*. Odessa, FL: Psychological Assessment Resources.)

Vigilance. The ability to monitor the environment over extended periods for infrequent target stimuli. [L. *vigilans*, wakeful, from *vigere*, to be vigorous, lively.]

Vineland Adaptive Behavior Scales. A questionnaire used to assess personal and social competence from birth through adulthood. Three versions of the Vineland Scales are available: the Interview Edition, Survey Form; the Interview Edition, Expanded Form; and the Classroom Edition. All three versions cover four domains of adaptive behavior: Communication, Daily Living Skills, Socialization, and Motor Skills. In addition, an optional Maladaptive Behavior domain is included in the Survey and Expanded Forms. (Sparrow, S.S., Balla, D.A., and Cicchetti, D.V. 1984. *Vineland Adaptive Behavior Scales*. Circle Pines, MN: American Guidance Service.)

Viscosity. An interpersonal style characterized by cohesive and "sticky" behavior that produces prolonged verbal contact. Speech is repetitive and circumstantial. This has been described in a small number of epilepsy patients.

Visual agnosia. *See* Agnosia. [Late L. *visualis*, visual, from L. *visus*, sight.]

Visual constructional impairment. A disturbance in visually guided constructional activity (i.e., constructional apraxia). Many favor the term over "constructional apraxia" because it is a theoretically neutral operational definition that does not imply a neurobehavioral cause.

Visual field. The total area of vision.

Visual field defects. Areas of blindness or altered vision within the visual field. They can be caused by lesions of the retina, optic nerve and tract, lateral geniculate body, geniculo-calcarine pathway, and striate cortex of the occipital lobe.

Visual Form Discrimination. A multiple-choice test of visual perception that employs a matching procedure. The stimulus to be matched contains three geometric designs, two of which are major elements and a smaller peripheral element. This can be conceptualized as a multiple-choice version of the Benton Visual Retention Test in which the stimulus figures remain present. (Benton, A.L., Sivan, A.B., Hamsher, K.deS., Varney, N.R., and Spreen, O. 1994. *Contributions to Neuropsychological Assessment. A Clinical Manual,* 2nd ed. New York: Oxford University Press.)

Visual neglect. Neglect restricted to the visual modality.

Visual Object and Space Perception Battery (VOSP). A measure of object and space perception that has eight subtests. Incomplete Letters requires the identification of degraded letter stimuli. Silhouettes measures object recognition. Object Decision deals with perceptual difficulty that is distinct from word-finding problems. Progressive Silhouettes presents silhouettes of the same object at different angles. Dot Counting measures spatial scanning. Position Discrimination addresses the ability to discriminate between two spatial positions. Number Location is a measure of spatial discrimination. Cube Analysis measures the perception of complex spatial relationships. All subtests are untimed. (Warrington, E.K. and James, M. 1991. *Visual Object and Space Perception Battery.* Bury St. Edmunds, Suffolk, England: Thames Valley Test Co.)

Visual paralexia. *See* Paralexia.

Visual Reproduction. A subtest from the Wechsler Memory Scale (WMS, WMS-R, WMS-IIII) assessing memory for simple designs. The original WMS included only an immediate recall of the Visual Reproduction designs. The Visual Reproduction subtest from the WMS-R and WMS-III contains both an immediate and a delayed recall. It is a supplemental WMS-III subtest.

Visual Search and Attention Test. A measure of visual scanning and sustained attention that is composed of cancellation tasks. In two practice trials a letter or symbol that matches the target is crossed out. The two selective cancellation tasks require the patient to cancel blue *H*'s and blue slashes from an array of letters or symbols printed in blue, green, or red ink. (Trenerry, M.R., Crosson, B., DeBoe, J., and Leber, W.R. 1990. *Visual Search and Attention Test.* Odessa, FL: Psychological Assessment Resources.)

Visuomotor apraxia, ataxia. *See* Optic apraxia; Balint's Syndrome.

Visuo-Motor Integration Test (VMI). A test of visual perception and visual construction that is intended primarily for preschool and elementary school children. The test involves copying geometric designs that increase in complexity according to a developmental difficulty gradient. Also called the Beery Visuo-Motor Integration Test. (Beery, K.E. and Buktenica, N.A. 1989. *Developmental Test of Visual-Motor Integration.* Odessa, FL: Psychological Assessment Resources.)

Visuo-spatial sketch pad (scratchpad). *See* Memory (working memory).

Vitamin deficiency disorders. A disorder resulting from a chronic low level of vitamins, typically vitamins in the B group. The most common central nervous system disorders result from lack of vitamin B_1 (thiamine), which produces Wernicke-Korsakoff's syndrome and vitamin B_{12}, which leads to white matter lesions in the nervous system and may be associated with mood disturbance, dementia, and psychosis. [L. *vita,* life; *amine, am*monia + *-ine.*]

Von Economo's disease (encephalitis). (Constantin von Economo, Austrian neurologist, 1876–1931). *See* Postencephalitic parkinsonism.

Voxel. The three-dimensional volume element corresponding to three pixel placements for a given slice thickness in MRI. "Voxel" is derived from volume element.

W

Wada Test. A technique used to assess cerebral language lateralization and memory function that involves administration of sodium amobarbital through the internal carotid artery. Multiple language and cognitive tasks are presented during the period of hemispheric anesthesia. Impairment on cognitive tasks suggests representation of those functions in the hemisphere being anesthetized. This is not a standardized test; different epilepsy surgery centers use different tasks, different amobarbital doses, and different performance criteria. Brevitol is used instead of amobarbital in some centers. (Wada, J. and Rasmussen, T. 1960. Intracarotid injection of sodium Amytal for the lateralization of cerebral speech dominance: Experimental and clinical observations. *J. Neurosurg.* 17:266–282.)

WAIS-R as a Neuropsychological Instrument (WAIS-R NI). A formal modification of the Wechsler Adult Intelligence Scale-Revised that is designed to maximize qualitative information about problem-solving approaches that a person uses to complete the WAIS-R. Although the WAIS-R NI does provide quantified information, comprehensive norms are unavailable. The standard administration and scoring of most WAIS-R subtests have been altered for the WAIS-R NI, although in most cases the traditional WAIS-S scaled scores can be calculated. In addition, three subtests not found in the WAIS-R are included: Sentence Arrangement, Spatial Span, and Symbol Copy. Sentence Arrangement requires the subject to make a sentence from words that are mixed up. The Spatial Span subtest measures forward and backward span with increasing block tapping sequence lengths that the subject reproduces. Symbol Copy involves copying the WAIS-R symbols from the Digit Symbol test subtest as quickly as possible, and thus eliminates the additional step of Digit Symbol translation. (Kaplan, E., Fein, D., Morris, R., and Delis, D.C. 1991. *WAIS-R NI Manual.* San Antonio: The Psychological Corporation.)

Wallerian degeneration. (Augustus V. Waller, British physiologist, 1816–1870). Atrophy of the distal part of neurons after being severed from the proximal part. Wallerian degeneration is often associated with trauma, infarction, or tumor infiltration.

Warrington Recognition Memory Test. *See* Recognition Memory Test.

Watershed zones. Border zone of *anastomoses* between the territories of two major cerebral arteries. A significant drop in blood pressure (or anoxia or carbon monoxide poisoning) will reduce the supply of oxygenated blood to where the two arterial distributions overlap. These areas become infarcted along with the contiguous distal branch territories of the arteries involved. Watershed lesions may isolate the Broca-Wernicke language axis, resulting in transcortical aphasia.

WC. Worker's Compensation.

Wechsler Individual Achievement Test (WIAT). An achievement test for assessing oral expression, listening comprehension, reading, spelling, arithmetic, and writing. One strength of the WIAT is that many individuals in the standardization sample also completed the Wechsler Intelligence Scales for Children-III (WISC-III). Consequently, ability-achievement discrepancy statistics on the same cohort have been computed. The WIAT

166

is designed for ages 5–19 and includes the following subtests: Basic Reading, Mathematics Reasoning, Spelling, Reading Comprehension, Numerical Operations, Listening Comprehension, Oral Expression, and Written Expression. (*Wechsler Individual Achievement Test* 1992. San Antonio: The Psychological Corporation.)

Wechsler Intelligence Scales (W-B, WAIS, WAIS-R, WAIS-III and WISC, WISC-R, WISC-III, WPPSI, WPPSI-R). (David Wechsler, American psychologist, 1896–1981). The Wechsler Intelligence Scales (WIS) are probably the most widely used tests of general cognitive abilities in neuropsychological assessment. Wechsler viewed intelligence as the ability to adapt, and saw the different subtests as different measures of intelligence rather than measures of different kinds of intelligence. The Wechsler Adult Intelligence Scale (WAIS) is the 1955 revision of the Wechsler-Bellevue test, which was first published in 1939. The WAIS was revised in 1981 (WAIS-R). In the WAIS and WAIS-R, six subtests comprise the Verbal IQ and five subtests comprise the Performance IQ. The Verbal subtests are Arithmetic, Comprehension, Vocabulary, Digit Span, Information, and Similarities. The Performance subtests are Block Design, Object Assembly, Picture Arrangement, Picture Completion, and Digit Symbol Substitution. The latest revision of the WAIS-R, the WAIS-III, published in 1997, adds new subtests (Matrix Reasoning, Cancellation) and factor-based composite scores. It can be used with individuals aged 16 to 89 years. The Wechsler Intelligence Scale for Children-III (WISC-III) is similar to the adult version and is appropriate for use with children ranging in age from 6 to 16 years.

The Wechsler Preschool and Primary Scale of Intelligence-Revised (WPPSI-R) is appropriate for children between 3 and 7 years of age. It is a downward extension of the WISC. The supplementary Sentences and Animal House subtests were developed to replace the Digit Span and Coding subtests of the WISC. Geometric Design replaces the Object Assembly and Picture Arrangement subtests (Wechsler, D. 1989. *Manual for the Wechsler Preschool and Primary Scale of Intelligence*, Revised. New York: Psychological Corporation; Wechsler, D. 1991. *Wechsler Intelligence Scale for Children*, 3rd ed. San Antonio: The Psychological Corporation; Wechsler, D. 1997. *Wechsler Adult Intelligence Scale*, 3rd ed. San Antonio: The Psychological Corporation.)

Wechsler Memory Scale (WMS; WMS-R; WMS-III). A widely used battery of tests to assess learning and memory. The original Wechsler Memory Scale (WMS) contained two versions that were intended to be parallel for repeated assessment, although most studies have demonstrated that the two forms are not equivalent. The original memory scale was criticized for including information in the summary score, the Memory Quotient (MQ), that was not considered a reflection of recent memory per se, for conceiving of memory as a unitary process, and for a lack of explicit scoring criteria. The Wechsler Memory Scale-Revised (WMS-R), published in 1987, addressed many of the problems with the original version, although it too was criticized, in part because of its standardization on relatively few subjects. The Wechsler Memory Scale-III (WMS-III), published in 1997, provides a larger pool of tests so that summary scores can be developed from measures with demonstrated sensitivity to brain impairment. Many individuals in the WMS-III standardization sample also completed the Wechsler Adult Intelligence Scales -III (WAIS-III). Consequently, ability-memory discrepancy statistics on the same cohort have been computed.

The WMS-III has 11 subtests; six comprise the core battery and five are considered supplemental. The WMS-III is used to explore three general content areas: verbal auditory memory, visual nonverbal memory, and attention and concentration. The Auditory/Verbal Memory Domain consists of Logical Memory, Verbal Paired Associates, and Word List. Logical Memory is a prose-passage recall task for two paragraphs; the second paragraph is presented twice and thus contains two learning trials. Verbal Paired Associates is a paired associate task containing only difficult word-pair associations. Word List is a supplemental test that contains an interference task in addition to standard learning trials. The Visual/Nonverbal Memory Domain contains Visual Reproduction, Memory for Faces, Dots, and Family Pictures. Visual Reproduction is a supplemental test for the WMS-III; it assesses recall of simple geometric designs. Memory for Faces is a measure of nonverbal memory for faces, Dots assesses spatial location memory, and Family Pictures tests memory for everyday activities. The Attention/Concentration Domain contains Mental Control, Spatial Span, Digit Span, and Letter-Number Span. Mental Control is a measure of mental tracking and manipulation of familiar sequences and is a supplemental test; Digit Span and Spatial Span are traditional measures of length of auditory and visual working memory; Letter-Number Span is a task in which letters and numbers are presented in a mixed-up order, and the task is to first state the numbers in ascending order and then to state the letters in alphabetical order. (Wechsler, D. 1997. *Wechsler Memory Scale*, 3rd ed. San Antonio: The Psychological Corporation.)

Wernicke's aphasia. *See* Aphasia syndromes.

Wernicke's area. (Carl Wernicke, German neurologist, 1848–1904). The posterior one-third of the superior temporal gyrus (Brodmann's area 22) that is concerned with phonemic decoding and encoding.

Wernicke's disease. (Carl Wernicke, German neurologist, 1848–1905). An acute phase of the Wernicke-Korsakoff syndrome that involves nystagmus, gaze paresis, ataxia, and confusion. Patients are disoriented, apathetic, unable to engage in meaningful conversation, and are amnestic. The etiology is B_1 (thiamine) deficiency most commonly seen in alcoholism. Treatment is with thiamine, and neurologic symptoms other than amnesia show great improvement following therapy. Also called Wernicke encephalopathy.

Wernicke's encephalopathy. *See* Wernicke' disease.

Wernicke-Korsakoff syndrome. (Carl Wernicke, German neurologist, 1848–1905. Sergei Korsakoff, Russian psychiatrist, 1853–1900). A syndrome seen in chronic alcoholism or malnutrition associated with B_1 (thiamine) deficiency. It is characterized acutely by Wernicke's disease and chronically by Korsakoff's disease. After the acute disease stages, patients display IQs in the average range but have a significant anterograde and retrograde memory impairment and demonstrate motivational difficulty. There are often impairments on visual-perceptual and frontal executive tasks. Patients may fail to demonstrate a *release from proactive interference*. Lesions are present in the midbrain, cerebellum, mammillary bodies, and thalamus. Lesions in the dorsomedial nucleus of the thalamus are thought to play a primary role in the anterograde memory impairment.

Wernicke-Lichtheim model. A brain-based model of language function first developed by Wernicke (1974) and subsequently systematized by Lichtheim (1885) in which normal function is associated with an underlying neural pathway that includes the input/output functions with clear interrelationships between other cortical language areas. Aphasia subtypes were explained by reference to where in the pathway damage occurred. In addition, previously unobserved language syndromes (e.g., conduction and transcortical aphasias) could be predicted. (Wernicke, C. 1874. *Der aphasische Symptomenkomplex: Eine psychologische Studie auf anatomischer Basis*. Breslau: Cohn and Weigert. In: *Wernicke's Works on Aphasia: A Sourcebook and Review*, (G.H. Eggert, trans.). The Hague: Mouton, 1977; Lichtheim, L. 1885. On aphasia. *Brain*, 7:433–484.)

West syndrome. (Charles West, British physician, 1816–1898). An encephalopathy of infancy characterized by infantile spasms, arrest of psychomotor development/mental retardation, and hypsarrhythmic EEG (high-voltage slowing and multifocal spikes).

Western Aphasia Battery (WAB). A language test battery with a summary score that provides an Aphasia Quotient (AQ). The tests are selected for all grades of aphasia severity but present no difficulty to a patient with intact language. Four oral language subtests (spontaneous speech, comprehension, repetition, and naming) are used to assess the severity and the type of aphasia. When reading, writing, praxis, drawing, block design, calculation, and *Raven's Coloured Progressive Matrices* scores are added, a Performance Quotient (PQ) is obtained. The combination of AQ and PQ yields the Cortical Quotient (CQ), a summary of cognitive function. (Kertesz, A. 1982. *Western Aphasia Battery.* New York: Grune & Stratton.)

Western blot. A blood test for infectious agents including HIV.

Whiplash. An acceleration extension injury of the cervical spine; popular term for an acute cervical sprain.

White matter. Axonal sheath of myelin that gives brain tissue a white appearance (white matter). Cell bodies are unmyelinated and thus give tissue a gray appearance (gray matter).

Whole word reading. Reading based on identifying a word as a whole rather than by segmentation.

Wide Range Achievement Test (WRAT). A test of academic achievement in single word reading, spelling, and arithmetic. Although grade equivalents are available, less reliance is placed on these scores than in the past. The reading subtest is a common approach to estimate the premorbid level of function since reading is considered to relatively resistant to the effects of diffuse brain impairment. (Wikinson, G.S. 1993. *WRAT3 Administration Manual.* Wilmington, DE: Wide Range.)

Wide Range Assessment of Memory and Learning (WRAML). A battery of verbal and visual memory tests designed for children between the ages of 5 and 17 years. Four indices are obtained from nine subtests: Verbal Memory, Visual Memory, Learning, and General Memory. Delayed recall can be obtained from Verbal Learning, Visual Learning, Sound Symbol, and Story Memory subtests, and recognition memory can be obtained for Story Memory. The number of specific subtests administered varies as a function of the child's age. (Adams, W. and Sheslow, D. 1990. *WRAML Manual.* Wilmington, DE: Jastak Associates.)

Williams syndrome. (J.C.P. Williams, 20th century New Zealand cardiologist). A genetic disorder of metabolism producing a characteristic "elfin" facial appearance, supra valvular aortic stenosis, marked visual-spatial deficits, and often mild to moderate mental retardation. Also known as infantile hypercalcemia.

Wilson's disease. (Samuel Alexander Kinnier Wilson, British neurologist, 1878–1937). An autosomal recessive disorder resulting from a defect in copper metabolism. The manifestations include an involuntary movement disorder and hepatic insufficiency/cirrhosis. The disease initially presents with personality changes, particularly mood changes, and progresses to dementia. Copper deposition in the cornea leads to the development of a pigmented copper ring (*Kayser-Fleischer ring*) at the outer margin of the cornea, and although not pathognomonic, this sign is strongly suggestive of this diagnosis. Also called hepatolenticular degeneration.

Wisconsin Card Sorting Test (WCST). A measure of hypothesis testing, abstract reasoning, and ability to shift and maintain the cognitive processes necessary for correct responding. Several version of the test exist. Each test consists of cards, each containing one to four symbols (triangle, star, cross, circle) printed in red, green, yellow, or blue. The subject is asked to place each card under one of four other cards—one red triangle, two green stars, three yellow crosses, and four blue circles—according to a principle that must be deduced from examiner feedback indicating whether or not the cards have been correctly sorted. The sorting principle changes multiple times during the test. Difficulty in changing sorting strategy, difficulty in maintaining a new sorting strategy after it has shifted, and the tendency to make perseverative responses are measured. Nelson (1976) modified the standard version by deleting all redundancies from the card packs and informed subjects when a shift in category was to be made. The Milwaukee Card Sorting Test, another modification, requires subjects to verbalize their strategy before sorting.

The WCST is often regarded as a test of frontal lobe function. Performance, however, may be disrupted by both anterior and posterior cerebral regions, and it may be unaffected by large frontal lobe lesions. Thus, the WCST is better viewed as a complex measure of executive functioning that is not linked to a single brain region but rather relies on the integration of multiple neural areas, including frontal lobes. (Grant, D.A. and Berg, E.A. 1948. A behavioral analysis of degree of impairment and ease of shifting to new responses in a Weigl-type card sorting problem. *J. Exp. Psychol.* 39:404–411; Nelson, H.E. 1976. A modified card sorting test sensitive to frontal lobe defects. *Cortex* 12:313–324; Osmon, D.C. and Suchy, Y. 1996. Fractionating frontal lobe functions: Factors of the Milwaukee Card Sorting Test. *Arch. Clin. Neuropsychol.* 11:451–552.)

Witzelsucht. Facetious, disinhibited, inappropriately euphoric affect that may be associated with frontal lobe pathology. The term "Witzelsucht" was coined by Hermann Oppenheim (1858–1919). [G. *Witz*, wit, joke; *Sucht*, a mania, obsession.]

WNL. Within normal limits. Colloquial and humorous expression for "we never looked."

Wonderlic Personnel Test. A test of problem-solving ability used primarily by business and governmental organizations to evaluate job applicants. It consists of 50 multiple-choice and short-answer items. This test items consist of verbal, mathematical, analytical, and pictorial stimuli and provide a rough estimate of IQ. (Wonderlic, E.F. 1992. *Manual of the Wonderlic Personnel Test and Scholastic Level Exam* II: Libertyville, IL: Wonderlic Personnel Test, Inc.)

Woodcock-Johnson Psychoeducational Battery. A standardized test battery with three parts: Tests of Cognitive Ability, which measures visual matching, auditory blending, concept formation, and reasoning; Tests of Achievement, which measure reading, mathematics, and written language skills; and Tests of Interest Level, which assess tendency toward scholastic orientation. (Woodcock, R.W. and Mather, N. 1989. *Woodcock-Johnson Tests of Achievement.* Allen, TX: DLM Teaching Resources.)

Word attack. A reading strategy in which a string of letters is subjected to segmentation before they are read.

Word blindness. *See* Alexia/dyslexia, acquired; Alexia without agraphia.

Word class effects. Differential performance of aphasic patients that is related to word type or class. Broca's aphasics, for example, omit more function words (grammatical or connecting words) than content words (nouns and verbs). Patients with reading disorders may make more errors reading abstract nouns than reading concrete nouns.

Word deafness. *See* Pure word deafness.

Word frequency effects. Differential performance of aphasic patients that is related to word frequency of occurrence. In general, high-frequency words are less vulnerable to errors in comprehension, expression, reading, and writing than low-frequency words.

Word salad. A mixture of words and phrases that lacks any comprehensive meaning or logical coherence. Associated with Wernicke's aphasia and schizophrenia.

Working memory. *See* Memory.

Working Memory Index. A measure from the Wechsler Adult Intelligence Scale-III (WAIS-III) and from the Wechsler Memory Scale-III (WMS-III) that is designed to reflect the ability to manipulate information in short-term immediate memory. Different subtests from the two scales contribute to the index. For the WAIS-III, the index is derived from performance on the Arithmetic, Digit Span, and Letter-Number Sequencing subtests. For the WMS-III, it is based on performance from the Letter-Number Sequencing and Spatial Span subtests; Digit Span is an optional WMS-III subtest and does not contribute to the index. The Working Memory Index is similar to the Freedom from Distractibility Index from the Wechsler Intelligence Test for Children-III (WISC-III).

X

Xanthochromia. Yellow discoloration of cerebrospinal fluid (CSF) due to the presence of blood that has been there long enough, i.e., for at least 1 day, to begin undergoing hemolysis. Typically associated with subarachnoid hemorrhage. [Gr. *xanthos*, yellow; *chroma*, color.]

XRT. X-ray therapy.

XXY syndrome. *See* Klinefelter's syndrome.

XYY syndrome. A chromosomal abnormality resulting from nondysjunction of the sex chromosomes that leads to cerebral migrational abnormalities and maturational delays. An increase in aggressiveness in XYY males was suggested by early reports but later brought into question.

Y

Yerkes-Dodson law. A relationship between anxiety and performance in which performance is facilitated by mild anxiety, but after a certain point increasing anxiety produces a rapid performance decline. This relationship is expressed graphically as an inverted-U function. (Yerkes, R.M., and Dodson, J.D. 1980. The relation of strength of stimulus to rapidity of habit formation. *J. Comp. Neurol. Psychol.* 18:459–482.)

Yohimbine. A neurotoxic alkaloid obtained from a tropical African tree, *Corynanthe yohimbe*. It is an anxiogenic substance that increases norepinephrine release, and it has been used in research to produce fear, anxiety, and panic attacks. [from Bantu *yohimb.*]

Z

Z score. A linearly derived standard score with a distribution mean of zero and a standard deviation of one.

Zebra. A colloquial expression for the diagnosis of a rare condition given a constellation of common clinical signs. For example, a diagnosis of sarcoidosis following Broca's aphasia is an example of a zebra since stroke is a much more likely etiology. The origin of the expression is obscure, but it is likely related to the fact that it is usually wrong to infer that a zebra rather than a horse is running by when hoofbeats are heard.